FAT AND THE BODY IN THE LONG NINETEENTH CENTURY

Meanings, Measures, and Representations

EDITED BY
AMY J. SHAW AND V. LYNN KENNEDY

Fat and the Body in the Long Nineteenth Century

Meanings, Measures, and Representations

UNIVERSITY OF TORONTO PRESS
Toronto Buffalo London

Toronto Buffalo London
utorontopress.com
Printed in the USA

ISBN 978-1-4875-5339-5 (cloth) ISBN 978-1-4875-5340-1 (EPUB)
ISBN 978-1-4875-5341-8 (PDF)

Library and Archives Canada Cataloguing in Publication

Title: Fat and the body in the long nineteenth century : meanings, measures, and representations / edited by Amy J. Shaw and V. Lynn Kennedy.
Names: Shaw, Amy J. (Amy Jeannette), 1972– editor | Kennedy, V. Lynn, 1970– editor
Description: Includes bibliographical references and index.
Identifiers: Canadiana (print) 2024041909X | Canadiana (ebook) 20240419111 | ISBN 9781487553395 (cloth) | ISBN 9781487553418 (PDF) | ISBN 9781487553401 (EPUB)
Subjects: LCSH: Obesity – Social aspects – History – 19th century. | LCSH: Overweight persons – History – 19th century.
Classification: LCC RA645.O23 F38 2025 | DDC 362.1963/98009034–dc23

Cover design: Val Cooke
Cover image: iStock.com/clu

We wish to acknowledge the land on which the University of Toronto Press operates. This land is the traditional territory of the Wendat, the Anishnaabeg, the Haudenosaunee, the Métis, and the Mississaugas of the Credit First Nation.

This book has been published with the help of a grant from the Federation for the Humanities and Social Sciences, through the Awards to Scholarly Publications Program, using funds provided by the Social Sciences and Humanities Research Council of Canada.

University of Toronto Press acknowledges the financial support of the Government of Canada, the Canada Council for the Arts, and the Ontario Arts Council, an agency of the Government of Ontario, for its publishing activities.

Canada Council for the Arts | Conseil des Arts du Canada

ONTARIO ARTS COUNCIL
CONSEIL DES ARTS DE L'ONTARIO
an Ontario government agency
un organisme du gouvernement de l'Ontario

Funded by the Government of Canada | Financé par le gouvernement du Canada | Canada

Contents

Section III: Cultural Representations and Constructions

Section IV: Imperialism, Colonialism, and the Body Politic

Illustrations, Figures, and Tables

Illustrations and Figures

Tables

Acknowledgments

Several years ago now, while doing research in the archives, Amy Shaw texted her friend and colleague an odd line from a letter she had found. A soldier at war was telling his family about how he was being teased for his weight gain and eagerly hoping that it was actually true. Lynn Kennedy, doing her own research and sitting amidst nineteenth-century advice manuals for mothers hoping for fat babies, had, it turned out, been collecting her own statements about nineteenth-century views on fat and the body. Perhaps unexpectedly, she responded with a plan. So this book is born from Lynn's ability to see connections, and Amy's tendency to say yes to things. Of such pairings are both terrible misadventures and exciting new projects made. This book, we hope, is the latter.

It is so largely because of the support of many people. The contributors to this collection have shared ideas and scholarly expertise, and have persevered through a long process with grace and humour. Thanks also to Len Husband, who took a chance on a manuscript about something few had tackled before, and the rest of the team at University of Toronto Press for their work in bringing it to publication. Barbara Porter ably shepherded it through its last stages, and Gillian Scobie's copy-editing helped keep us in line. We are grateful to two anonymous readers for taking the time to read the manuscript and provide thoughtful advice that improved it. Timothy Pearson took on the task of indexing a book that ranges across continents and classes and art forms and brought it together masterfully. (Really our index is great: Foucault and freakshows and Fat-Ten-You!) Thanks to our supportive colleagues at the University of Lethbridge, to Mustafa for early advice, and to the Laurier Centre for the Study of Canada for its support.

Thanks also to all the local coffee shops that fueled this project with croissants and so, so many lattes, and let us sit and discuss comma placement for hours on end.

And, of course, to our families. Thanks to Lynn's dad, Jerry, who is always supportive, and who shares a long-standing interest in food with her as they talk about interesting meals made and eaten; and to Amy's dad, Colin, who always worries "can you write about that?" Thanks to Damon, who has had to have more conversations about nineteenth century bodies with his mother than is reasonable. And thanks to Nick, even though he's wrong to prefer "overtones" to "connotations."

Our final thanks goes to friendship. What began when two new grad students shared an office many years ago has grown into a relationship that has enriched and sustained so much. This book is just one of its many fruits (but definitely not a banana).

FAT AND THE BODY IN THE LONG NINETEENTH CENTURY

Introduction

The modern reader encountering T.C. Duncan's 1878 work *How to be Plump* might at first believe it to be a parody. Why, they might wonder, would anyone either need or desire a manual for increasing their weight? Yet in the preface to this work, Duncan insisted that many nineteenth-century readers, particularly women, frequently queried of themselves: "How shall I get fleshy? I would give the world to be as plump as Miss – !" while others exclaimed "I would give a dollar a pound for more fat!" Yet by the mid-twentieth century, and carrying on into the present, such attitudes are seemingly obsolete, replaced by a common understanding that fat is an evil that must be fought, a peril to the body both in terms of health and aesthetics. Working to understand the much more complicated and diverse ways that the English-speaking world viewed fat in the nineteenth century, this collection helps us envision numerous, frequently competing, meanings that have been assigned to the fat body in the past.[1]

An article on the development of the bathroom scale written for a popular audience observed that "White America has always denigrated corpulence as a sign of immorality and sin."[2] Such a view of fat as an absolute evil fits the way that the fat body is frequently portrayed in contemporary society. Interestingly, however, there is an equally common supposition that in the past fat was viewed quite positively, and it is only contemporary society that has warped this acceptance of the corpulent body. Christopher Forth, in his recent work on the cultural meanings of fat through time, posits that the "lipophobia" of our current society has led many to "subscribe to some version of the idea that the history of so-called obesity is the story of 'how what was good became ugly and then bad.'" Yet he argues that this construction leads many contemporary scholars "to overlook the multiple and sometimes contradictory ways in which bodies may be conceived and experienced at any given time."[3] The broad scope of Forth's work, across millennia, helps to suggest that the concern with the body generally, and with fat in particular, has been a constant theme across time, while what the fat body might mean was shaped by the larger context in which it existed. Often there were complex, even contradictory, ways of assigning meaning. Focusing on the nineteenth century, a time of immense flux in the views of the body and society, provides a particularly good understanding of how these ideas about corporality and the adipose body have been socially constructed.

Historians of most eras have for a very long time disembodied their subjects, concerned more with ideas and actions than the physicality of the individual or group taking these actions or thinking these thoughts. This is particularly true for the eighteenth and nineteenth centuries, for which the realms of ideas and economics have been of central historiographical focus. Only in the last few decades has the body itself gained a history, leading to the physical presence being understood as "constructed historically and inscribed with political, social, and cultural meanings."[4] Body size – fatness and thinness – has emerged as an important subfield in this scholarship addressing the body, but because historians are always shaped by the issues and concerns of their own era, a large number of these works have focused specifically on dieting and the struggle to be free of fat, particularly in the twentieth century when such matters were becoming a growing concern. One of the first and most important studies of the history of dieting and its effect on views of the body was Hillel Schwartz's *Never Satisfied,* which explored the various interpretations of the body and attempts to control it through the management of weight. Writing in 1986, Schwartz lamented that "the absence of an analytical tradition is almost startling, given more than a century of failed diets."[5] A decade later, Peter Stearns took up this challenge. Looking for the origins of the perception that fat was a negative attribute that must be corrected through diet and exercise, Stearns begins his study in the late nineteenth century, arguing that "Concern about weight and dieting is not timeless; its origins are modern and can be quite precisely traced. It is also, at least in the form it took, not inevitable. Forces in the past created a need for change and formed a culture still very much in operation today."[6] Stearns compares historical attitudes in the United States with those in France, providing important insight into how views of the body are not absolute, but shaped by the cultural and historical context in which they are embedded. Wendy Mitchinson's work on dieting in Canada also shows that "place matters," describing this nation's own complex relationship to trying to control the fat body in the twentieth century.[7]

Most of the early work that situated the fat body as the focus or object of dieting, rather than as significant in and of itself, was embedded in, if not always accepting of, the negative cultural assumptions about fat. Mitchinson, however, takes a more nuanced approach to the discussion, especially the intersections of past attitudes toward fat with the more recent developments in "fat studies" that call on historians to take "an aggressive, consistent, rigorous critique of the negative assumptions, stereotypes, and stigma placed on fat and the fat body."[8] This call to action has been most clearly laid out in the collection of essays assembled by Esther Rothblum and Sondra Solovay into *The Fat Studies Reader*. In the introduction, entitled "Fat Studies: An Invitation to Revolution," fat acceptance advocate Marilyn Wann argues that one cannot be neutral when discussing fat because "every person who lives in a fat-hating culture inevitably absorbs anti-fat beliefs, assumptions, and stereotypes, and also inevitably comes to occupy a position in relation to power arrangements that are based on weight."[9]

Amy Erdman Farrell's *Fat Shame: Stigma and the Fat Body in American Culture* skillfully balances political engagement while placing attitudes toward fat in their specific and unique historical context.[10] The essays in our collection, situated in the long nineteenth century, also suggest that focusing solely on negative attitudes or representations of the fat body misses the more complex understanding of this subject in specific times and places. The fat body is neither simply good nor bad but represented in myriad and complex ways.

The many changing meanings assigned to the fat body over time have been more frequently emphasized in works that look well beyond the twentieth century for cultural representations of fat. Christopher Forth's *Fat: A Cultural History of the Stuff of Life* spans prehistory to the modern era, emphasizing that weight was only one (fairly recent) way of looking at fat and the body, with ideas about status, politics, religiosity, even mysticism superseding mere physical weight; and further, that these interpretations of body size varied, shifted, and co-existed in often complex, even contradictory, ways. In the ancient world, a fat body could signify nobility, privilege, and abundance, but also stupidity or an insensate personality. Similarly, in the late nineteenth century, even as fat was becoming less and less acceptable for certain individuals, the barrel-chested captain of industry remained a symbol of opulent success, although attitudes were again beginning to shift.

Forth notes that "this ambiguity regarding male corpulence persisted throughout the nineteenth century, providing a rather tense back-story to colonial engagements with fat overseas."[11] As imperialists increasingly othered and racialized the fat body, fat became less acceptable in western society. Sabrina Strings's study *Fearing the Black Body: The Racial Origins of Fat Phobia* traces this gradual shift in attitudes about weight, race, and beauty, beginning in the Renaissance and coming to a peak in the late nineteenth century, again asserting that attitudes toward fat and the body occur in culturally specific contexts.[12]

The historiography of fat as a social and cultural marker during the twentieth century has grown significantly in the last decade. This scholarship suggests some of the key questions about representation and ambiguous meanings of the fat body. Wendy Mitchinson, Jenny Ellison, and Deborah McPhail, together and separately, have provided important insights into the linkages between understandings of the social and political meanings of fatness in post-Second World War Canada. McPhail's work demonstrates the connections between discussions of fat bodies and national preparedness during the Cold War, while Ellison's work specifically focuses on the linkages between feminism and fat activism in the last third of the twentieth century. Sociologist Deborah Lupton takes an international focus in her book *Fat*, "a book about why the fat body is so reviled, the target of such intense discussion and debate about ways to reduce its size down to socially and medically acceptable dimensions." All of these works provide excellent models for tying the fat body to the broader context in which it exists. The chapters in this collection, focused on the long nineteenth century, suggest similar contextual concerns that introduce more fluid conceptionalizations of the meanings of fat before the dominant themes that have shaped understanding of fat in the twentieth century had been established.[13]

The long nineteenth century, extending from the late eighteenth century to the First World War, was a period of great change in the English-speaking world, making it a liminal period in the understanding of fat and the body. Broader social and cultural developments, including industrialization and urbanization, the growing prominence of science and medicine, and the forces of imperialism all played a role in how the body was viewed, both as a physical entity and as a symbolic vessel. Considering the developments in this era provides both a foundation for understanding current views about fat and the body as well as important insight into the values and viewpoints of the nineteenth century itself, and the body's role in constructing both individual and group identities.

We perhaps imagine the changes created by industrialization leading into and through the nineteenth century most often as written on the landscape, marked by the appearance of large factories and growing urban slums. But these developments were written on the body as well. Body size and weight, and the views surrounding these issues, often became a symbol of the growing class divide. On the one hand, consumer goods, particularly processed foods and sugar, were increasingly available. This abundance, combined with increasingly sedentary white-collar work, meant that the growing middle class was literally growing – increasing in girth as well as in political and economic power. Fat, once the domain of the wealthy, was being democratized (and thus rendered less desirable in some eyes). But it would only be at the end of the nineteenth century that the at least apparently plumper middle class would become a real concern for social commentators, spurring the interest in weight control and diets that so shaped the subsequent era. For much of the nineteenth century, this increasing body weight could be characterized as a sign of success, with the great girths of wealthy businessmen celebrated in popular portrayals of the rise of big business.

The rotundity of these successful magnates could be readily contrasted with the masses of industrial workers who lived on the edge of starvation. Low wages and boom and bust cycles left many in dire poverty, and their new residency in urban slums made acquiring food even more difficult than for those who remained in the countryside. This led many social reformers to decry the deplorable conditions of these factory workers' lives, evidenced by their waiflike bodies and underdeveloped children. Demographers have determined that the undernourished condition of many mothers in urban industrial settings may have been a major factor in the appallingly high infant mortality statistics during this era.[14] Also contributing to the high death rates in all age groups was the widespread prevalence of tuberculosis that, while most remarkable in crowded industrial areas, knew no bounds of class, race, or gender. This disease ran rampant, killing as many as four million people in England and Wales alone in the last half of the nineteenth century.[15] Poor nutrition made people particularly vulnerable to this disease, also known as consumption or "the wasting disease" for what it did to its sufferers. There is little wonder that in the midst of this epidemic, plumpness, rather than thinness, became associated with health.

Another key development of the nineteenth century that profoundly affected ideas about fat and the body was the growing centrality of science, and particularly the field of medicine. If the moderately adipose body had long been equated with health, the growing field of medical science increasingly saw it as doctors' role to quantify, and attempt to control, what exactly the healthy body should look like, using aggregate measurements and statistical formulae. It had not always been thus. Originally, measuring of the body had been aimed at understanding the averages and ranges of human physiology, just as Enlightenment scientists had became deeply interested in measuring and categorizing all elements of the natural world. One of the most influential men in the field of anthropometrics was Belgian astronomer and statistician Adolphe Quetelet, who used the height and weight measurements of both children and adults to establish the qualities of the "average man." Quetelet's work would become the basis for the body mass index (BMI) still widely in use. At about the same time, Pierre Charles Alexandre Louis developed his "numerical method," suggesting that biometry be used for clinical purposes. But medical interest in such studies remained relatively small until the second half of the nineteenth century. The American Civil War would provide one of the first large-scale opportunities to systemically collect data. Actuary Benjamin Gould, under the auspices of the United States Sanitary Commission, measured the weight and height, as well as the head circumference and other bodily lengths of over a million recruits in the Union Army, correlating this data with information about race, age, and region of origin. In the post-Civil War era, insurance companies began to make use of these anthropometrical statistics to predict longevity, tying "normal" weight to health. Henry Bowditch, a Harvard professor of physiology, and Charles Roberts, an English surgeon and reformer, both turned their attention to measuring children's heights and weights in the last decades of the nineteenth century, suggesting a clear link between weight, development, and health. The great growth in public education during this era not only made children a particular focus of those interested in statistical measurements, but also of the developing physical education movement that began to seek to monitor and control the physical development of children.[16]

Physicians, as suggested above, were particularly interested in the measurements of the human body. The medical community was also in the process of professionalizing during the nineteenth century, using scientific rhetoric to gain respect for their professional authority. As S.E.D. Shortt shows, there was a growing concern about health matters among middle-class Victorians, but as doctors claimed professional authority, "normal physiology and the pathological conditions of the body were, it now appeared, areas of expert knowledge no longer accessible to the layman." Statistical measurements became part of this rhetoric, and at a remarkably rapid rate the "average" became the "normal" and then anything outside of that range becoming "abnormal" or deviant, and increasingly associated with the "other."[17]

Throughout the nineteenth century, the most important idea for scientists, doctors, and most laypeople seems to have been an avoidance of extremes. Moderation was the desirable outcome, although how exactly to define moderation remained a matter of debate. Sociologist David J. Hutson, in an examination of medical journals, health reform literature, and popular magazines from the nineteenth century, finds that weight was represented as being on a spectrum rather than constituted by an ideal number. Most commentators advocated a moderate plumpness or leanness, while extremes of either corpulence or gauntness could create concern about compromised health. Hutson concludes that "the symbolic position held by weight constitutes a more complicated phenomenon than previously believed."[18]

The myriad words to describe this goal of moderation – plumpness, corpulence, leanness, gauntness – suggests some of the slipperiness of language about this bodily state in the nineteenth century. The choice of language reflected the social position of both the speaker and the subject, reflecting contextual perceptions as much as any particular size or weight, and did not necessarily carry the moral judgments we now associate with such words. The modern focus on measuring and the predominance of the body mass index has linked the use of certain words – obese, overweight – to a numerical formula, giving them an aura of precision. Yet scholars, including Deborah Lupton, have contended that the use of such terms both reflects and shapes medicalized understandings of the body, and such language has "become increasingly political and contentious" in contemporary usage.[19] We have chosen to use "fat" in this collection not so much as an activist position but as a term that would have been widely used and understood in the nineteenth century. Further, the wide variety of other words describing the body in individual chapters reflects the multifarious ways of seeing and interpreting the body in this era.

Ultimately, moderation was viewed as optimal by most people in the nineteenth century not only because of its links to health, but because of a connection between certain body types and particular character traits or behaviours. Increasing institutionalization in the nineteenth century – prisons, hospitals, asylums, schools – created a venue for scientific studies focused on measuring and weighing, and statisticians and social commentators frequently turned correlations into causation when it came to body size. Many responded to the anxieties brought on by the myriad changes occurring in the nineteenth century with an effort to measure and thus control. In the age of social Darwinism, perceived connections between extreme fatness or thinness and "deviancies" such as immorality or criminality abounded.

The links between body size and "otherness" were just as easily turned to the project of imperialism, which was another central theme within the nineteenth century. Virtually all European nations, and the United States too, sought to acquire territory all over the globe. Claiming this land inevitably resulted in attempts to control the populations already there. Colonization raised important questions about power, race, and the control of resources and many of these themes were both physically and symbolically written on the bodies of both the colonizers and the colonized. Indeed, well before the nineteenth century, differences in body types as well as skin colour had been called upon to justify colonization, particularly in Africa. Through much of this history, Europeans had emphasized the fatness of the African people they encountered, with the implicit, and often explicit, belief that the valuing of fat bodies in various African cultures marked their lack of civilization and self-control in comparison with the more svelte European frame. As colonization became a central project of most English-speaking nations, power was frequently expressed through the control of resources, including food, so that the power relations between the colonized and colonizer produced bodies either emaciated through starvation or fattened by the spoils of empire, often flipping the existing narratives around body size while still maintaining a sense of embodied otherness.[20]

Shifting ideas about appropriate body shapes and sizes, then, were affected by a variety of trends that took place, unevenly, throughout the English-speaking world in the long nineteenth century. These included the abundance and privation brought about by industrialization, which imprinted itself on the bodies of those who toiled in its factories and those who reaped the benefits of its wealth. The growing strength of the middle class, whose claims to power were based on ability and rectitude rather than birth, was expressed partly through bodily evidence of self-control and moderation. Nineteenth-century imperialism brought westerners into contact with other bodies and cultures, and supported the ideological imperative to show why slim, white, self-controlled bodies were the epitome of civilization, and the justification for western dominance. The trend to quantification is also key. The process of professionalization of physicians and social scientists was premised partly on their expressed certainties about what constituted health and normality and racial superiority. Growing institutionalizion – of schools and prisons – gave the opportunity to measure and weigh groups of people and to quantify physical manifestations of "deviance." All the efforts to consolidate power that characterized the nineteenth-century West – including in terms of ethnicity, race, gender, and class – used the language of fatness and thinness, and sometimes the literal control of food, as part of their arsenal.

The essays in this collection all situate themselves in the major changes and developments occurring in the nineteenth century that were shifting the world as people knew it. The contributions represent scholarship from numerous disciplines, including history, sociology, philosophy, and anthropology; and they use a wide variety of sources, including philosophical treatises, popular and medical journals, personal letters, art prints, material culture, statistics, newspapers, cartoons, and photographs. This diversity is important in representing the full spectrum of the ways to consider fat and the body both as approached by scholars and by the historical actors themselves, well beyond the singular focus on dieting, weight control, and health. Although each of these approaches represents a unique perspective, they also contain threads of similarity that tie them to the broader context of the nineteenth century.

Section I considers the epistemological discussions of fat and the body. Current discussions of body size tend to view fat as an individual issue of health and self-control, but in the nineteenth century, philosophers, medical commentators, and social reformers were just as likely to posit group character traits often linked to metaphysical and moral rather than physical well-being. Kristen Hardy's essay examines how biomedical language developed to categorize certain bodies and groups as abnormal or pathological through the writings of philosophers like Michel Foucault. Similarly, Bessie Rigakos and Wesley Bishop focus on three social reformers of the Progressive Era whose works functioned to link body size to particular moral traits and characteristics, gradually enshrining the negative view of overweight individuals that would become dominant by the mid-twentieth century.

Section II suggests how weights and measures became the default way of understanding this subject. These authors use studies of different groups to show shifts from qualitative to quantitative approaches to understanding the body becoming predominant. Lynn Kennedy's essay focuses on fat babies, tracing how qualitative assessments of healthy plumpness shifted to a nearly obsessive monitoring of every ounce gained or lost, largely linked to the increasing intervention of doctors and parenting manuals promoting scientific motherhood. Conor Heffernan introduces the physical culture movement, one of the first groups to conscientiously measure themselves. Men like Eugen Sandow and Bernarr Macfadden taught members of the general public to monitor and control their body size through the use of exercise and diet regimes, setting the trend for what would follow in the twentieth century. The essay by Luiza Antonie, Kris Inwood, and Hamish Maxwell-Stewart takes a different methodological approach by looking at the actual measurements of men held in Canadian prisons at the end of the nineteenth century. The use of these demographic sources suggests some of the challenges of relying on the numbers when discussing weight in historical context.

Section III focuses on cultural sources, such as art, material culture, literature, and photography, considering how such representations shaped broader understandings of the fat body. These cultural representations affirm the complex envisioning of fat and the body in the long nineteenth century as neither entirely positive nor negative. Freya Gowrley studies the artistic and material representations of Daniel Lambert, who turned his immense body size into a form of celebrity. The material legacy of Lambert suggests that the fat body could be a source of some fascination in this era. Tatiana Konrad explores the symbolic uses of fat and thin bodies in literature through an in-depth analysis of Joseph Conrad's *Heart of Darkness*. The portrayals of these bodies mirrored the complex views that Europeans of this era had of both Africans and those who colonized the African continent to plunder its resources. Nsima Udo flips that mirror in his examination of the mbopo fattening ritual in Nigeria. Looking at this ritual through the photos taken by European anthropologists and through the cultural production of the Ibibio/Efik women who underwent this ritual reveals the complexity of cultural representations of fat in the long nineteenth century.

Section IV continues some of the themes of colonization discussed in the previous section but through the lens of politics and the drive for empire that led to war in the late nineteenth and early twentieth centuries. Bonnie Miller situates her discussion in the lead-up to the Spanish-American and Philippines War, examining how the cartoon portrayals of the shifting girth of Uncle Sam reflected larger attitudes about imperialism and the control of global resources. Amy Shaw looks at the War in South Africa, occurring at about the same time, through the letters of Canadian soldiers. Their discussions of food and fat show the ways weight functioned as a shorthand that tried to tie families together across hemispheres, and expressed the power of the British Empire.

Although richly diverse in focus, sources, and methodology, these chapters, taken together, suggest a number of key themes and ways of envisioning fat in the long nineteenth century. First, they generally suggest that the meaning of fat in this era was often tied to group identity rather than being an individualized "problem." Many of these essays suggest the conflicted and complex moral meanings assigned to the fat (or thin) body. Fat was neither clearly good nor clearly bad during this era; rather, it depended on whose body was being judged, who was doing the judging, and the particular context involved. This suggests the important linkages to ideas about race, gender, and class that shaped interpretations and representations of fat bodies, interlinkages that intensified as imperialism and colonialism turned these ideas into embodied political symbols.

Together, the essays in this collection begin to suggest the very complex visions of fat and the body that existed in the English-speaking world in the long nineteenth century, and to offer multivariant approaches, methodologies, and conclusions for understanding this. These diverse essays suggest multiple lenses through which people in the past looked at and understood their bodies. The overarching conclusion of this collection is that there was no *one* way of seeing the body in this era. Weight was a concept in flux, its changing attitudes shaped by science, culture, and politics. The fat body could undoubtedly be subjected to social judgments, but not in ways that necessarily reflect current values and debates. Rather, fat bodies held their own sets of meanings that reflected the context and concerns distinctive to the time in which they lived.

NOTES

1 T.C. Duncan, *How to be Plump: or Talks on Physiological Feeding* (Chicago: Duncan Bros., Pub, 1878), iv.
2 Kelsey Miller, "The Completely Bonkers History of the Bathroom Scale," *Elemental*, 15 Feb 2021, elemental.medium.com.
3 Christopher E. Forth, *Fat: A Cultural History of the Stuff of Life* (London: Reaktion Books, 2019), 8–9, and 242.
4 Jane Nicholas & Patrizia Gentile, eds., "Introduction," in *Contesting Bodies and Nation in Canadian History* (Toronto: University of Toronto Press, 2013), 3.
5 Hillel Schwarz, *Never Satisfied: A Cultural History of Diets, Fantasies and Fat* (New York: The Free Press, 1986), 4.
6 Peter N. Stearns, *Fat History: Bodies and Beauty in the Modern West* (New York: New York University Press, 1997), ix.
7 Wendy Mitchinson, *Fighting Fat: Canada, 1920–1980* (Toronto: University of Toronto Press, 2018), 19.
8 Mitchinson, *Fighting Fat*, 9.
9 Marilynn Wann, "Foreward: Fat Studies: An Invitation to Revolution," in *The Fat Studies Reader*, ed. Esther Rothblum and Sondra Solovay (New York: New York University Press, 2009), xi.
10 Amy Erdman Farrell, *Fat Shame: Stigma and the Fat Body in American Culture* (New York: New York University Press, 2011).

11 Forth, *Fat: A Cultural History*, esp. ch. 2, and 219 and 222.
12 Sabrina Strings, *Fearing the Black Body: The Racial Origins of Fat Phobia* (New York: New York University Press, 2019).
13 Jenny Ellison, Deborah McPhail, and Wendy Mitchinson, *Obesity in Canada: Critical Perspectives* (University of Toronto Press, 2016); Deborah McPhail, *Contours of the Nation: Making Obesity and Imagining Canada, 1945–1970* (University of Toronto Press, 2017); Jenny Ellison, *Being Fat: Women, Weight, and Feminist Activism in Canada* (University of Toronto Press, 2020); Deborah Lupton, *Fat,* 2nd ed. (Routledge, 2018), 2.
14 Robert Millward & Frances Bell, "Infant Mortality in Victorian Britain: The Mother as Medium," *The Economic History Review* 54 (Nov., 2001), 699–733; W. Peter Ward & Patricia C. Ward, "Infant Birth Weight and Nutrition in Industrializing Montreal," *American Historical Review* 89 (Apr., 1984), 324–45.
15 John Firth, "History of Tuberculosis. Part 1 – Phthisis, Consumption and the White Plague," *Journal of Military and Veterans' Health* 22 (June 2014): 32; Achim Schwenk & Derek C. Macallan, "Tuberculosis, Malnutrition and Wasting," *Current Opinion in Clinical Nutrition and Metabolic Cure* 13, 4 (July 2000): 285–91.
16 Michael S. Shimkin, "The Numerical Method in Therapeutic Medicine," *Public Health Reports* 79, no. 1 (Jan. 1964): 1–12; James Allen Young, "Height, Weight, and Health: Anthropometric Study of Human Growth in the Nineteenth-Century American Medicine," *Bulletin of the History of* Medicine 53, no. 2 (Summer 1979): 214–43; Amanda M. Czerniawski, "From Average to Ideal: The Evolution of the Height and Weight Table in the United States, 1836–1943," *Social Science History* 31, no. 2 (Summer 2007): 273–96; Patricia Vertinsky, "'Weights and Means': Examining the Surveillance of Fat Bodies Through Physical Education Practices in North America in the Late Nineteenth and Early Twentieth Centuries," *Journal of Sport History* 35, no. 3 (Fall 2008): 449–68.
17 S E.D. Shortt, "Physicians, Science, and Status: Issues in the Professionalization of Angle-American Medicine in the Nineteenth Century," *Medical History* 27 (1983): 51–68.
18 David J. Hutson, "Plump or Corpulent?: Lean or Gaunt? Historical Categories of Bodily Health in Nineteenth-Century Thought," *Social Science History* 41, no. 2 (Summer 2017): 284.
19 Deborah Lupton, *Fat*, 2nd ed. (New York: Routledge, 2018), 3, 27–32.
20 Sabrina Strings, in *Fearing the Black Body* (2019), provides an excellent introduction to the way Europeans viewed the bodies of Africans and how this shaped their views of fat. James Daschuk, *Clearing the Plains: Disease, Politics of Starvation, and the Loss of Indigenous Life* (Regina: University of Regina Press, 2013) suggests how the control of resources, particularly food supplies, was used for political purposes, in this case in a North American context.

SECTION I

Epistemologies and Philosophies

How we talk about fat matters. The focus on the so-called obesity epidemic in the twentieth and twenty-first centuries has flattened out the narrative surrounding weight to focus almost exclusively on health issues. The term "overweight" implies a standard or normative weight from which one has deviated. The focus is thus on a number that goes up and down with gains and losses. All of these language choices suggest a very specific, medicalized construction of the body, but the chapters in this section show that these are epistemological choices, which developed and altered over time reflecting larger social beliefs and purposes.

In chapter 1, Kristen Hardy examines some of the historical and philosophical bases for a changing view of the body specifically as it relates to size and weight. Notably, she reveals how biomedical language has functioned to define some bodies as "abnormal" or "pathological" with defining the normative body becoming a particular project of nineteenth-century social theorists based on their understandings of class, race, and especially gender. Their constructions ultimately justified the medical community's own intercession in matters related to body weight. In this framework, by the mid-twentieth century being "overweight" had become established in the collective imagination as a medical condition. Understanding these epistemological developments provides a foundation for understanding the social, cultural, and political ways of looking at fat and the body discussed in the other sections of this collection.

In chapter 2, Bessie Rigakos and Wesley Bishop also offer an examination of the philosophical underpinnings of social understandings of fat, specifically how weight became a moral issue intertwined with ideas about race, gender, and deviant behaviour. Focusing on the Progressive period of the late nineteenth and early twentieth century, their study suggests how the rise of the expert, a reliance on measurement and categorization, and a reverence for efficiency all contributed to conceptions of fat and the body. By examining three Progressive Era experts – Ella Adelia Fletcher, Cesare Lombroso, and Guglielmo Ferraro – Rigakos and Bishop demonstrate how corporal measurements became markers of not only health but of social "fitness." While the fat body may be associated with laziness and lack of control in the twenty-first century imagination, these commentators of the late nineteenth and early twentieth century went further, drawing links between the fat body and criminality, prostitution, and moral turpitude, all tied to ideas about race, gender, and class. But rather than being inherent or self-evident linkages, this chapter suggests just how these attitudes toward fat and the body were intentionally constructed, and their lingering effects on what we now perceive as idealized bodies. How experts and social commentators talked about fat mattered.

1 The Enfleshment of Difference: Medicalizing and Gendering the Fat Body in the Nineteenth Century

KRISTEN A. HARDY

"There is no objective pathology." – Georges Canguilhem[1]

The western biomedical tradition has been, and continues to be, characterized by a collection of discourses and practices brought into being, sustained, and fostered through particular social, cultural, political, and economic forces that are characteristic of its globally distributed, historically situated sites of emergence.

To appreciate how, over the course of the nineteenth century, fatness came to be seen as a problem and as a fundamentally gendered phenomenon, we need to understand something of the broader and deeper social and cultural forces that have acted on bodies. The emergent biomedical system was a pivotal player here, but not only in the narrow sense of health-care institutions and services. As sets of specialized knowledges and practices, supported by claims of their ability to accurately comprehend bodies and successfully intervene in their functioning, the biological sciences and medicine were, and are, inherently pervaded by power. As sociologist Peter Conrad has written in his study of the medicalization of modern societies, "the key issue remains definitional – the power to have a particular set of (medical) definitions realized in both spirit and practice."[2] In particular, delineating specific embodied states as "abnormal" or "pathological" and in need of professional intervention and correction is a key manifestation of how this power operates at the most fundamental levels of human experience.

Modern biomedicine has contributed significantly to pathologizing bodies deemed "fat," characterizing them as appropriate sites for such intervention. The specialized terminology of contemporary medicine – "overweight," "obese," "morbidly obese" (now slightly softened to "severely obese") – has been created and periodically redefined to cast particular bodies as fundamentally "not normal" (or *non-normate*) by virtue of their weight, size, and/or shape. This categorization speaks to the importance which, over time, has come to be attached to measuring and quantifying the degrees of otherness of certain bodies.

A substantial collection of research has emerged in recent decades seeking to critique biomedical paradigms of fatness; taken together, these trajectories of scholarship offer an incisive critique of historical and contemporary discourses and practices about and toward fatness and "weighted" bodies. Scholars such as Paul Campos,[3] J. Eric Oliver,[4] Michael Gard and Jan Wright,[5] and Lindo Bacon[6] are among those who have produced widely read and well-received critiques of the often-flawed science and the partisan motivations behind the constitution of the "obesity epidemic" as an object of socio-medical fixation in the late twentieth and early twenty-first centuries. Other researchers, among them Susan Bordo,[7] Kathleen LeBesco,[8] Sander Gilman,[9] and Sabrina Strings,[10] have emphasized the broader and intersecting social forces at work in the constitution of the fat body as "abnormal," "undesirable," and "diseased" that developed, particularly over the course of the nineteenth century. Gilman's and Strings's respective works have been particularly groundbreaking as examples of "game-changing" intersectional research – Gilman in his consideration of antisemitism as a key force in the pathologization of the fat body, and Strings in her sustained examination of the role of race and, particularly, efforts to establish white supremacy in western historical conceptions of fatness across spheres ranging from art to medicine.

Medical interest in fat bodies has much earlier precursors – Hippocrates (c. 460 BCE – c. 370 BCE) and Galen (129 CE – c. 200 CE) – were among the first physicians on record to cast fatness as a "condition," which they attributed to an imbalance of the humours (the balance of internal fluids once believed to control physiology).[11] Sporadic attention was given to "corpulence," "adiposis," or "obesity" by a variety of western practitioners over the course of the millennia that followed.[12] However, the epistemological changes of the eighteenth and nineteenth centuries – specifically, our frameworks of beliefs about how bodies and minds can be accurately understood – coupled with shifting societal concerns, significantly shaped the manifestations of this biomedical interest that would fully come to fruition in the twentieth century. Under this new regime of medical perception, the medical gaze could discern particular tissue configurations as abnormalities, and fat became a medical condition. During the nineteenth century in much of Western Europe and North America, the management of embodied conditions of difference also became intimately and explicitly linked to social class – to the symbolic health of the bourgeoisie – and the collective well-being of the nation. This shift presented medicine with the possibility of seeing fat as a *necessarily* problematic presence within bodies which threatened society collectively, and especially the elites within it. And, as Strings has explored through a sociologically informed lens, these bodily differences are also bound up with racial hierarchization, particularly the legacy of the transatlantic slave trade and questions of the "nature" of Black people and their bodies.[13]

The cultural representations of fat bodies through image and text do not, historically or presently, exist in isolation from the gendered discourses that have influenced professionalized medicine, as well as many other sociocultural spheres. Fat bodies have long been constituted and "disciplined" through biological and medical thought and practice in ways that frequently reflect the presence of binary sex-stratified bodily and behavioural ideals, which are themselves rooted in specific histories and ways of seeing. Increasing scholarly attention in a number of fields has been devoted to fat subjects' constitution, specifically in how they deviate from essentialized norms of sex and gender; however, scant historically oriented work exists on this subject. Most studies of this genre, rather, attend to present-day social constructions, representations, and experiences of fatness and gender;[14] a much smaller number of sources focus on gendered bodily norms during specific periods of the twentieth century.[15] Only select authors, however, grant sustained attention to sex/gender and fatness as manifest in earlier historical periods, particularly in the nineteenth century when these concepts were in some flux.[16]

Working from an approach that recognizes the contributions of the biological sciences, medical institutions, political interests, socioeconomic stakes, popular culture, and fat subjects themselves, this chapter examines some of the ways in which these agents and forces participated in the medicalized enactment of the nineteenth-century fat body as a fundamentally sexed and gendered entity. More specifically, drawing upon the theoretical work of a number of scholars, including Michel Foucault's "archaeological" study of the modern biomedical establishment,[17] Sander Gilman's work on the psychosocial pathologization of physical difference,[18] Thomas Laqueur's investigation of the evolution of western practices of sex differentiation,[19] and Annemarie Mol's conception of bodies and conditions as enacted in "multiple" fashion,[20] I wish to consider how particular historical shifts in epistemology and sociopolitical thought have participated in casting certain "sized" and "weighted" bodies as deviant, not simply in relation to an abstract model of health, but in specific, *gendered* ways.

The very notion of a *normate body* – the assumption that bodies ought to conform to an identifiable standard configuration and that other varieties of embodiment are, to a greater or lesser degree, deviant or abnormal – is predicated, according to Foucault, upon a particular "regime of truth."[21] Truth regimes are components of a particular *épistème*, the historically and culturally specific framework used to make intelligible statements about phenomena.[22] (This concept is somewhat similar to Thomas Kuhn's famous notion of "paradigms" in science,[23] though more expansive in its scope of cultural applicability.) Such *épistèmes*, in Foucault's reading, are subject to shifts and changes over time, with new ones emerging into dominance while others wane in prominence and authority.[24]

In *The Birth of the Clinic: An Archaeology of Medical Perception*,[25] Foucault locates one such epistemic "rupture," or emergence of a novel paradigm within western thought, in late eighteenth-century France, when modern clinical medicine was ushered into existence in the aftermath of revolutionary societal changes. This development was made possible, he argued, by and through the particular organization of knowledge and perception that emerged during this period, which was linked with the shift from Catholic-run charitable institutions to large, modernized teaching hospitals.[26] A new, pathology-focused "anatomo-clinical" perspective blossomed in such spaces during the nineteenth century, superseding the previously dominant "classificatory" medical regime – which Foucault characterizes as identifying sets of abstract "disease states" that existed apart from their actual, unique, embodied variations, and as focused upon static, essentialized illness "pictures." This novel way of thinking about illness and health care spread throughout Western Europe and to North America, as the construction of large teaching hospitals became increasingly commonplace and offered what was to gradually emerge over the course of the nineteenth and early twentieth centuries as the only fully credentialled form of biomedical education.[27] The characteristic "way of seeing" fostered within these environments emphasized the physician's penetrating perception of the truth of health and illness through a sense-based encounter with disease as manifest within the body of the patient, using sight, touch, even smell.[28] Specifically, Foucault identifies the clinical crux of this change as the privileging of *le regard*, the "pure gaze" of the doctor, rendering visible – and, in turn, making communicable to colleagues and pupils – the true character of bodies and their conditions. He notes a shift in attention toward discerning observable tissue changes in disease, and the increasing importance conferred upon the physician's discernment of *signs* (rather than patient-reported *symptoms*) as characteristics of this regime of the gaze.[29] Yet, in anatomo-clinical medicine, Foucault explains,

> the sign no longer speaks the natural language of disease; it assumes shape and value only within the questions posed by medical investigation. There is nothing, therefore, to prevent it being solicited and almost fabricated by medical investigation ... To establish these signs, artificial or natural, is to project upon the living body a whole network of anatomo-pathological mappings: to draw the dotted line of the future autopsy.[30]

Foucault's use of "the future autopsy" here is not metaphorical; dissection came to assume a central place in medical education and practice throughout the nineteenth century – leading to the notorious cadaver trade in Britain and America[31] – and symbolizing, for emerging physicians both on the continent and in Europe's settler colonies, a significant break from previous approaches, which were increasingly deemed outdated and in imminent danger of being eclipsed by Parisian-style hospital medicine.[32] As multisensory engagement with the body's interior after death became de rigueur for allopathic doctors, so their clinical practice reflected a parallel emphasis on diagnosis through searching and often invasive physical examination of their still-living patients. In a very tangible sense, then, medical professionals participated in creating specific pathologies out of the diverse assemblage of parts, tissues, and conditions of the embodied subject, and, in so doing, solidified the consignment of authority about bodies to the external "expert" observer. This would become significant as biomedicine came to value what could be seen by the doctor – including fat – over what was reported by the health-care seeker.

Paralleling these historical changes in the nature of medical perception that accompanied the rise of the teaching hospital was the unfolding of a sociopolitical trajectory, explored by Foucault in his later work, that functioned to manage subjects via regulating life itself. Modern "biopower" operates by the state deploying coordinated efforts to support and protect human lives – to "make live," in Foucault's terminology – juxtaposed against the ability to selectively kill, or "make die," once wielded by the sovereign ruler.[33] As Foucault notes in the first volume of *The History of Sexuality*, two major facets of this biopower are clearly discernible in the modern era, (1) anatomo-politics and (2) biopolitics.[34]

The first of these, the development of an *anatomo-politics* of the individual body, emphasized the exercise of disciplinary power to optimize the usefulness (to others, and especially to systems) and docility of embodied subjects. Building upon this theme, the eighteenth century witnessed the rise of the "bourgeois body," whereby this emerging social class, lacking the aristocracy's claims to a blood-based superiority – linked to both class and race – became focused instead upon the creation of a body that "looked to its progeny and the health of its organism"[35] for power and perpetuity. The bourgeoisie's emphasis was not, Foucault maintains, on actually maximizing labour capability, but rather upon the political and economic *symbolism* of those bodies which signified physical health, strength, and longevity.[36] Such "precious" bodies required that great care and concern be expended to maintain them, and provided a fertile ground for experts to intervene in the practices of health. And such symbolically healthy bodies, in the cultural framing of the time, were not fat.

Second, and even more closely coterminous with the rise of clinical medicine, was the late eighteenth-century emergence of *biopolitical* strategies, which, in supplementing disciplinary practices, sought to manage the health of populations on an aggregate level, coming to take the form of "public health." Biopolitical power operates, in Foucault's conception, via technologies of the "regularization" of embodied subjects,[37] moving toward what disability studies researcher Lennard Davis has termed a "utopia of the norm."[38] In this paradigm, statistically determined standards for bodies become established as morally laden aspirational ideals – a problematic situation for those whose bodies defied such standards, regardless of their actual subjective perception of illness or wellness. Governing the population through cultivating the health and vitality of the collective has, further, often been expressed through twinning discourses of nationalism together with those of science, crafting the body politic through biomedically politicizing bodies. Public health thus surfaced as a matter of intense sociopolitical concern in the nineteenth century, with the increasing medicalization of the populace acting to produce and justify a regime of surveillance and behavioural control. Of particular interest were society's lower classes, whose moral and physical hygiene were perpetually suspect and conceived of as posing not just a threat to themselves and their much-needed labour power, but to the social body as a collectivity.[39] (And, as historical photos of working-class and underclass people from nineteenth-century Europe and North America attest, fat bodies were not rare among these groups.)

But the bodies that served as the objects of medical investigation, disciplinary control, and biopolitical governance during this era were inscribed with another socially consequential distinction – that of sex. In an engaging study of the shifting perception of categories of bodily difference in western thought and practice, historian Thomas Laqueur locates a fundamental change in western ways of conceptualizing sexed bodies roughly around the eighteenth century.[40] Examining an extensive collection of historical texts and illustrations on science and medicine, Laqueur posits a transition from a "one-sex" worldview, prevalent from at least classical antiquity, in which males and females were conceived of as variant manifestations of a single body prototype (with differing genital configurations representing homologous structures), to an increasing dominance of a fundamentally "two-sex" model. With the growing influence of the latter perspective, male and female subjects became increasingly conceptualized as wholly different from one another, a distinction that was attributed to supposedly immutable biology.[41] In this respect, Laqueur's work constitutes an important and nuanced critique of the classic Beauvoirian model of biological sex versus socially constructed gender.[42] Laqueur observes:

> No discovery or group of discoveries dictated the rise of a two-sex model, for precisely the same reasons that the anatomical discoveries of the Renaissance did not unseat the one-sex model: the nature of sexual difference is not susceptible to empirical testing. It is logically independent of biological facts because already embedded in the language of science, at least when applied to any culturally resonant construal of sexual difference, is the language of gender.... Two incommensurable sexes were, and are, as much the products of culture as was, and is, the one-sex model.[43]

Although eschewing a simplistic causality, Laqueur maintains that this epistemic change – like those identified by Foucault – was intimately linked with the broader sociopolitical context of the times. In particular, with faith in a divinely constituted cosmic order faltering, establishing biological bases for patriarchal ideas and practices helped those ideas to endure alongside secular, post-Enlightenment ontologies and social-contract-based politics. Thus, Laqueur asserts, a cisgender woman's purported inferiority became securely grounded in her incommensurable biology, solidifying male control over key social, cultural, political, and economic spheres through the powerful discourses of science and medicine.[44]

In bringing to light the constructed nature of the two-sex model, Laqueur's work extends and enhances Foucault's own conclusions concerning the historical change in ways of seeing that made possible subsequent developments in scientific perceptions of the body. The shift toward locating the basis of physical *and* social differences and structures of inequality in anatomical configuration, rather than in a religiously justified social order that appeared increasingly antiquated within the rapidly industrializing world, was an important precondition for biomedical discourses about particular varieties of embodiment to emerge in subsequent centuries, which would eventually manifest in particular perceptions and conceptions of fatness and of the female body.

The specific ways in which putative sexual differences have been used to support a modern androcentric social order have been explored at some length by science historian Londa Schiebinger in her influential monograph *Nature's Body: Gender in the Making of Modern Science*.[45] In particular, Schiebinger's work makes evident the intimate linkages between scientized sexism and racism justified by similar discourses. During the eighteenth century, European women, and non-Europeans of both sexes – particularly those of African descent – were objects of especially close attention from practitioners of the biological sciences. This spate of interest was sparked in part by the challenges that these groups posed within increasingly democratized societies, both in the metropole and the colonies, whose dominant members nevertheless fervently sought to protect the exclusivity of white men's political rights.[46] As both sex- and race-based varieties of anatomically justified hierarchy gained increasing cultural dominance (a phenomenon that would flourish more fully during the nineteenth century), the authority of those who laid claim to relevant scientific knowledge widened in scope as well as in potency. Of the consequences of this historical trend, Schiebinger writes: "Increasingly, questions of ethics (particularly those concerning equality) were taken to stand or fall on the findings of anatomists."[47] In other words, "expert" knowledge of bodies strongly influenced dominant conceptions of the capacities, natures, and rights of men and women and of racial and ethnic groups. In this regard, Schiebinger's analysis dovetails nicely with Foucault's conclusions on the growing role and changing nature of scientific and medical expertise, as well as with Laqueur's assertion of an emerging sexual differentiation of human subjects that was rooted in anatomical structures.

While there was a strong political investment in establishing that the "natures" of white women and non-white men were rooted in their biology to justify inequalities (including denying female rights and personhood, and rationalizing enslavement and other forms of sociolegal inequality, respectively), an intense interest in the comparative anatomy of African women (particularly the Khoekhoen, or so-called Hottentots discussed further in chapters 2 and 6) and their white European female counterparts also flourished; genital features, pelvis configurations, and distributions of body fat in breasts and buttocks preoccupied western medico-scientific men.[48] As Sander Gilman and, subsequently, Sabrina Strings have each stressed in their respective work on race, gender, and weight, Black women and their ostensibly "overdeveloped" fleshy bodies came to represent sexual surfeit, further emphasizing the "natural" modest and non-passionate character of the white bourgeois lady.[49] White women of the lower classes in Europe fared midway between these points, with "African-like" physical characteristics alleged to prevail in the "degenerate" working-class prostitute.[50] Both the accumulation of fat and, particularly, its apportionment in a manner that emphasized secondary sexual characteristics, marked certain classed and raced bodies as improper and inferior.[51] In an ironic twist, those female-identified bodies with prominent female-coded secondary sexual characteristics were often deemed to fall outside of feminine bodily norms.

By the height of scientific racism and comparative anthropometric study in the latter decades of the nineteenth century, physiognomy had gained a reasonably well-entrenched respectability, and the discernment of character from bodily form found a prominent place within "progressive" science.[52] While the ideas did not go unchallenged, mainstream medical literature often plainly linked physical features, particularly those of women, with mental "aberrations" or supposed deficiencies of the will (nymphomania and homosexuality were prominent among such maladies).[53] In other cases, men were the principal object of concern; Jews were popular nineteenth-century targets of gendered and racialized psychobiology, with their supposed predisposition to certain physical qualities – fatness among these – taken as evidence of the essentially effeminate character of Jewish males.[54] Whether the specific objects of anthropometric study were features considered to be inborn traits (such as ear, nose, and skull shape) or those that were ostensibly the consequences of behaviour (such as a "peculiar plumpness" among sex workers, posited to be the result of a life of leisure and excess),[55] bodies most certainly did matter – and the matter comprising bodies was increasingly situated by nineteenth-century medical science at the foundation of deeper human differences.

As these examples suggest, ways of seeing bodies shaped the possibilities of their interpretation. Granted, few of the developments in pre-twentieth-century biomedical epistemology could be said to require any *specific* stance toward particular bodies based solely upon how their sexual organs were configured or how much fat tissue they had and how it was distributed. However, social, cultural, and political trends and contestations exerted significant torque upon both theoretical discourses of biomedicine and concrete encounters with scientized subjects, shaping the meaning ascribed to various bodies.

Such intersections of sex, race, and bodily form also call our attention toward an important consideration: constituting bodies is inevitably a "multiple" enterprise. Illuminating here is the work of political theoretician and medical ethnographer Annemarie Mol. In her study of atherosclerosis in a contemporary Dutch medical centre, Mol has investigated the ways in which a given disease, as a singular named phenomenon, is generated in clinical practice through a variety of disparate but coordinated "enactments" by various agents. These agents, including the afflicted subject and various specialists and medical technicians, draw on unique sets of experiences, make diverse assumptions, use different technologies and forms of evidence, and work toward distinct goals.[56] Mol cautions that, inevitably, the "technicalities" of scientific and medical practice "depend on social matters: practicalities, contingencies, power plays, traditions."[57] Her work is part of a broader tradition of scholarship that attends to the practice of diagnosis as a socially and culturally constructed phenomenon, and as a site for both collaboration and contestation over bodies and their normate or non-normate (or, "normal" or "abnormal") statuses.[58] As Mol's study demonstrates, even the most resolutely "scientific" of medical classifications involves engaging multiple discourses, frameworks, forces, and parties to produce an intelligible body.

But let us turn back again specifically to fatness. In the nineteenth century, clearer and pervasive discursive linkage between fatness and pathology emerged reflecting the foundational roles of new ways of seeing and multiple contributors toward establishing "disordered" bodies. Given that fat – neither an "irregular" variety of bodily matter in and of itself, nor generally a symptomatic "illness" – would not likely be presented to a physician as a *symptom* (a health complaint) except in rare instances, the emphasis on *signs* (observable or measurable changes in body or behaviour) discerned by the medical "expert" was a prerequisite for the wholesale pathologization of fatness itself. In identifying disease-specific tissue types, post-mortem pathological studies of tumours and other growths and infiltrations of the era often involved the descriptor "fatty," both of their visual and tactile character;[59] this suggests an intriguing possibility that the increasingly central role granted to anatomical examination in medicine may have actually fostered a facile conflation of pathological fat-like substances with other types of fat accumulations on and in the living body, even if the latter did not produce symptomatic dysfunction. (We can still observe this slippage today, with cholesterol's presence within the arteries and visible fat accumulations in various bodily regions both described in the language of "fatty" deposits, despite their very different physiological roles and effects.)

Although neither of the twin aspects of biopower made the pathologization of fat bodies inevitable, they, like the epistemic culture of clinical medicine, provided further ground for it to emerge, with both individuals and collectivities serving as loci and foci of attention. The meme that "fatness signified wealth," often casually dropped into present-day discussions of pre-twentieth-century western social contexts, obscures the more complex class politics toward which Foucault's work gestures. While few eighteenth- and nineteenth-century bourgeois subjects would have wanted to be confused with underfed and overworked farm-turned-factory labourers, they also did not seek to be conflated with the "idle rich" of the hoary aristocracies. (One would do well, in this connection, to recall the French Revolutionary cry, "The people against the fat.")[60] Cultivating an association with *industry* gave a distinctive moral cast to the bourgeoisie's wealth and power, with an implicit self-justification of *earned*, not inherited, abundance. The image of the frivolous, lackadaisical, and overfed effeminate aristocrat was the very antithesis of the energetic masculine industrialist; this juxtaposition, coupled with the growing anatomo-political stress on controlling the habits and practices of the body, carved out a space for the emergence of the *body-as-project*. In the case of male citizens of the European colonial powers, this emphasis became increasingly interlinked with the theme of "imperial masculinity," with its stress upon a cultivated physique as an essential aid to moral discipline. British officers in nineteenth-century India, for instance, were berated for their increasing "unmanliness," shamefully evinced in part by their fleshy bellies.[61] Together, all of these developments laid fertile ground for negative readings of fat bodies, particularly those of men, as insufficiently disciplined, unsuitably self-indulgent, and inappropriately gendered. These concepts are explored in more detail in the chapters by Conor Heffernan and by Amy Shaw later in this volume.

Nineteenth-century biopolitical strategies also opened up the possibility of attempting to regularize bodies on a collective scale along a variety of axes, including gender and weight conformity. The historical precursors to contemporary norms of "biocitizenship" (or national belonging based on meeting or pursuing prescribed biological criteria) meant that sex and fatness, each by this point constituted as meaning-laden biological markers, could serve as a twinned pair of meeting points for the dual branches of biopower. This was particularly true insomuch as nationalistic concerns were themselves profoundly gendered. As Gilman observes, campaigns for weight modification through diet and/or other means became a way

> to intervene so as to improve the private life of the individual and thus the health of the nation. These two qualities were regularly linked. There were claims that morbid obesity impacted on the health of the mother and child, and thus weakened the state. Others believed that fat people could not fulfill their civic and military duty and became a drain on the state. The obese, from at least the mid-nineteenth century on, were seen as a danger to themselves as well as to others.[62]

Both the fat woman and the fat man possessed bodies that could be read as evidence of their failure as biocitizens, but in sex-specific ways to which each was bound by anatomical destiny. While "obese" females were thought to procreatively endanger the health of the nation and the race (the upkeep of which served as the female counterpart to the "white man's burden"), "excessively" fleshy males also fell outside of the bounds of normative – that is, economically and socially generative – masculinity, and it was feared they would induce a collective vulnerability in the populace. Thus, not only was fatness understood to impair both sexes, early anti-fat reasoning and rhetoric simultaneously acted to reaffirm disparate gender roles on the basis of biology, vesting men's biopolitical value in their *production*, and women's in their *reproduction* (or perceptions thereof).

In spite of their minimal relevance for ordinary clinical practice, medical interest during this period was particularly aroused by cases of exceptional or "monstrous" obesity, with photos and descriptions of extraordinarily corpulent individuals circulated via physicians' textbooks.[63] Such bodies were represented as curiosities on account of their uncommonness, but also – as the "monstrous" label suggests – as objects of anxiety for transgressing social norms and boundaries and lacking the "restraint of the will" that their weight was often believed to betoken. Though most reported cases were male (including Daniel Lambert, who became famous for his girth in eighteenth-century England, as discussed by Freya Gowrley later in this volume), the fascination with these unusually fat bodies mimicked the voyeurism shown toward the supposedly remarkable anatomies of African women – providing a revealing glimpse at intersections among practices of spectacularization (the making of certain subjects into "spectacles") and fetishization of racialized, sexed, and "weighted" bodies in western culture. As some fat female bodies failed to "perform" femininity in ways deemed proper, so too did certain fat male bodies spill over the bounds of the expected norms of white heterosexual masculinity, and both attracted the attention of medical science in part for their gender non-conformity.

Addressing the connection between such "unsettling" bodies (including fat bodies) and pathologization, Gilman marshals the insights of psychoanalytic theory:

> Order and control are the antithesis of "pathology." "Pathology" is disorder and the loss of control, the giving over of the self to the forces that lie beyond the self. It is because these forces actually lie within and are projected outside the self that the different is so readily defined as the pathological. Such definitions are an efficient way of displacing the consciousness that the self, as a biological entity subject to the inexorable rules of aging and decay, ultimately cannot be controlled.[64]

Gilman's reading of pathologization through the lens of psychodynamic processes provides a useful tool for understanding how "monstrous" bodies could be made to serve as the repository for the anxieties of a medical community whose ability to exercise control over disease and death was far from faultless, within a broader cultural context in which un/disciplined bodies and behaviour were invested with great symbolic value. As Black African bodies became the screen on which the sexual excesses disavowed by white European observers were projected, "monstrously" fat individuals performed a similar role for medical scientists and practitioners who sought membership within the "restrained and industrious" social classes in abjuring gastronomic gluttony and enervated sloth.

Not only the exceptional body drew the attention of experts by mid-century, however, but also the "project" of constructing the *normate* body. The rise of statistical medicine in Western Europe during this period brought with it an interest in correlating weight mathematically with other population characteristics – particularly height – and ushered in a discussion of establishing norms for clearly determining an individual's status as "overweight" or not.[65] The novelty of this interest is corroborated by the fact that the first scale designed for use in clinical settings was not manufactured until 1865.[66] As anthropometry sought to transform past physiognomic practices into "legitimate" science, computing population-wide norms, as well as differentiating quantified bodies by factors deemed culturally relevant (such as race, sex, class, ability, size, and configuration of tissues), became increasingly important tools for its widespread application. The captive populations of prisons were a prime location for such experimentations at quantification and control, as Antonie, Inwood, and Maxwell-Stewart explore in chapter 5 of this volume.

The "modern fetish for precise, standardized measurements"[67] only gradually came to be applied to body mass on a wide scale, with insurance tables toward the end of the century being among the first attempts to institutionalize a normative pattern of height/weight figures.[68] Such tables would figure among the most important instruments in strategies for weight-based biopolitical management later in the twentieth century. While efforts to establish normative values for fatness – outside of the comparative anthropometric study of particular body parts – remained largely in their infancy during most of the nineteenth century, these tables further solidified the legitimacy of sex-based anatomical divisions. As a result, as quantified corpulent subjects entered the realm of norm-based clinical medicine, they did so in progressively bifurcated streams as "fat men" and "fat women."

The other dimension of the physiognomic legacy in biomedicine is an aesthetic one: the discursive linkages cultivated between health and "attractiveness," and, correspondingly, between illness and "ugliness." While characterizing bodies in this manner long predates the nineteenth century, the rise of the norm-enforcing, biopolitical regime of health during this period lent such efforts a refined and legitimated character and a new impetus. In the medical philosophy of the day, as Gilman has written,

> the healthy is the beautiful, is the erotic, is the good, for it leads to the preservation and continuation of the collective. This is the norm against which the deviant is to be measured. The deviant is ill and is therefore ugly and evil ... The ugliness of the deviant may be overtly evident upon first glance, may appear over time, or may be evident only to the 'trained eye' of the physician/aesthetician.[69]

Not merely "unpleasant," the realm of the ill is further cast as actively *dangerous*, "always attempting to colonize the world of the healthy."[70] Health, beauty, and good citizenship thus emerge as powerfully intertwined constructs.

Within the medical-aesthetic evaluation of the body, Gilman notes, fatness occupied an ambivalent status. With regard to the female form, body fat could point, paradoxically, both to normalcy and to deviance. While, as noted above, racialized and classed women, such as the African Khoekhoen and European sex workers, were thought to be physiognomically marked by an "unnatural" fatness, the "healthy and beautiful" white bourgeois lady could also be recognized by her moderate, "attractive" plumpness, which signalled her capacity to aid in the healthy reproduction of the nation and the race.[71] Given that fatness could thus be read as a sign of vitality *or* degeneracy, it was imbued with an element of deception and, by extension, threat. However, within the anatomo-clinical framework, the ability to distinguish between these states was vested in the physician, who, as Foucault maintains, came to be perceived as exercising a form of trained, "essentially demystifying" sense perception,[72] revealing the truth of disease that remained obscure to the uninitiated layperson. Unlike those aforementioned males whose "monstrous" fat bodies made their otherness evident to all onlookers, the *ambiguous* voluptuosity of women necessitated the expert eye to discern life-giving health or species-defiling disease within their fleshy bodies. That the "diagnosis" commonly followed lines of race and class should be of no great surprise; given a racist and patriarchal tradition of objectification, in which bodies sexed as female have so often served as passive metonymies for broader social and political phenomena, the *meaning* of women's fat was of the utmost importance.

Given this context of increasing concern over non-normate bodies, it is not surprising that, toward mid-century, the notion of fatness as a medical disorder universally in need of remedial treatment began to take hold in many western nations. The first decades of the 1800s had witnessed the refinement of classificatory medicine's earlier attempts at analysing fatness, resulting in formulations of specific pathology-based understandings of fat tissue and the mechanisms of its accumulation.[73] Christoph Wilhelm Hufeland (1762–1836), a noted German physician, included within his 1828 treatise on medical practice a thoroughly pathologized understanding of "excessive" fat accumulation, asserting that it acted to

> impede the functions of the part concerned; and when it is universal, to embarrass motion, to overload the individual, to molest the whole economy, to oppress the circulation, to obstruct secretion and excretion; to dispose to external erysipelatous inflammations and abscesses; [and] finally, transition into cachexy and dropsy.[74]

Thus, fat and fatness by this point had started to become conceptualized as a clear and present danger to health, in and of itself, with decided pathological effects.

Nineteenth-century therapeutics directed toward the fat body, however, initially remained little changed since the days of ancient Greece (with the notable addition, as was common in the era, of mercurial treatment), and medical intervention into fat accumulation continued to be rare throughout the early 1800s.[75] In fact, one of the earliest overt efforts at expounding a systematic "treatment" of fatness is to be found, not in professional medical literature, but in an immensely popular pamphlet penned by William Banting (1797–1878), an English undertaker and coffin-maker. Banting developed an enthusiasm for "slimming" as a cure for various aliments after he lost a substantial amount of weight by adhering to a reduced-carbohydrate diet, as laid out in his 1863 *Letter on Corpulence*.[76] However, his system of dietary restrictions – "Bantingism," as it came to be popularly known – had a complex and troubled association with the medical profession. The weight-reduction approach described in his writing was inspired by the advice of Banting's physician, William Harvey, who drew on then-novel discoveries about how sugars and starches were metabolized. Yet, the pamphlet's success inspired vocal concern among some whose authority was threatened by this opening of health-related guidance and care to non-professionals.[77] In spite of Banting's repeated overcautious admonitions to only make such dietary changes under a physician's guidance, medical men still expressed disdain for the advice of this uncredentialled workingman who blurred boundaries between doctor and patient; the complaints clearly reveal a presumption of professional and class privilege among the medical community by this time. Indeed, it was nineteenth-century Britain that witnessed the rise of the "doctor-hero," much celebrated in popular culture, and entrusted with both knowledge of physique and moral leadership – an image that was to spread widely as new biomedical achievements changed once-incurable ailments into treatable inconveniences.[78] It is notable that Banting reports that he himself had not thought to look to his supposedly "incurable" girth to remedy his hearing loss or other health issues, until his physician suggested a connection.[79] Thus, the association of fat/ness with systemic pathology commenced, in Banting's case, through the expert gaze, as befits the medical regime of the period.

Literary scholar Joyce L. Huff has observed that Banting's method, while not the only Victorian attempt to cast corpulence in this fashion, held particular appeal because "the type of body that Banting documented, addressed, and came himself to embody was particularly well-suited to the forms of disciplinary power that appeared in the nineteenth century."[80] Crucially, she observes that Banting's reading of the body presents it as dynamic through ongoing tissue growth and decay; as capable of quantification and measurement for the sake of normalization; as in need of constant, unremitting management through the exercise of the will; and as culturally legible in terms of an individual's values, practices, and personal development.[81] It is evident that Banting's work is thoroughly predicated on many of the epistemic premises identified by Foucault – the framing of "disease" as the particular, observable configuration of specific tissues; health conditions presented as diagnosable through the perception of signs visible only to the gaze of the expert doctor; the body represented as a project requiring an internalization of disciplinary regimens; and the establishment of a normate body to which the populace at large was exhorted to conform.

The highly sex-stratified nature of Victorian society resulted in much overtly gendered self-improvement literature, including that concerning health and domestic remedies. Banting's pamphlet, though lacking the gendered mandate in the title of some contemporary texts for "ladies" or "gentlemen," nevertheless implicitly frames the advice therein as directed toward a male reader, by including a regularizing height/weight chart based solely on men's physical data and approving a fairly liberal use of hard liquor. Yet, perhaps more compelling than these points is the fact that the author consistently discusses fatness and weight loss in terms of his own subjective perceptions of bodily conditions, sensations, and experiences. What is comparably absent, in contrast with much of women's literature on health and lifestyle from the nineteenth century, is the body described as an aesthetic object of external perception. While evidence of the medical gaze is certainly present in Banting's text, the author demonstrates little interest in his own physical appearance or that of others – contrary to that witnessed in the more-professionalized and male-dominated scientific studies of the bodies of white women and of both men and women of colour.[82]

Banting was not alone in presenting his diet in a masculine frame. As historian Hillel Schwartz has noted, British and North American "public dieters" during most of the century were rarely female, and male exponents of weight loss tended to frame their slimming quest as "a muscular, willful act … a romance, an unburdening, a freeing up, a moral athleticism."[83] Schwartz contrasts this stance with the simultaneously discounted weight-loss attempts of women, commonly thought by men to be mere affect or vanity, as well as the more thorough medicalization of female bodies. He notes that, given the latter fact, "women's reducing had to be spoken of in terms of fluids, internal secretions and sexual ichor, as if womb and stomach were identical twins."[84] Complementing these gendered and sexed views was the sociopolitical stock placed in western women's bodies and behaviour to uphold the purity and repute of the "white race" in the context of colonial empires.[85] The shaping of female fat, therefore, was less an exercise in self-modification than it was a professionalized effort at restraining deviant bodies. Indeed,

> since it seemed that a woman's fluids were not completely under her control, women were to be cured of corpulence by intervention, by an imposed order and extrinsic technique. Hence the male insistence (today still) that women dieters are exasperatingly uncooperative and cannot will their own transformation.[86]

This orientation, notes Schwartz, left a lasting imprint on medical views of bodies, and provides a vivid example of the extent of the cleavage between the "two sexes" of Laqueur's model. Not limited to a distinction between sets of reproductive organs, the anatomic bifurcation of the body into male and female, when twinned with gendered notions of character and will, was to become an all-encompassing lens for encounters with bodies, including with their size, weight, and configuration of tissues. For example, Schwartz observes that

> very fat men in Western society have been represented most often as gluttons or monsters, very fat women as patients or freaks ... [thus] fat men contract diseases of the stomach and joints (as gluttons) or diseases of the heart (as monsters). Fat women endure glandular disturbances (as patients) and the misfortunes of heredity (as freaks). Men suffer from solidity and largeness: the paunch, the swollen heart. Women suffer from fluidity and smallness: the hormones, the chromosomes. The condition of fat men is reparable because more tangible and accessible; women's fat is intransigent because constitutional, deep and ultimately historical.[87]

The "active" monstrosity or excess attributed to the fat male subject, and the objectification of the fat female as the "passive" patient (unlike, for example, the patient-as-advisor model of Banting), with a body in need of – if perpetually resistant to – external control, remains deeply embedded within the cultural logic of biomedicine, as manifest in research and clinical settings, as well as in popular discourses of health and fat/ness. The continuing propensity of western biomedical practitioners to diagnose such ailments in distinctly sexed and "weighted" ratios (even when statistical data may not support these distributions) reflects the deep and abiding entrenchment of the nineteenth-century gendering and sexing of fat.

Schwartz's analysis brings us full circle, as it were, to Peter Conrad's remark, cited early in this chapter, that the power of medicalization is, at its root, "definitional." The constitution of selected subjects as "normal" and others as "deviant" depends on delineating specific criteria by which to mark out both centre and periphery. Further, it demands a discursive power that must justify and maintain its authority and hegemony – a task much more readily and securely accomplished through the institutionalized perpetuation of the epistemologies, discourses, and practices that constitute its characteristic "regime of truth." In defining fat bodies as pathological and in need of professionalized intervention, *all* bodies are brought further within a regime of diagnostic reasoning, where weight and size are always subject to being measured and evaluated against a set of norms. As these norms themselves are unstable, shifting, and responsive to broader sociocultural currents, all embodied subjects come to exist within a suspenseful indeterminacy of sorts, in which anyone may potentially be deemed "abnormal."

And yet, all bodies are not equally vulnerable in this regard. The disparities in the medicalization of fat bodies nuance Foucault's general explication of the development of the anatomo-clinical medical regime. While the clinical gaze achieved a dominant role in the pathologization of fat bodies over the course of the nineteenth century, it was also embedded with gendered, racialized, and classed epistemic dimensions, resulting in fat subjects being perceived and managed in diverse ways.

Fat men, as Gilman notes, were made to embody the "dangers" of fatness even in texts targeted at female readers during the nineteenth century.[88] This was made possible by a cultural context in which males have tended to function as the unmarked normative prototypes for humanity, and the prevalence of the notion that a "hobbled masculinity"[89] endangered the collective well-being of the species (and more particularly, the interests of the white upper classes). Yet, in medical discourse, most nineteenth-century fat white men were at least fortunate enough to retain some degree of active subjectivity in relation to their bodies, even if it was often deployed to seek conformity with socially and medically reinforced ideas of weight. Fat female bodies, for their part, were more consistently rendered as objects and pressed to bear a surplus of meaning, reducing women's already-limited agency within a medicalized regime of truth and power/knowledge. The interlacing of existing constructions of female irrationality and obstinacy with biopolitical goals for managing and healthfully reproducing the state, placed corpulent women at a further disadvantage under the anatomo-clinical gaze. Yet, as fatness was medicalized along lines of sex and gender, the latter were simultaneously co-constituted by discourses and practices relating to fatness. Fat tissue and its distribution within individual bodies and among human populations increasingly emerged as a crucial component of the multiple enactment of sexed bodies and gendered subjectivities.

NOTES

1 Georges Canguilhem, *The Normal and the Pathological*, translated by Carolyn R. Fawcett and Robert S. Cohen (New York: Zone Books, 1991 [1972]), 226.
2 Peter Conrad, *The Medicalization of Society: On the Transformation of Human Conditions into Treatable Disorders* (Baltimore, MD: John Hopkins University Press, 2007), 8.
3 Paul Campos, *The Obesity Myth: Why America's Obsession with Weight is Hazardous to Your Health* (New York: Gotham Books, 2004).
4 J. Eric Oliver, *Fat Politics: The Real Story Behind America's Obesity Epidemic* (New York: Oxford University Press, 2006).
5 Michael Gard and Jan Wright, *The Obesity Epidemic: Science, Morality and Ideology* (London: Routledge, 2005).
6 Lindo Bacon, *Health At Every Size: The Surprising Truth About Your Weight*, 2nd ed. (Dallas, Texas: BenBella Books, 2010).
7 Susan Bordo, *Unbearable Weight: Feminism, Western Culture, and the Body* (Berkeley, CA: University of California Press, 1993).
8 Kathleen LeBesco, *Revolting Bodies? The Struggle to Redefine Fat Identity* (Amherst: University of Massachusetts Press, 2004).
9 Sander L. Gilman, *Fat: A Cultural History of Obesity* (Cambridge: Polity Press, 2008).
10 Sabrina Strings, *Fearing the Black Body: The Racial Origins of Fatphobia* (New York: New York University Press, 2019).
11 See Sander Gilman, *Fat Boys: A Slim Book* (Lincoln: University of Nebraska Press, 2004), 35–45. See also Gilman, "Fat as Disability: The Case of the Jews," *Johns Hopkins University Press* 23, no. 1 (Spring 2004): 46–60, https://10.1353/lm.2004.0003.
12 See George A. Bray, "Obesity: Historical Development of Scientific and Cultural Ideas," *International Journal of Obesity* 14 (1990): 909–26.
13 While these connections are too substantial and extensive to devote adequate attention to in the context of this chapter, the reader is strongly encouraged to consider Strings's *Fearing the Black Body* in conjunction with the argument presented here, for a richer picture of these racializing histories of fatness.
14 For examples, see McKinley 1999; Braziel 2001; Kent 2001; Mosher 2001; Murray 2004; Bell & McNaughton 2007; Rice 2007; and Monaghan 2008.
15 See Saukko 1999; Shieff 2001; and Jutel 2009.
16 See Schwartz 1986; Gilman 2004; Mitchinson 2018; and Strings 2019.
17 Michel Foucault, *The Birth of the Clinic: An Archaeology of Medical* Perception (New York: Pantheon, 1973).
18 Much of Gilman's work deals with these themes, and the reader is directed to the bibliography for Gilman's relevant works.

19 Thomas Laqueur, *Making Sex: Body and Gender from the Greeks to Freud* (Cambridge, MA: Harvard University Press, 1992).
20 Annemarie Mol, *The Body Multiple: Ontology in Medical Practice* (Durham: Duke University Press, 2002).
21 Following the lines of Foucault's influential analysis, any given society is characterized by (1) particular "types of discourse which it accepts and makes function as true" (1980, 131); (2) means and mechanisms for distinguishing "true" knowledge from invalid or unintelligible statements about the world; and (3) criteria for vesting authority over truth in certain persons and institutions. Such a truth regime is created, sustained, and extended via its intimate imbrication with systems and structures of power – leading Foucault to argue for the indivisible pair "power/knowledge" as the key factors in the constitution of subjects (ibid.).
22 Michel Foucault, *The Archaeology of Knowledge*, trans. A.M. Sheridan Smith (London: Routledge, 1989 [London: Tavistock, 1972]), 211.
23 Thomas Kuhn, *The Structure of Scientific Revolutions*, 2nd ed. (Chicago: University of Chicago Press), 1970.
24 For a more detailed account of Foucault's notion of *épistémè*, see Michel Foucault, *The Order of Things: An Archaeology of the Human Sciences* (New York: Pantheon Books, 1970).
25 Foucault, 1973.
26 *The Birth of the Clinic*, like much of Foucault's work, focuses specifically on the French context; it is clear from his other writings and, particularly, interviews that Foucault intended his analysis to apply in a broader sense, including other parts of Western Europe and North America, insomuch as these societies partook in a high degree of cultural exchange, particularly within the realm of medical study and practice.
27 This trend toward a tightly controlled credentialized system was solidified in the early twentieth century in the United States and Canada with the issuance of the Flexner Report in 1910, funded by the Carnegie Foundation.
28 See *Birth of the Clinic*, ch. 1 ("Spaces and Classes"), 3–21.
29 See *Birth of the Clinic*, ch. 7 ("Seeing and Knowing"), 107–23. Importantly, Foucault notes that "the medical gaze embraces more than is said by the word 'gaze' alone. It contains within a single structure different sensorial fields. The sight/touch/hearing trinity defines a perceptual configuration is tracked down by markers, gauged in depth, drawn to the surface, and projected virtually on the dispersed organs of [the patient or] the corpse" (*Birth of the Clinic*, 164).
30 *Birth of the Clinic*, 162.
31 See Elizabeth T. Hurren, *Dying for Victorian Medicine: English Anatomy and Its Trade in the Dead Poor, c.1834–1929* (Hampshire and New York: Palgrave Macmillian, 2012).

32 See Rachel N. Ponce, "'They Increase in Beauty and Elegance': Transforming Cadavers and the Epistemology of Dissection in Early Nineteenth-Century American Medical Education," *Journal of the History of Medicine and Allied Sciences* 68, no. 3 (July 2013): 331–76.
33 Michel Foucault, *"Society Must Be Defended": Lectures at the Collège de France, 1975–1976,* trans. by David Macey (New York: Picador, 2003), 240–1.
34 Michel Foucault, *The History of Sexuality: An Introduction* (vol. 1), trans. by Robert Hurley (New York: Vintage Books, 1990 [New York: Pantheon Books, 1978]), 139–45.
35 Foucault, *The History of Sexuality*, 124.
36 Foucault, *The History of Sexuality*, 125.
37 Foucault, *"Society Must Be Defended,"* 252.
38 Lennard Davis, "Introduction: Normality, Power, and Culture," in *The Disability Studies Reader*, 4th edition (New York: Routledge, 2013), 2.
39 See Foucault, *History of Sexuality*, 146–50.
40 Thomas Laqueur, *Making Sex: Body and Gender from the Greeks to Freud* (Cambridge, MA: Harvard University Press, 1990).
41 Laqueur, *Making Sex* , 52.
42 Simone de Beauvoir's famous statement, "On ne naît pas femme: on le deviant," is often taken as marking the inauguration of the now-mainstream position that occupying a specific type of sexed body is not itself a determinant of a particular sort of gendered experience in society. See Beauvoir, *Le deuxième sexe* (Paris: Editions Gallimard, 1949), or the book's various English translations as *The Second Sex.*
43 Beauvoir, *Le deuxième sexe,* 153.
44 Beauvoir, *Le deuxième sexe*, esp. 154–8.
45 Londa Schiebinger, *Nature's Body: Gender in the Making of Modern* Science (Boston: Beacon Press, 1993).
46 See Schiebinger, *Nature's Body*, 183, and also Strings, *Fearing the Black Body,* ch. 7, "Good Health to Uplight the Race," 169–86.
47 Schiebinger, *Nature's Body*, 172.
48 See Schiebinger, *Nature's Body*, esp. chs. 4 and 6: "The Anatomy of Difference" and "The Hottentot Venus."
49 Sander Gilman, ch. 3: "The Hottentot and the Prostitute" in *Difference and Pathology* (Ithaca, NY: Cornell University Press, 1985), 76–108, and Strings, ch. 3, "The Rise of the Big Black Woman," 67–98.
50 Gilman, "The Hottentot and the Prostitute," esp. 94–108.
51 See Sabrina Strings, *Fearing the Black Body: The Racial Origins of Fatphobia* (NY: NYUP, 2019), for a detailed exploration of the complex racialized dynamics of this gendered phenomenon, which are, regrettably, outside of the scope of this chapter.

52 See, for example, the many works on race and physical constitution published in the *Journal* of the Anthropological Society of London (1863–1871).
53 See Gilman, *Difference and Pathology*, esp. 89–101.
54 See Gilman, "Fat as Disability: The Case of the Jews," *Literature and Medicine* 23 (2004): 46–60.
55 Gilman, *Difference and Pathology*, 94.
56 Annemarie Mol, *The Body Multiple: Ontology in Medical Practice* (Durham: Duke University Press, 2002).
57 Mol, *The Body Multiple*, 171.
58 For example, see J.F. Duchan and D. Kovarsky, eds., *Diagnosis as Cultural Practice* (Berlin: Mouton de Gruyter, 2005).
59 Examples of this labelling are provided by Foucault in *Birth of the Clinic*, 157.
60 Quoted in Gilman, *Fat Boys*, 3.
61 Gilman, *Fat Boys*, 107.
62 Gilman, *Fat: A Cultural History of Obesity* (Cambridge: Polity Press, 2008), 4.
63 Bray, 920.
64 Gilman, *Difference and Pathology*, 24.
65 Bray, 919.
66 Peter N. Stearns, *Fat History: Bodies and Beauty in the Modern West* (New York: New York University Press, 1997), 27.
67 Stearns, *Fat History*, 27.
68 Stearns, *Fat History*, 42.
69 Sander Gilman, *Picturing Health and Illness: Images of Difference* (Baltimore: The John Hopkins University Press, 1995), 66.
70 Gilman, *Picturing Health and Illness*, 66.
71 Gilman, *Picturing Health and Illness*, 62.
72 Foucault, *Birth of the Clinic*, 121.
73 See Bray, 917.
74 Quoted in Bray, 918.
75 Bray, 918.
76 William Banting, *Letter on Corpulence*, 4th ed. (London: Harrison, 1869).
77 Joyce L. Huff, "A 'Horror of Corpulence': Interrogating Bantingism and Mid-Nineteenth-Century Fat-Phobia," in *Bodies Out of Bounds: Fatness and Transgression*, ed. J.E. Braziel and K. LeBesco (Berkeley: University of California Press, 2001) 40.
78 See Roy Porter, *Bodies Politic: Disease, Death and Doctors in Britain, 1650–1900*, esp. ch. 10: "Victorian Developments," 250–71 (Ithaca, NY: Cornell University Press, 2001).
79 Banting, *Letter on Corpulence*, preface.
80 Huff, "A 'Horror of Corpulence'," 43.

81 See Huff, "A 'Horror of Corpulence'," 43–53.

82 See Strings, chapter 5, "American Beauty: The Reign of the Slender Aesthetic," 122–46, for a richer account of these racialized norms in nineteenth-century America.

83 Hillel Schwartz, *Never Satisfied: A Cultural History of Diets, Fantasies and Fat* (New York: Macmillan, 1986), 17.

84 Schwartz, *Never Satisfied*, 17.

85 See, for example, Mrinalini Sinha, *Colonial Masculinity*, ch. 1: "Reconfiguring Hierarchies: The Ilbert Bill Controversy, 1883–84" (New York: Manchester University Press, 1995), 33–68.

86 Schwartz, *Never Satisfied*, 17–18.

87 Schwartz, *Never Satisfied*, 18.

88 Gilman, *Fat Boys*, 5.

89 Gilman, *Fat Boys*, 19.

2 To Measure Skulls, to Measure Waists: The Nineteenth-Century Origins of Modern Health Standards

BESSIE RIGAKOS AND WESLEY R. BISHOP

The world would do well to remember the life of Sarah Baartman. Born in 1789 in South Africa, she relocated to Europe in the early 1800s to work as a performer.[1] Once there, she was routinely abused by her manager, who placed her in carnival-like performances. She was forced to dance and appear naked before Europeans so that the white audience members could gawk at her body. Of particular note among the media and audiences of the day was her buttocks. This racist exhibitionism would warrant a study even if the audience members were merely everyday folk. However, European scientists also viewed Baartman's performances and body. White researchers deemed Baartman's size and fat excessive and concluded that these features were "proof" that Black Africans, specifically Black women, were "inferior" due to their anatomy, proportions, and size. Europeans then labelled Baartman the "Hottentot Venus," and used her specific body to make broad generalizations about the alleged "fitness" and civility of all African people.

The racist project continued well after Baartman's death in 1815. A museum in France acquired her remains. Her skeleton, and a cast of her body, continued to greet visitors until the 1970s (Figures 2.1 and 2.2) when the South African government finally gained control of her body and laid her to rest in her home country.[2] As far as historical subjects go, Sarah Baartman is widely known, the subject of many scholarly and artistic studies. With dramatic films like *Venus Noire* (2010), she has even made her way into popular understandings of how body ideals – size, shape, and fat density – are based on notions of white supremacy and colonialism. Yet, despite her story being known and widely discussed in numerous historical and sociological texts, how often do people learn of this history and continue to count calories, fret over body size, and personally project onto themselves racist ideals of fatness and thinness?

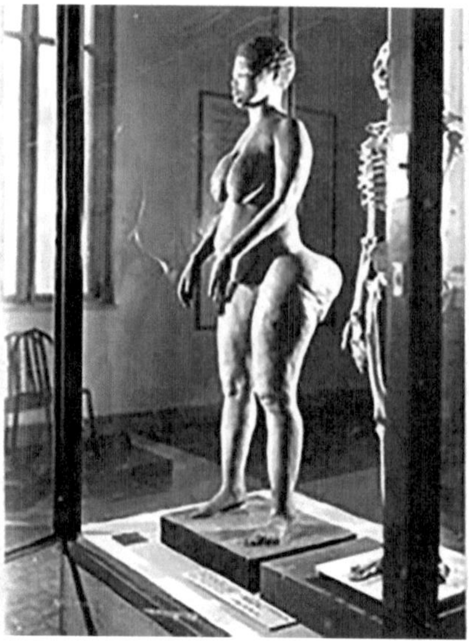

Figure 2.1. Sarah Baartman's bodily remains and cast in the *Musée de l'Homme (Museum of Man).* Baartman died in Europe in 1815, at around the age of twenty-six.

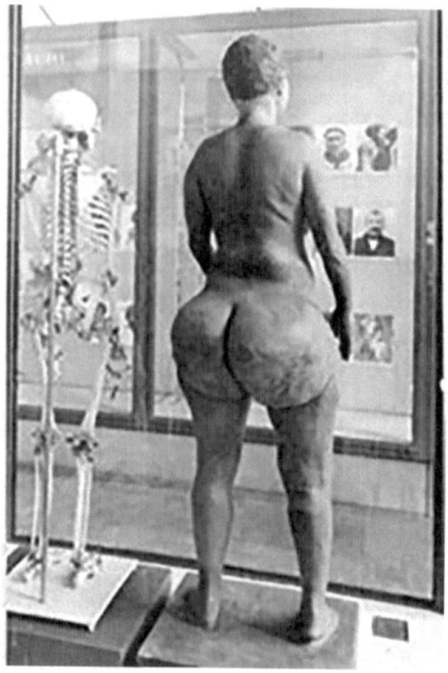

Figure 2.2. Europeans preserved Sarah Baartman's bodily remains for the purpose of arguing for white supremacy in terms of race and body size. Her remains would not be retrieved by the South African government until 2002.

This chapter attempts to clarify the misrepresentations of body ideals, specifically so-called deviant bodies and attitudes toward policing women's bodies, which had become firmly established by the beginning of the twentieth century. We argue that the deviant body has historically often been associated with marginalized persons. In the Progressive Era of the late nineteenth and early twentieth centuries, fat and body size became a central part of conceptualizing that deviancy, shaping contemporary attitudes about class, gender, and scientific beliefs about health. Examining the writings of three global Progressive Era scholars and social commentators – Ella Adelia Fletcher, Cesare Lombroso, and Guglielmo Ferrero – suggests that the same thinkers and movements who often measured skulls to determine alleged mental "fitness" also measured waists to determine health ideals. Their methods aimed to create not merely a standard of medical health, but a set of norms to judge a person's potential civil and criminal qualities.

The phenomenon now known as "fatphobia," and the racist classification of bodies in the long nineteenth century, was of wide concern among thinkers and activists in the Progressive Era. We have selected three figures – Fletcher, Lombroso, and Ferrero – to show how certain thinkers shaped these ideas. Our aim in this chapter is to show that anti-fat bias did not rest on sound medical reasoning but rather was shaped by cultural attitudes, poorly defined, and flimsily defended. Indeed, "medicine" and "cultural biases" were often indistinct concepts during this era. This is evident when comparing Fletcher, a popular inspirational writer, and Lombroso, a medical researcher, who, despite these differences in approach present their arguments in very similar ways based almost entirely on rhetoric. The only major difference was that Fletcher took arbitrary measurements and codified many of the biases of the nineteenth century under a veneer of science. We have also included Ferrero because his work provides a better understanding of the emergence of fatphobia and its adoption in subsequent generations. Ferrero, a historian and writer who had married into Lombroso's family, popularized many of these ideas. His thinking was taken seriously enough that in 1908 he was invited to visit Theodore Roosevelt in the White House. Journalists described Ferrero's impression of the president: "Roosevelt denounces physical as well as moral sterility … The President believes that a glorious civilization is in store if we can preserve intellectual refinement from eclipse by luxury, which will happen if we invoke primitive energy to create an eternal civilization."[3]

Ferrero's work shows us how these ideas of the ideal human body, and their relation to health, both personal and social, continued on after the initial writings of figures like Lombroso. Also, given Ferrero's wide acceptance and his connection with other major figures of the period, we see in these three figures how these ideas originated, continued, and eventually dominated.

Eventually, these ideals of human fitness led to prescribed social norms of what a "civilized" and well-regulated body should be. Efforts to achieve this ideal involved policing or controlling and stigmatizing bodies, especially women's bodies. This tension is seen clearly in the various sections of the Progressive Era reform movements that portrayed fatness as a signifier of capitalist excess and greed. Images, typically of white men with bulging bellies, were used throughout the long nineteenth century to signify an individual's class status. Through much of the nineteenth century, fat was a marker of successful capitalism and a signifier of wealth and ability, as discussed by Conor Heffernan in this volume. During the Progressive Era, some social commentators began to argue that fatness was a result of taking more than

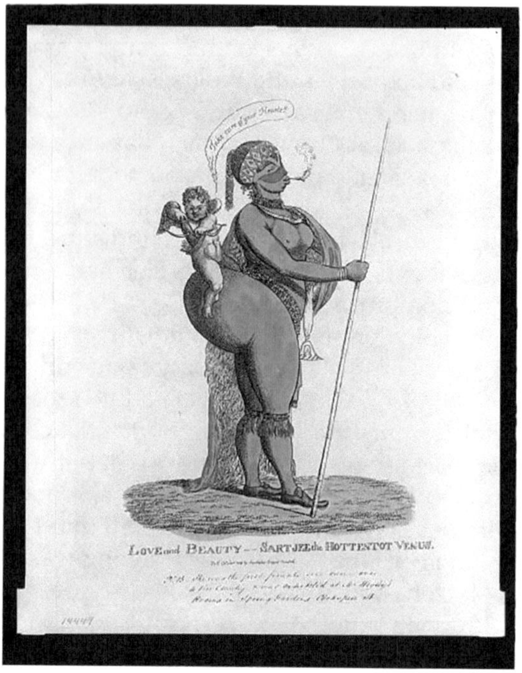
Take care of your Heart!
LOVE and BEAUTY -- SARTJEE the HOTTENTOT VENUS.

Figure 2.3. Print of a mostly naked Sarah Baartman created in 1811. The image of the cupid says, "Take care of your heart."

what was warranted, thereby impoverishing the masses. The visceral image of fatness, therefore, served as a way that activists and commentators simultaneously struggled for greater economic equality while also furthering the marginalization of particular peoples.[4]

There is no shortage of examples of these stereotypes of fat people tied to race and capitalism. What we see in Figures 2.3 and 2.4 are representations of bodily connections between savagery and capitalism. In Figure 2.3, there is the racist stereotype of the "African savage," and in Figure 2.4 is the engorged white capitalist of western modernity. Found in the middle of the two images would be a Progressive Era ideal of fitness and responsible civic behaviour. People of colour were often depicted by white European and American media as living in a state of savagery, incapable of civilization, let alone moderation. Their bodies revealed them as diametrically opposed to the Progressive ideals of self-control, virtue, and self-guidance. Capitalism and modern consumption could also pose a problem, however, in that their excesses produced a body type similar to that of the supposed savage. The key then, to

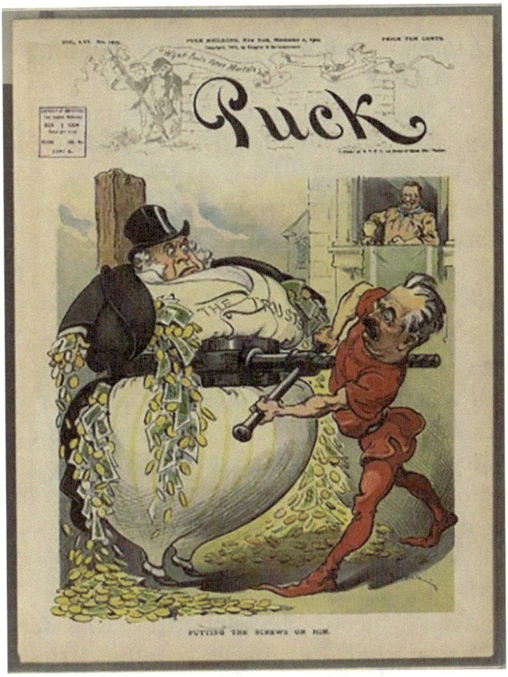

Figure 2.4. 1904 cover of *Puck* magazine with then-secretary of Commerce and Labor George B. Cortelyou attacking the excesses of corporate capitalism. Theodore Roosevelt, the progressive reformer turned president, watches approvingly. Fatness is equated with both greed and violating good democratic government. Captioned: "Putting the screws on him."

this Progressive Era thinking, was strict moderation, virtue conceived through the ability to regulate oneself and prevent a descent into either savagery or gluttonous excess. As is further discussed by Bonnie Miller in chapter 9, a "good" citizen, one who was capable of self-regulation and civic responsibility, was a person who could maintain a "good" physical body.

This attention to the virtues of moderation did not just decry fat, but also eschewed excessive thinness. Throughout the nineteenth century, there was much evidence that medical researchers also worried that bodies, specifically women's bodies, could be too slender, which also created concern and the need for policing. As Sabrina Strings argues, the weight of women became a regulation issue for medical professionals in the late nineteenth and early twentieth century. If women were to become too thin or too fat, there could be substantial social and cultural consequences. Education by experts seemed to be required. "The weight of American women represented, to many, a national black eye," Strings writes. "But was it truly the case, as was often suggested, that these women were simply nutritionally uninformed? Given the right information would they gain in flesh, and by proxy, in health, strength, and beauty?"[5]

The scope of Progressivism means that the answers to these questions depended on region, individuals, and the decade within the Progressive Era. Yet even when accounting for these differences, one can see the emergence of an understanding that connected people's failings in civic life to the shape and size of their body. More specifically, as the Progressive Era reached its apex in the beginning decades of the twentieth century, fatness took on new emphasis in demarcating unfitness for civil life. Scientists and researchers of this period created not only a set of cultural norms about health but also eugenic programs that classified and labelled specific body types, particularly fat bodies, as both criminal and a danger to civil society. The surest way to ensure the maintenance of regulated bodies was, of course, to forcibly police them through eugenics.

The term "eugenics," meaning "well born," was coined in 1883 by Sir Francis Galton, a respected British scholar and cousin of Charles Darwin, to "indicate a program of planning and rationalization of human reproduction, aimed at the biological improvement of the species."[6] This version of the eugenics movement peaked in the late nineteenth and early twentieth century, but its roots stretched back to antiquity; perhaps most infamously, Plato's *Republic* presented a society in which the state monitored human reproduction.[7] The Spartans also ensured that only the most robust babies would survive by bathing them in wine and exposing them to harsh elements. Likewise, according to ancient Roman law, children who were born defective must die. Seneca, the Roman philosopher, wrote that "We put down mad dogs; we kill the wild, untamed ox; we use the knife on sick sheep to stop their infecting the flock; we destroy abnormal offspring at birth; children, too, if they are born weak or deformed, we drown. Yet this is not the work of anger, but of reason – to separate the sound from the worthless."[8] These classical ideals prescribed vigorously regulating the biological nature of human populations, and went on to inform the writings, research, and policies of nineteenth-century thinkers. What is of particular note here is that the standards that these commentators, ancient to modern, used to demarcate superior and inferior bodies were not consistent with one another or over time. Rather, these thinkers used the idea of eugenics as a way to organize their own ideal society. Nineteenth- and early twentieth-century eugenicists did the same, suggesting that inferior people, which was a judgment explicitly based on criteria such as body size (both too small and too large), perceptions of strength, and membership in particular classes, be discouraged from reproducing because that would ultimately destroy a society. Eugenics was the justification for carrying this out by explicitly policing bodies, with the social and subjective aspects of the movement combined with standards of "health" created by Progressive Era thinkers like Ella Adelia Fletcher, Cesare Lombroso, and Guglielmo Ferraro.

Ella Adelia Fletcher was a late nineteenth-century American spiritualist and philosopher who wrote several books and many articles on health, beauty, the soul, and natural healing. Fletcher's work is particularly important for understanding the way white supremacists compared other cultures' views of beauty and particular body types with the broader culture of the late nineteenth and early twentieth centuries. As Christopher E. Forth has argued, medical researchers from the long nineteenth century shared as much with spiritual and fashion writers as they did medical health researchers.[9] This can be seen in Fletcher's writing in 1901, where she stated:

> There are some tribes in Central Africa where the perverted taste for excessive corpulence is carried to such an extent that the 'beauties' have to be supported when they walk abroad, their flesh hanging like pendent bags from their arms and legs … One is driven, involuntarily, to draw a parallel between the physical distortions cultivated among savage races and the follies of Fashion which give temporary vogue to equally as absurd deformities; a proof that there is a lingering taint of the savage and barbarous which civilization has not yet succeeded in exterminating. But it is daily becoming a greater sin to commit offenses against true beauty, because more and more our opportunities are widened for the acquirement of knowledge which supplies us with the data necessary to distinguish between the true and the false.[10]

Fletcher argued that overindulgence did not only reflect different cultures but that it was a remnant of all past cultures, and therefore pointed toward western civilization's past. This past could be returned to, with savagery replacing any semblance of progress that western civilization had made, if society remained unchecked. This fear was mostly aimed at the existence of fat bodies, unregulated bodies, bodies that did not conform to the nineteenth and early twentieth-century European ideals of beauty and restraint. In *The Philosophy of Rest* (1900), Fletcher continues this line of reasoning, arguing that the entire modern age was guilty of giving in to excess. "We seem to be engaged in a warfare with time, whom we would annihilate," she wrote, "when ninety-five men and women out of every hundred struggle to make their days thirty hours long."[11] The key was to imbue oneself with the spirit of regulation, moderation, and, ultimately, rest. "Cultivate repose and a critical faculty of selection. Live upon the heights and limit your desires to the high things, the great things of life."[12]

Of course, only some people were deemed capable of such an exercise, and therein lay the issue for broader society. Certain people were thought to be fundamentally incapable of the regulation needed for a healthy, attractive body. Fletcher, among many others, explicitly stated that these particular people were not white. Yes, white Europeans could fall into a state of savagery, but if they did, it was because they had regressed. This viewpoint posited women of colour as being in a state of permanent "barbarism" or "savagery," which white society had allegedly moved beyond but was permanently poised to fall back into. Since women of colour were incapable of this self-regulation, they were automatically unable to be fully respected members of the Progressive Era society. And, since white women, or even men, could return to this state, they required constant supervision.

This policing was not, according to Fletcher, only the responsibility of the state. Instead, white women and men could regulate themselves by practising behavioural control. Fletcher linked the mind and body using a pseudo-spiritual way of thinking. She argued for the cultivation of a so-called soul force, a mindset that regulated not only the body but also people's behaviours, energies, and psychological state. People's inability to self-regulate meant that they were either "savages" (typically non-westerners and people of colour) or modern people who had succumbed because their manifest unfitness had led to decadence. Soul force, Fletcher explained "is a force that to be effective must be recognized, and which waxes strong only under the favoring influences of cultivation," i.e., civilization and personal behaviour. Fletcher, most interestingly, given her attention to people's bodies, predicted that "materialists" would demand physical evidence, and she chastised those who would make such inquiries. "There are few who deny the divine origin of vital force, yet materialism blinds men to the fact that the soul, through its spirit, is the connecting link with that origin, and the ever-ready agent … [Of] increased strength and vitality to the whole being, physical as well as mental. Over the vast and mysterious sensatory organization of the body, and nervous system, it has absolute control."[13]

Fletcher was mainly a nineteenth-century cultural critic and self-help author. Her work fits into the broader push of marginalizing fat bodies, but by her own admission contained next to no real scientific evidence. Yet Fletcher's lack of proof did not mean that other Progressive Era thinkers would not attempt to use the auspices of science to justify their ideas. This can be seen with the writings of nineteenth-century Italian criminologist Cesare Lombroso.[14] Lombroso was influenced by German materialism, which sought objective fact; by Comtian positivism, which demanded scientific phenomena; and by a Darwinian biological evolutionary theory, which was later extended into the idea of social evolution by Herbert Spencer.[15] From this knowledge, Lombroso gained a new perspective and added to it the controversial dimension of eugenics and the notion of atavism or the hereditary deterioration that disrupts the process of human evolution.[16] His primary objective was not to intervene in the reproductive process, but rather to isolate antisocial criminals and segregate them from the rest of society. Lombroso developed a theory of deviance that argued that a person's bodily constitution indicated whether they were predisposed to criminality. Rejecting the idea that crime was a universal characteristic of human nature, Lombroso believed that certain strains of human populations inherited criminality. Physically deviant individuals were born criminals because they were regressions to an earlier, more primitive stage of human evolution. In developing his theory, Lombroso used the dichotomy of "good" and "bad" when making comparisons. For instance, when observing the physical characteristics of Italian prisoners ("bad") and comparing them with those of Italian soldiers ("good"), he concluded that the group of prisoners were, in fact, criminal, and thus "bad" because they were physiologically different.

The physical characteristics he used to identify prisoners relied mainly on body size, and specifically fat, but also included asymmetry of the face or head, large "monkey-like ears," enlarged lips, a twisted nose, excessive cheekbones, long arms, and excessive wrinkles on the skin. He concluded that any individual, male or female, with the physical makeup, mental capabilities, and instincts of "primitive man" was atavistic. Lombroso declared that men with a majority of these physical features should be marked as born criminals and segregated from others in society. Women, on the other hand, required fewer of these features to be born criminals. Lombroso used the results from his study of a "total of 1,033 observations on female criminals, 176 observations on the skulls of female criminals, 685 on the skulls of prostitutes, 225 on the normal women in hospitals, and 30 others also normal"[17] to draw conclusions favouring the superiority of men and further criminalizing the bodies of physically "deviant" women by introducing a control group of "normal" women, labelled as the "good" group. His flawed methods, which were both misogynistic and racist, marginalized this deviant group of women and established a standard for further oppressing certain body types.

The fat body, Lombroso argued, was one of the most visible signs of criminality and criminal tendencies. He stated that excessive weight and weight gain were seen in prostitutes, which he blamed on their "savage" and "primitive" nature, attributed to atavism. Lombroso further made the connection that fat prostitutes were physiologically comparable to African women, thus linking fatness to race. Fat was thus part of a menu of deviant traits that developed over time and peaked as a pejorative in the twentieth century. Lombroso's perception of the fat body was negative, and he argued that it was dangerous enough to warrant state-sanctioned policing. When we discuss fat in the twenty-first century, we are often still talking about this belief. Yet we need to understand that fat was nothing more than a random marker, intentionally chosen by turn-of-the-century researchers to delineate some bodies as deviant. It is not in self-care and health, but instead in criminality and punishment, disproportionately directed toward women of colour, that twentieth and twenty-first century fears of fat originate. To continue to fear, hate, and police fatness is as ethically justifiable as continuing to fear, hate, and police any of the other markers that Lombroso singled out.

As Dorie Klein wrote about Lombroso's book, *The Female Offender* (1903), "Lombroso described female criminality as an inherent tendency produced in individuals that could be regarded as biological atavisms, similar to cranial and facial features, and one could expect a withering away of crime if the atavistic people were prohibited from breeding."[18] Lombroso's theory of criminality gained popularity because his results supported contemporary prejudices, and because they relied on quantitative methods. These gave researchers the ability to duplicate the false science by merely generalizing their observations, including numbers, and deeming certain behaviours simply innate. Lombroso maintained that criminality, or unethical behaviour in general, was tied to in utero defects rather than agency or free will. In this way, Lombroso connected medical conditions to broader social actions, arguing that both were inescapable characteristics of particular body types. This served as a way for scientists following Lombroso to justify their cultural attitudes not as bigotry but instead as simple measurable science.

Lombroso attracted a circle of followers when he linked deviant biological and physical characteristics to those he labelled "bad" or "delinquent." But he is only one extreme of an anti-fat continuum; his science reinforced more general cultural beliefs about fat bodies. Lombroso's theories continue to influence contemporary researchers who have used his methods to explain that emotional, physical, and psychological differences distinguish the "good" group of women from the "bad" group and thus indicate biological inferiority.[19] Lombroso theorized that individuals developed differently according to sexual and racial categories, from the most highly developed: the white man; to the most primitive: the woman of colour.[20] He described physical characteristics or traits found among the "bad" group of women, such as moles, darker skin, more massive weight, and deviant height, wrinkles, white hair, etc., that would classify women of the atavistic type.

Lombroso analysed the body types of female criminals, concluding, based on his own and other's research, that "weight appears more often equal to or above the medium in thieves and murderers, but especially in prostitutes."[21] He added that "60 per cent of female poisoners, 59.4 per cent of prostitutes, 50 per cent of female assassins, and 46 per cent of female thieves, have a weight above the average"[22] while only a minority of criminals were below average weight. Focusing on the weight of prostitutes, Lombroso argued that they tended to have thicker thighs and larger calves than other women, asserting that prostitutes tended toward obesity. "This greater weight among prostitutes is confirmed by the notorious fact of the obesity of those who grow old in their vile trade, and who gradually become positive monsters of adipose tissues."[23] In these observations, Lombroso was linking fatness to what was alleged to be uncivilized. He attempted to argue that prostitutes were physiologically similar to African women, who he categorized as "savage" because of their virile, or masculine, nature, in comparison to white European women, whom he considered feminine. Using language similar to that which Europeans employed to describe Baartman, Lombroso wrote, "Hottentot, African, and Abyssinian women when rich and idle grow enormously fat, and the reason of the phenomenon is atavistic."[24] The fat body, Lombroso concluded, was a visible sign of criminality and criminal tendencies, a present threat to modern society.

In addition to linking fatness to promiscuity, Lombroso also linked fatness to hygiene by adding that "people living among these women and observing them every day have certified that this obesity only begins at about the age of 25 to 30 years."[25] He attributed this peculiarity to the "great number of hot baths which such women are accustomed to taking throughout the year, and, above all to their inactive lives and abundant nourishment."[26] Furthermore, "the lower orders of prostitutes, who are the fattest, do not take baths; and if their lives in the daytime are inactive, they are not so at night, when their wakeful hours are frequent and diversified by dances and orgies."[27] Here, Lombroso links fat bodies to laziness and uncleanliness.

In the same way that nineteenth-century Progressive Era reformers would claim capitalists were fat based on their class concerns, Lombroso reveals that aversion to fatness was less based on associated health concerns, and more on social perceptions of how particular body types consumed resources, responded to physical labour, and were able to regulate themselves as "good" modern citizens. For instance, "in Africa the standard of beauty consists in weight, to increase which, various artifices are resorted to, such as imbibing enormous draughts of milk and beer in a progressive ratio, until at last the venal women of those societies are simple monsters of obesity." Lombroso's language considered overweight women as not only criminal and savage but literally incapable of functioning in society according to Progressive Era ideals. Further, Lombroso argued, "[i]n prisons and asylums for the insane, the female lunatics are far more often exaggeratedly fat than the men." In other words, Lombroso dismisses non-western standards of beauty and equates fatness with both mental and physical pathology, as well as a "primitive" state of evolution.[28]

In 1893, Lombroso collaborated with Guglielmo Ferrero on a study of female criminality. *The Criminal Woman, the Prostitute, and the Normal Woman* was translated into English and became the first book ever written on women and crime. Ferrero was born in Portica, Piedmont, on 21 July 1871. While a law student at Pisa, Bologna, and Turin, his interests were in contemporary problems, an orientation confirmed by his first meeting in 1889 with Lombroso. Ferrero later married Lombroso's daughter. While Lombroso was the actual author of the text, Ferrero was instrumental in collecting notes and compiling data.[29]

Their central thesis was two-fold. They stated that women show fewer physical signs of criminality than men, but that the physically criminal female is unfeminine, unevolved in terms of gender, and twice as deviant as the physically criminal male. Lombroso and Ferrero argued that criminal women fall into two categories, the "born criminal" and the "degenerative" criminal. In making their argument for the existence of the "born criminal," they rejected the idea of agency as an explanation for why people are deviant. In other words, they based their typology of the female on degenerate types, suggesting that if she was a criminal, a prostitute, and fat, she was not reformable because she did not have control or agency over her body. They used physical characteristics of the "degenerate women" to support their theory that criminality was hereditary and that women were inferior to men. Lombroso and Ferrero wanted to show women as creatures that deviated from the male norm, or, as they articulated it, "If I must show that in mind and body woman is a male of arrested development, the fact that she is somewhat less criminal than he, and a little more pitiful, can compensate a thousand fold for her deficiency in the realm of intellect."[30]

In the first part of the text, "The Normal Woman," Lombroso and Ferrero focused on the female in the animal world, her anatomy, biology, psyche, and traits of cruelty, love, morality, and intelligence. They concluded that women were inferior to men because of particular physiological and biological characteristics. First, they argued that women were colder than men because, "The woman's heart, proportionate to her body size, seems a little smaller in volume than that of man; this is the effect of less work."[31] Also, women are of smaller stature: "In human races the woman is nearly always inferior to the man in height and weight, an inferiority that increases with age and civilization. Even in embryo the male is quite a bit larger at the same point in time than the female."[32] Next, they based their argument on aging: "White hair and baldness demonstrate delayed aging and, indirectly, lesser sensitivity in women compared to men."[33] Finally, women had smaller brains and skulls: "In general, according to all the authorities, and in all races, but more so in the civilized ones, the female skull is more childlike in capacity and shape than the masculine, and it is always inferior and always offers less variation than that of the male."[34] The authors assumed that these differences were significant in determining which body type was deviant, and also in classifying women's inferiority to men because they believed that their physiology was more similar to children than actual adults.

The authors continued to use their flawed theories and methods when determining which female body types were criminal. They argued that the brains of criminal women weighed even less than those of healthy women. Of the other physical differences between normal and criminal women, they suggested that their findings "do not amount to much"[35] but yet went on to suggest that criminal women were shorter than other women and that prostitutes were fatter and heavier than their counterparts, the "honest women." Other deviant and criminal-causing abnormalities among the criminals, and especially prostitutes, included cranial asymmetry; large lower jaws; moles; lack of, or enlargement of the nipple; and exaggerated development of the clitoris.

"Almost all anomalies occur more frequently in prostitutes than in female criminals, and both classes have more degenerative characteristics than do normal women," they explained. "Prostitutes are almost free of the wrinkles and other anomalies that create ugliness, but they have more marks of degeneration. Murderers, poisoners, and arsonists have the most prominent cheekbones, and women who commit infanticide show the largest number of asymmetrical faces and exaggerated jaws. On the whole, however, murderers – both those who use violence and poisoners – form a more degenerate type than do those who commit infanticide."[36]

The authors' research also preached the superiority of white people over other racial identities, in a way that had severe ramifications for people of colour. They used these theories to draw connections between people of colour, criminal behaviours, and body types. Ferrero believed that people of colour belonged to a sub-race because of their "primitiveness, laziness, and criminality."[37] He also wrote that a characteristic of Africans was that they could suddenly become extremely violent and quickly engaged in fits of rage. Again, links are made between race and savagery.

In comparison, Ferrero wrote that the Teutonic (German) race had gone through a similar experience when they, too, were considered "savage" and "atavistic." Still, because of what he saw as the evolutionary process, they were now civilized and hard-working. In other words, people of colour continued to exhibit the criminal characteristics associated with atavism, whereas the Germans had evolved. Taken together, these arguments provided a scientific outlook that dictated health norms. Ferrero argued, in an explicit warning to his readers, that body types that were not thin and fit threatened the peoples of Europe with a descent back to a state of savagery. Like Lombroso and Fletcher, Ferrero concluded that fatness was a threat to the very existence of civilization.

This work was widely embraced by many global scholars, who endorsed the belief of African inferiority, the innate "Black criminal," and the Black delinquent, as well as linking these stereotypes to perceptions of genetic inferiority. Ultimately, such ideas contributed to the "global racist eugenics movement, which was also targeted at racial and ethnic groups."[38] American sociological scholars W.E.B. Du Bois and Frances Kellor, whose theories explained race differences in delinquency, were the first to criticize this work, and later, European scholars, such as Dutch criminologist Willem Bonger, who believed in a causal link between crime and economic and social conditions, noted that the Lombrosian theory was ridiculous. Nevertheless, it is essential to remember that Lombroso and Ferrero's work – with its distinguishing of "bad" and "good" groups of bodies based on perceptions of biological inferiority, specific physiological characteristics, and blatant racism – continues even today to inform how society polices women's bodies regarding fatness, thinness, and weight, in general.

Although Lombroso did not explicitly rely on spiritual or cultural justifications for his work (attempting instead to provide "hard data" for his ideas), he nonetheless argued a similar, if not identical, line of thinking to Fletcher's. Lombroso maintained that many conditions (epilepsy, fatness, and criminality) were the result of fetuses not developing correctly and producing flawed humans with defective nervous systems. Lombroso provided charts of data, quantifying his hatred of fat people, and the differently abled. Fletcher insisted that "men and women are wont to ridicule the assertion that the mind influences the nerves, simply because the fact cannot be given an anatomical demonstration; but I beg you, be not so dogmatic with reference to things about which you are profoundly ignorant."[39] However, both argued that the state not only could but should target those who did not comply with ideal body types. The very existence of fat people served as a dire warning that western civilization could return to savagery via overindulging.

In conclusion, we need to understand the historical development of ideas that permeate our present moment. How did fatness come to be a pejorative? How have movements to decrease oppression helped and hindered that development? And most important, how can we know the history of that development in such a way that we can identify, refute, and construct new conceptions that do not marginalize, stigmatize, and oppress fat people? This is no small task, and as is often the case with histories aimed at altering our perceptions of "good" and "bad" bodies, it will require a protracted engagement with present-day people who have vested large amounts of intellectual capital into the belief that their body's size equates to a moral component, and therefore, affords them a certain amount of privilege. It will mean engaging a range of industries that have profited enormously from people's desire to reach a specific body size, peddling ideas of "self-control" strikingly similar to the so-called soul force. In that vein, we acknowledge the ongoing work that fat activists have undertaken and offer this essay as an entry into the broader movement of needed diverse-body acceptance.

NOTES

1 The exact details of her contract, and the level of coercion in forcing her to perform, has been a subject of debate among historians. For more see, Clifton C. Crais and Pamela Scully, *Sara Baartman and the Hottentot Venus: A Ghost Story and a Biography* (New Jersey: Princeton University Press, 2009). Baartman is variously called Sarah, Sara, and Saartjie. In this text we have chosen to use Sarah Baartman following the advice of the Saartjie Baartman Centre for Women & Children, www.saartjiebaartmancentre.org.za.
2 Image of Sarah Baartman's remains on display at France's "Museum of Mankind." "The Saartje Baartman Story," *Hadithi Africa*, accessed 1 December 2019. https://hadithi.africa/2019/09/10/the-saartjie-baartman-story/.
3 "Theodore Roosevelt Interpreted by Historian Ferrero," *Sun-Journal* (Lewiston, Maine), 21 December 1908.
4 Christopher Crupper, "Love and Beauty – Sartjee the Hottentot Venus." October 1811. Library of Congress. Date accessed: 1 December 2019. https://www.loc.gov/pictures/item/2007680266/. Udo J. Keppler, "Putting the Screws on Him." November 1904. Library of Congress. Date accessed: 1 December 2019. https://www.loc.gov/item/2011645581/.
5 Sabrina Strings, *Fearing the Black Body: The Racial Origins of Fat Phobia* (New York: New York University Press, 2019), 3.
6 Francesco Cassata, *Building the New Man* (Budapest: Central European University Press, 2011), 9–10.
7 David J. Galton, "Greek Theories on Eugenics" in *Journal of Medical Ethics* 24, no. 4 (August 1998): 263–7.
8 Seneca, *Moral and Political Essays, Book 1, XV*, trans. J. Cooper (Cambridge: Cambridge University Press, 1995).
9 Christopher E. Forth, "Fat, Desire and Disgust in the Colonial Imagination," in *History Workshop Journal* no. 73 (Spring 2012), 231.
10 Ella Adelia Fletcher, *The Woman Beautiful* (New York: W.M. Young & Co., Publishers, 1899), 28–9. The long subtitle of Fletcher's work is particularly illuminating, "A Practical Treatise on the Development and Preservation of Woman's Health and Beauty, and the Principles of Taste in Dress."
11 Ella Adelia Fletcher, *The Philosophy of Rest* (New York: Dodge Publishing Company, 1900), 11.
12 Fletcher, *The Philosophy of Rest*, 22–3.
13 Fletcher, *The Philosophy of Rest*, 29.
14 Cesare Lombroso and William Ferrero, *The Female Offender* (New York: D. Appleton & Company, 1895). There is some uncertainty as to when

his book, *The Female Offender*, was published in the US. We do not know who initiated the publication, who translated it, or whether the impetus came from England (where the book was published simultaneously by Unwin) or from someone in the States. We also do not know the size of the initial print run, which would indicate the book's anticipated reception. However, we do know that the New York publisher D. Appleton published *The Female Offender* in 1895 and reprinted it three times before Lombroso's death in 1909. That indicates remarkable interest in a book on what was at the time an unfamiliar topic and one considered "less important" than criminal man. Nicole Rafter, "Lombroso's Reception in the United States" in *The Eternal Recurrence of Crime and Control: Essays in Honour of Paul Rock*, ed. David Downes, Dick Hobbs, and Tim Newburn (Oxford: Oxford University Press, 2010): DOI:10.1093/acprof:oso/9780199580231.003.0001.

15 Marvin E. Wolfgang, "Pioneers in Criminology: Cesare Lombroso (1825–1909)" in *Journal of Criminal Law and Criminology* 52, no. 4 (November–December 1961): 361–91.

16 Although atavism assumes a biological predisposition to evil, the principle of social defence, based on the institutional practices of segregation, prevention, and control, still fell within Lombroso's definition of eugenics.

17 Cesare Lombroso and William Ferrero, *The Female Offender*, ed. Douglas Morrison (New York: D. Appleton and Company, 1895), 47.

18 Dorie Klein, "The Etiology of Female Crime: A Review of the Literature," in *Issues in Criminology*, 8, no. 2 (Fall 1973), 4.

19 For instance, contemporary researchers John Cowie, Valerie A. Cowie, and Eliot Slater argued that certain traits, such as body size, may lead to aggressiveness. In 2017, psychologists reviewed previous studies and used meta-analysis to evaluate whether there is evidence of a relationship between "overweight/obesity" and physical aggression in children and adolescents. A systematic search of studies that reported the effect of overweight/obesity (in the form of body mass index) on physical aggression was conducted. A total of twenty-three studies were identified, representing data from 255,377 participants. The results indicated that children and adolescents who doctors label as overweight were more physically aggressive than their average-weight or smaller peers. Finally, a nine-year longitudinal study examined aggressive/depressive symptoms in ninety larger and average weight children. The researchers argued that overweight children demonstrated an increase of aggressive symptoms over time. These results highlight how well into the twenty-first century people are using body size to determine behaviour, as well as the importance of considering not just body size but the social effects of stigmatizing fat bodies.

20 Dorie Klein, "The Etiology of Female Crime: A Review of the Literature" in *Issues in Criminology* 8, no. 2 (Fall 1973), 8.
21 Anna Krugovoy Silver, *Victorian Literature and the Anorexic Body* (Cambridge: Cambridge University Press, 2002).
22 Lombroso, *The Female Offender*, 53.
23 Lombroso, *The Female Offender*, 50.
24 Lombroso, *The Female Offender*, 114.
25 Lombroso, *The Female Offender*, 113.
26 Lombroso, *The Female Offender*, 113.
27 Lombroso, *The Female Offender*, 114.
28 Lombroso, *The Female Offender*, 114.
29 While serious scholars and students will rightly discard the arguments and scientific validity of these writings, we must contemplate their continued importance. Sexism, racism, and biological determinism still influence our social institutions, academic worlds, and popular culture. Lombroso and Ferrero's writings offer insight into the early influences of the social sciences upon our daily and scholarly lives.
30 Lombroso and Ferrero, *Criminal Woman*, 14.
31 Lombroso and Ferrero, *Criminal Woman*, 46.
32 Lombroso and Ferrero, *Criminal Woman*, 46.
33 Lombroso and Ferrero, *Criminal Woman*, 57.
34 Lombroso and Ferrero, *Criminal Woman*, 50.
35 Lombroso and Ferrero, *Criminal Woman*, 125.
36 Lombroso and Ferrero, *Criminal Woman*, 134.
37 Shaun L. Gabbidon, *Crimininological Perspectives on Race and Crime* (New York: Routledge, 2010), 13.
38 Gabbidon, *Crimininological Perspectives on Race and Crime*, 16.
39 Fletcher, *The Philosophy of Rest*, 30.

SECTION II

Weights and Measures

Few people knew what they weighed in the nineteenth century. Nobody kept a scale in their homes that they stepped on daily to monitor pounds gained or lost. Body size was marked by adjectives – thin, plump, puny, healthy – rather than numbers. But by the mid-twentieth century, weight had become equated to a number that was closely monitored and judged. The chapters in this section suggest some of the ways that the measurements of body size shifted from a quantitative to a qualitative assessment, and how an interest in statistical averages developed into a normative standard that labelled all those outside the increasingly narrow range "deviant." The chapters in this section consider how the measuring of weight became a marker of health among various groups, and how historians might use both qualitative and quantitative sources to understand the broader meaning of body size.

The nineteenth century was a period in which scientific categorization and expertise was taking an increasingly central role in all areas of life and when medical professionals increasingly claimed authoritative knowledge. Lynn Kennedy's chapter explores how, over the course of the nineteenth century, advice literature aimed at mothers, frequently written by physicians, increasingly focused on measuring the weight of infants, becoming an early indicator of the shift from qualitative to quantitative assessments of health and well-being. The introduction of infant formula, and doctors who now specialized in infant care, began to require a careful and quantifiable assessment of weight gain or loss, changing the meaning society applied to both healthy infants and "good" mothers.

The physical culture movement explored in the chapter by Conor Heffernan took the size and weight standards developed by scientists and physicians and used them to self-police their own bodies. Early body builders such as Eugen Sandow and Bernarr Macfadden developed exercise and diet regimes, first to perfect their own physiques, and then to sell their ideas to the public. Their writings and complementary merchandise became an early precursor to the diet and exercise industry that would become such a fundamental part of understanding weight and the body in the twentieth century. The emphasis on measurements that had gradually developed over the course of the nineteenth century was becoming part of the narrative, albeit still for a small, particularized group of practitioners, who had begun to measure and monitor their bodies using these quantitative figures as a mark of both health and success.

Although weight has now become axiomatically linked to measurement – to the modern mind, weight is a number from which multiple conclusions are drawn – little historical quantitative data exists before the twentieth century. While an increasingly insistent discussion of weight at the beginning of the twentieth century and an immense growth in the diet industry have led to a general sense that people were getting fatter, was that actually true? The chapter by Luiza Antonie, Kris Inwood, and Hamish Maxwell-Stewart uses data from the Canadian prison population in the late nineteenth century to consider statistical changes in body size over time, suggesting some methodological approaches to the existing data, and alerting historians to some of both the possibilities and cautions of talking about weight quantitatively in the nineteenth century. Measuring weight and assessing its meaning was not so easy as stepping on a scale and recording a number – for either the historical actors concerned with their health or for the historian attempting to understand the physical realities of the past.

3 "All young things are fat if they are in health":[1] The Shift from Qualitative to Quantitative Assessments of Infant Weight in the Nineteenth-Century United States

V. LYNN KENNEDY

In 1913, Julia Clark Hallam, a suffragist and prolific author on numerous subjects, wrote a manual for mothers. Under the heading "Important Data," she provided detailed instructions on how to weigh and measure infants. She chided mothers for buying "elaborate and expensive garments" for their babies rather than purchasing a quality scale to take these measurements, arguing that the latter purchase would "result in greater ultimate good for the baby" by allowing mothers to closely monitor weight gain or loss. Such an intense focus on an infant's weight may not seem particularly unusual for twenty-first-century readers since regular monitoring has become commonplace, beginning with including the newborn's weight in most birth announcements. But while a "fat baby" has, over the course of centuries, served as a marker of infant health, discussions of infant weight, beginning in the nineteenth century, gradually shifted from qualitative to quantitative assessments, mirroring shifts in the medical community's involvement in neonatal care and the related understanding of what characterized a "good" mother and a healthy infant. This chapter examines the changing rhetoric of child-care experts in the United States over the course of the nineteenth century from qualitative to quantitative, and how it influenced a broader understanding of infant health and the meaning of fatness, as these experts, particularly doctors, sought to establish their authority in judging both infants and mothers.[2]

The Progressive Era that emerged in the United States in the late nineteenth and early twentieth centuries has generally been associated with an increasing faith in experts to solve all kinds of social ills. Experts such as social scientists and doctors relied on measuring, monitoring, and statistical analysis to assess and solve problems. The

American government also established numerous agencies to collect statistics and to put the advice of these experts to work, including the Public Health Service, which concerned itself with the bodies of the nation. But, as discussed by Rigakos and Bishop in this volume, while the Progressive Era represented a new apex of measuring the human body, it did not emerge out of nowhere. From the seventeenth century onward, various "experts" had been writing about the body, its weight, and how it might be controlled.[3] And while the Progressive Era enshrined the development of scientific parenthood in the creation of the Children's Bureau in 1912, "expert" parenting advice also had a long history in the United States.[4] By the mid-nineteenth century, medical doctors had begun to make claims to expertise and professionalism, as advising new mothers on infant care became one of the ways to exert this authority.[5] Mothers had long been charged with the responsibilities of maintaining the well-being of their infants, but as quantitative measures became more common, authority also seemed to shift, at least partly, to the experts, who could claim a knowledge of standards and norms (while still allowing mothers to be blamed for infants who failed to meet these newly standardized markers, whether too fat or too thin).[6]

Qualitative Assessments of Infants in the Early Nineteenth Century

The child-care manuals written during the first decades of the nineteenth century place little emphasis on the measuring of infants – words such as "weigh" or "weight" rarely appear in relation to assessing the well-being of a newborn. The focus of many of these manuals was more on the moral health of the infant than on the physical. Lydia Sigourney's popular *Letters to Mothers* (1839) is representative of the sentimental tone that emphasized the mother's duty to nurture the spiritual and moral well-being of her infant. In a period of high infant mortality and limited medical knowledge, preserving the physical health of children often seemed a tenuous task. High mortality rates combined with a religious fatalism had long created a degree of resignation about infant death. Increasingly, however, a cultural celebration of maternal love also entailed blaming mothers when things went wrong either morally or physically. Parents had long turned to family members and ministers to negotiate the tumultuous waters of infant care; in the nineteenth century, they also turned to doctors and other experts.[7]

Yet even the early child-care manuals written from a more medicalized perspective, such as *The Female Monitor, Consisting of a Series of Letters to Married Women on Nursing and the Management of Children* (1801) by Hugh Smith, and *The Maternal Physician: A Treatise on the Nurture and Management of Infants* (1818) written by "An American Matron," provided few instructions for weighing or measuring an infant, nor did they regularly use terms such as fat, thin, plump, or puny to describe the infant body. Dr William P. Dewees's popular work, *Treatise on the Physical and Medical Treatment of Children* (1829), included an extensive index with entries for "weaning" and "worms" (two key issues in infant weight gain), but had no entry for "weight" itself.[8] Nor did those who actually delivered babies place a particular emphasis on measuring the weight of the neonate. In the United States, most births throughout the nineteenth century occurred at home with the assistance of female relatives or a midwife. Scales were not common pieces of equipment in most households at this time; caring for the life and needs of mother and newborn was the primary focus of the birth attendants; seeking out a scale or other measuring device to weigh the newborn only occurred in extraordinary circumstances, such as the arrival of an unusually large or small child.[9]

The rather lackadaisical attitude of these experts toward taking measurements was reflected in the actions of the general public in the first half of the nineteenth century. Parents, mirroring the published language of experts, typically announced the arrival of a newborn with qualitative observations about the infant's size rather than with a specific weight or measurement. In 1806, for example, Rosalie Calvert of Maryland wrote to her sister, "I am pleased to announce the birth of a big baby girl who is in excellent health, as am I." The closest she came to a quantitative assessment was in the comparative observation she made a month later, that this baby was "much more robust than any of my other children at the same age." Two years later, Calvert made a similar comparative evaluation of another newborn, this time a son, who, she noted, "is much bigger than my other children at this age." Such comparisons, however, did not include a precise measure of how much bigger, or any clear demarcation of what might be considered "average" or "normal" in the size of these infants.[10]

Instead of a reference to an abstract numerical standard, mention of the size of a newborn was combined with a qualitative judgment; either the child was "fine," meaning both well-looking and appearing healthy, or it might be observed that the child was "puny" and thus perhaps not destined to survive. William Pollock, for example, wrote from Illinois in 1839 that his day-old daughter was "a fine large hearty child." And in 1831, Betty Cole of Virginia similarly recorded that a week-old child was "said to be the largest & finest child ever seen," concluding that "Mother & child are both doing well[.]" South Carolina attorney and future congressman William F. Colcock used more evocative language in an attempt at humour in describing the small size of his newborn nephew in 1834, writing to his father that the new arrival was "about the size of a kitten & is as ugly as he has by paternal inheritance a right to be." Later in his letter Colcock added:

> However as tall oaks fr. little acorns grow he may yet attain sufficient height when he arrives at maturity, to sit to table without the aid of a backgammon box to assist his understanding. I give you this minute description of this 12-barley-corn-ling stranger because Tom & Eliza charged me not to laugh at him – & I take you know, twice as much pleasure in doing what people beg me *not* to do as in doing what they beg me *to* do.

While providing a description that clearly indicated the smallness of this infant, the closest that Colcock came to using a quantitative measure was the reference to a barleycorn, which was a small English unit of length equal to about a third of an inch, and here he almost certainly used it facetiously. His use of humour was undoubtedly meant to allay the fear in this situation that such a small infant might not grow into a strong child. But whether mocking the smallness or complimenting the fineness of an infant, in the early decades of the nineteenth century the size of newborns was almost entirely described in qualitative terms.[11]

As the child progressed from infancy, assessments of their growth continued to be largely qualitative in the first several decades of the nineteenth century. Rosalie Calvert, who had referred to her newborn as "a big baby girl," would continue to use this same qualitative language when, just over a year later, in December of 1807, she referred to the now-toddler as being "as strong and robust as a little savage, mischievous and always in motion," conveying a healthy, vigorous development without mentioning a specific weight. Indeed, scales capable of weighing a toddler remained even rarer than those available to measure a newborn, for whom the grocer's scales might sometimes be called into service. Scales intended to weigh farm produce or shipping goods could certainly be used to weigh a larger child, but this would have been more of a novelty than a regular occurrence. In general, a language of fat and thin, large and small, plump and puny, substituted for specific measurements in assessing the growth and development of both infants and growing children.[12]

This is not to say that weight did not weigh heavily on some parents. A child's "failure to thrive" was of great concern for parents. A too thin infant or toddler seemed to suggest that the child might suffer from a lack of the reserves of flesh necessary to weather both the ordinary trials of childhood, such as teething, as well as more threatening childhood diseases, such as measles and chickenpox. Dr Hugh Smith warned in 1801 that "it is entirely owing to the weakness of their bodies, that children cut their teeth with so much difficulty, and that it is attended with fever, convulsions, and death." A healthy amount of fat could thus be viewed as a prophylactic against a child literally wasting away.[13] But while a failure to gain or maintain weight might be caused by numerous factors, the fault was commonly laid with the mother not providing adequate or proper nutrition for the child. And yet there was little that either a mother, a doctor, or any other expert could do in the first decades of nineteenth century if an infant or child did not remain healthy or grow fat – few measures, and no measuring, could be of assistance for the child who failed to thrive.

Increasing Quantitative Measures at Mid-Century

In the mid-nineteenth century, a growing focus on medical training and scientific knowledge began to change the emphasis experts placed on measuring and statistical norms. Increasingly, weight, and weighing, were identified as important elements in monitoring the health of an infant. Not inconsequentially, in the same decades American doctors began to seek more substantial professional recognition, forming the American Medical Association in 1847 to regularize the educational requirements of entry into their profession. In 1848, Dr Charles Meigs, who taught at Jefferson Medical College in Philadelphia, decried those "who, while they style themselves doctors, are really not members of the Scholar vocation, and of course not physicians."[14] Physicians who trained in the latest scientific methods at the many emerging medical schools turned their attention to dispensing medical advice to their patients, including mothers of infants and young children who worried about "normal" growth and development, although the answers they offered often remained inconclusive in this era.

Works such as Dr Stephen Tracy's *The Mother and Her Offspring* (1853) began to demonstrate a clear interest in measuring the neonate's weight, offering the observation that "the ordinary length of the child is from 19 to 21 inches, and its weight from 7 to 9 pounds." These suggested averages, which increasingly came to dominate the medical discourse as the century progressed, may have been drawn from the work of European statisticians, who had begun to make a study of the measurements of people, including newborns, to determine the mean sizes of the population in terms of weight and height. Yet Tracy also observed that "often the size is influenced by causes not very easily explained," thus suggesting that the use of these quantitative measures was not fully entrenched, nor regarded as an absolute standard. Further, Tracy made no specific recommendations to mothers about measuring or monitoring their own infants in order to make comparisons to the statistical averages. Nonetheless, his discussion of specific figures does indicate a shift that was beginning to take hold in measuring the newborn's weight.[15]

More generally, among medical and child-care experts an emphasis on quantitative measurement was taking firm root. In 1868, a British publication provided extensive information on measurements, including a table that aggregated the weights of 3,000 infants, drawing the conclusion that "the normal weight of a mature new-born infant is not less than 6 nor more than 8lbs, the average weight being 6½ or 7 lbs, the smaller number referring to female and the higher to male infants." This new emphasis on what was "normal" was an important development in the rhetoric of child care. Most of the American guides published in the late nineteenth and early twentieth century also began to include some discussion of average birth weights, and often a chart or table correlating age and weight. Gradually, any deviation from this norm became a matter of concern.[16]

Some parents did begin to follow the lead of doctors and other experts, with evidence of weighing and measuring newborns beginning to appear in letters and diaries, although these figures were inconsistently given and still balanced with qualitative discussions of size and health. New father Arthur Ritchie boasted of his newborn son, delivered in July of 1843: "He is a fine stout little fellow." He also noted that the infant "weighed just after birth 10 ¾ lb." Similarly, Henry Lesesne of Charleston remarked on the arrival of a new family member who "weighed 13 pounds the day he was born."[17] The unusually large size of these infants may have prompted their weighing. Yet such notations also suggested the beginnings of a transition in which the measurement of a newborn's weight became increasingly common as part of the announcement of a birth, and, by the end of the century, requisite.

At mid-century, among most parents, however, qualitative assessments continued to co-exist, if not completely overshadow, any quantitative information linking health and fatness. "What can any one say of a Baby four months old," Mary Lowndes queried in 1850, "she is very fat." Elizabeth Fisher of Philadelphia wrote of her six-month old daughter, in December of 1840: "She is now so very rosy, & *so* heavy;" she similarly wrote in 1842 of her second daughter, who was just beginning to teethe, that she was "fatter every day, & grows uncommonly fast." More than two decades later, Tryphena Fox wrote from Louisiana of her baby son Frank: "He is now three weeks & three days old & as fat & hearty as any Mother could wish." In 1875, Fox similarly labelled her toddler son Burt "a great, stout looking fellow." Heaviness, heartiness, even stoutness, were meant to convey a positive healthfulness; unfortunately, not all infants garnered such robust appraisals. A relative of Cary North Pettigrew described Pettigrew's infant son, writing, "I never saw a smaller or feebler infant, his face is about as large as a good sized squash." The writer cautioned the recipients of this letter that they must say nothing about the size of the child because his mother "thinks her baby a fine child, & I don't think likes him to be thought small or puny." But whether positively or negatively, mothers, family, and friends continued to make qualitative evaluations of infants and their development. Throughout these decades, qualitative assessments of size lingered as the norm among parents for discussing their infants.[18]

Mahala Roach, a resident of Vicksburg, Mississippi, represented the newer quantitative trend that was emerging. She kept extensive diaries in the 1850s in which she recorded the arrivals of her last two children, specifically notng their birth weights. She wrote on 2 May 1859, that the child she had given birth to that day, named James, "weighs 7½ pounds and seems healthy." Her previous child, John, born in July of 1856, however, was recorded as weighing only 3½ pounds, and she noted "he is a delicate, poor baby," although remarkably he did survive into adulthood. Roach also recorded the birth of her brother's daughter, who "weighed 9½ lbs, and is quite fat," and the birth of the child of an enslaved woman named Henrietta, "a fine large baby boy, weighing 10 ½ pounds[.]" Roach was a middle-class, urban resident who evinced an interest in adopting new technologies. She was, for example, the proud owner of a sewing machine, a technology that had only recently become widely available for purchase. This openness to new innovations may have made Roach particularly receptive to the messages doctors and child-care experts were increasingly putting forward about the importance of weights and measures in the mid-nineteenth century. Notably, she also recorded several incidents in her diary when she walked to the local depot to use their scales to weigh herself (since home scales were not yet available). While Roach almost always continued to combine qualitative assessments with her quantitative information, increasingly careful measurements would be pushed by physicians and child-care experts, and recorded by parents, in the late nineteenth century.[19]

Feeding the Infant and the Increasing Role of the Expert

The introduction of infant formula in the 1870s changed expectations about the feeding and fattening of babies, and rapidly expanded doctors' claims to expertise in the area of child care. It also solidified the practice of measuring and weighing of infants as a standard method of monitoring an infant's health. For most of history, the only sustenance that ensured that infants would thrive and grow fat was human breast milk. When a mother either could not, or, on rarer occasions, would not, feed the child herself, it became a direct threat to the baby's health. In such situations, another source of nourishment had to be found if the child was to survive, a fact recognized in the extensive discussion of alternative feeding methods that frequently appeared in parenting and medical manuals in the early nineteenth century.

Despite the suggestion of potential substitutes, however, most early experts continued to advise breastmilk as the most healthful means of feeding an infant. In 1829, William Dewees's *Treatise on Physical and Medical Treatment of Children* made an unequivocal statement on the importance of this method of feeding:

> We have assumed as principles, and as we think upon broad and well established data – 1st, that the mother is the proper and only source from whence a child, until a certain period, should derive its nourishment; 2d, that every woman, caeteris paribus, is able to furnish it; 3d, that no other nourishment, is so entirely proper, as the milk of a healthy mother.[20]

Indeed, throughout much of the nineteenth century, the main question for mothers was not whether they should nurse their own infants, but at what point they should wean the child to ensure the health of both themselves and their baby. Lydia Sigourney, whose writing took a decidedly sentimental tone, counselled her readers to "be not anxious to abridge this halcyon period." Physicians generally took a more prosaic tone, but in the first half of the nineteenth century they largely agreed on a prolonged period of breastfeeding as the best means of maintaining a fat and thus healthy infant. Dr Thomas Ewell conceded that some babies could thrive if weaned as early as four months, but recommended that, when possible, mothers should continue nursing for at least nine months as this would "have the effect of greatly enlarging our puny breed of men and women." Many physicians in the latter decades of the nineteenth century continued with such recommendations, including Dr Louis Starr, who in 1894 advised breastfeeding until some time between the tenth and twelfth month as long as the mother's health remained "robust and the child steadily grows and gains flesh[.]" The main concern was that weaning should be done when adequate replacement nutriments, especially fresh milk, were available, which usually meant avoiding particularly warm weather or periods when epidemic or endemic diseases might endanger the child's health. The key indicator in such situations would be the weight of the child.[21]

The second-best option for feeding an infant throughout most of the century was the hiring of a wet nurse, an option usually only available to those with the resources, and the luck, to find an appropriate candidate. Employers of wet nurses, and those offering their services, both often relied on advertisements and word of mouth to locate a match that could offer the necessary nutrients as well as a degree of compatibility between nurse, mother, and infant in this most intimate of interactions. Sometimes this demanded what the employers viewed as a sacrifice on their part to accommodate the nurse. In 1856, for example, South Carolinians Henry and Harriet Lesesne required the services of a woman named Mary Dodge to feed their infant. They were thus forced to accede to her demand that she keep her baby with her. Remarking on the trouble this caused them, the Lesesnes asserted that they would have fired her if they could, but their own child was too feeble to do without the sustenance she offered, and so "she nurses both of them." Their observation that Dodge "has her own infant up here it has grown very fat & is the picture of health," both illustrates, and seems oblivious to, the fact that if Dodge had had to leave her own child to nurse her charge (the fate of many, if not most, wet nurses) then her infant would not have fattened but instead faced a precarious chance of survival deprived of its own mother's milk. Fat babies very often marked an embodied privilege – both in terms of the availability of pre- and postpartum care, and as a mark of the value ascribed to the infant by social structures and choices – some babies were apparently more important, and thus fatter, than others.[22]

Eliza Middleton Fisher faced a different dilemma with a wet nurse, but one that also contemplated the value of this service to infants and their families. Fisher's daughter seemed to become too attached to the wet nurse hired to care for her and ensure she gained the appropriate amount of weight. Fisher eased her psychological angst about this close relationship by likening the nurse to an Alderney, or dairy cow, while claiming for herself the role of moral nurturer. Fisher undoubtedly recognized the important contribution that the nurse made to the child's health and well-being; she had herself nursed her baby "5 or 6 times" a day, while supplementing these feedings with "three wine glass fulls at a time of milk & water," explaining to her mother that she found this method preferable to using a bottle "which required great attention and care to keep it clean." Fortunately, using this augmented feeding schedule had ensured that the baby "flourishes & fattens famously."

But while her own efforts signified a maternal devotion, the wet nurse's contributions to ensuring her daughter thrived were reduced to a mere physicality, and a transactional process.[23]

While Eliza Fisher noted the difficulties of keeping the feeding equipment safely clean, the more significant problem was what should go into these bottles (or wine glasses) to ensure babies received the proper nutrition. In the early part of the nineteenth century, parenting manuals frequently provided recipes for infant food that combined cow's milk and water, as well as, sometimes, sugar and/or a paste made of bread called pap. William Dewees, however, decried the addition of this latter ingredient as deleterious to the infant's health. Virtually all authors before the 1870s, regardless of the pages devoted to these feeding methods, continued to emphasize the truth that there really was no proper substitute for breastmilk if the child was going to fatten and thrive. And sadly, many "hand-fed" babies did not fare well. Anne Webb observed in 1840 that the five-month-old daughter of a relative was "not so healthy," providing the explanation that "she has had to nurse her with the sucking bottle." Historian Jacqueline Wolf avers that "If human milk was wholly unavailable, the baby almost always died."[24]

Thus, when commercial infant formula began to be available in the mid-1870s, it came as a relief to many mothers who put their trust in the doctors and scientific experts who manufactured it. Most of the earliest breastmilk substitutes were expensive and medical professionals had to intervene to determine and order the proper formulation. The earliest versions were adaptations of cow's milk prepared in labs that sought to balance the ratios of fat and protein content (hence formula) to improve the infant's ability to digest this food. Later, powdered formula, meant to be added to cow's milk or water, and canned condensed milk, provided options for a wider market. Advertising for the companies producing this infant formula soon sought to win over mothers and doctors alike to the use of their specific product, appealing to both science and threats of underfeeding, notably evoking the puny baby long feared by parents. A 1902 advertisement for Eskay's, one such manufacturer of infant food, displayed a picture of emaciated twins juxtaposed with an "after" photo in which the twins have been, ostensibly, made fat – healthy and happy – through their product (Figure 3.1).

In reality, however, the results of these early feeding supplements were decidedly mixed, both in their ability to appeal to consumers and in their ability to nurture healthy infants. Until at least the 1920s, impure milk and water supplies and limited access to refrigeration still made the use of artificial feeding perilous for infants. Nonetheless, more and more people gradually embraced the use of these products

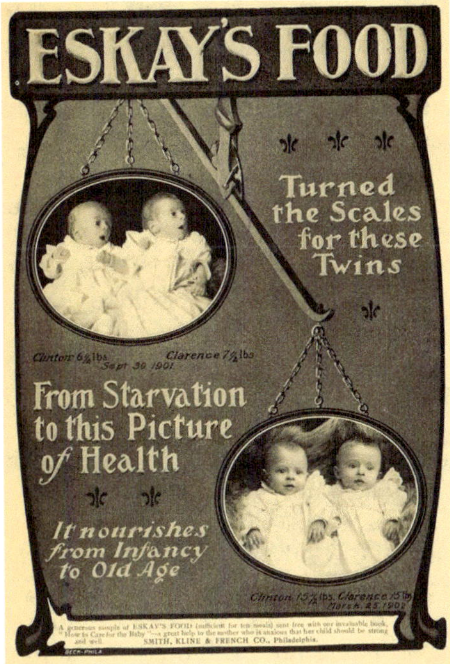

Figure 3.1. Eskay's 1902 Ad, oldmainartifacts.wordpress.com/2015/04/24/eskays-albumized-food-philadelphia-pa/.

out of either necessity or convenience. While some doctors warned against the potentially dire consequences, and the false security of the apparent fattening they offered, others embraced this scientific solution to an age-old problem of undernourished infants. Dr Louis Starr might be counted among the skeptics, asserting in 1894 that "infants fed upon condensed milk, though fat, are pale, lethargic and flabby, although large, are far from strong; have little power to resist diseases; often cut their teeth late, and are very likely to drift into rickets." Indeed, well into the twentieth century doctors blamed the large number of infant deaths on the fact that mothers could not or did not breastfeed. Starr's comments further represented the paradoxical dilemma for all mothers – fat babies were good, but not too fat; and even more frightening, fat might provide only the illusion of health, masking an underlying puniness. In all cases, mothers must carefully monitor their infants for signs that something was going wrong.[25]

Notably, the advent of commercially available infant food occurred at about the same time as pediatrics became established as a distinct specialty, putting a new focus on the particular diseases of childhood. The increasing use of infant formula also undoubtedly contributed to the growing emphasis on weighing and measuring babies, with quantification and statistics required to monitor the correct amounts and formulations of substitute foods, again providing an aura of scientific authority to doctors and other child-care experts. And yet, despite the increased medical involvement, the messages about just how to ensure a healthy baby remained mixed. The one thing most of society could agree upon was, whether too skinny or too fat, the blame should probably be placed on something the mother did, or perhaps did not do, in caring for her infant.

The Triumph of Quantification and Celebrating the Fat Baby

For many people in the nineteenth century, a fat, rosy baby had become a marker of not only a healthy infant, but of a baby properly tended by a doting mother. J.P. Crozier Griffith counselled the readers of *The Care of the Baby* that "A healthy and well-developed new-born infant should be plump and firm, with its bones well-covered with a soft and extremely delicate skin." T.C. Duncan went further, arguing that "The importance of fat are physical, mental and moral. A child well nourished, fat and fair, grows rapidly and develops easily and finely; while a child thin of flesh (fat) grows feebly and develops poorly and with a struggle."[26] So prevalent were such sentiments about the benefits of fat in the infant throughout the nineteenth century that often individuals felt a compulsion to apologize, or at least explain, if they believed that a baby did not possess adequate amounts of body fat to meet the social and medical standards. Early in this period, for example, Mary Custis's aunt wrote of a baby that was "not very fat, but very healthy," presumably believing that one might not assume the latter given the former. Elizabeth Perry described her son Willy as "not inclined to corpulency, but rather slender delicate, at the same time manly." Such notations sought to offer assurances that although these children were not fat, they could indeed still be healthy, vibrant, and even "manly."[27]

There is, in the twenty-first century, a substantive link in the medical literature between low birth weight and health complications for the neonate, often continuing on into childhood.[28] British physician and author of *Infant Mortality*, George Newman, made this connection explicit in 1906, writing: "The importance of the weight of an infant as a criterion of its health and progress is well known. Indeed, the weight is often the only criterion as to whether the infant is improving in health or not." Similarly, the American physician Louis Starr asserted in 1894 that "To be robust the newly-born infant must have a certain average length and weight. The length varies between 16 and 22 inches and the weight between 6 and 8 pounds." Such medical assertions linking size to robustness or health reflected not only newly developing scientific orthodoxy, but what parents had intuitively believed and expressed throughout the nineteenth century – that a fat baby was a healthy baby.[29] Historical demographers who have attempted to understand the reasons for high infant mortality rates in the nineteenth century have also drawn links not only between low birth weights and high infant mortality, but between low birth weights and poor maternal health, particularly in the emerging urban industrial centres. These demographic findings offer countervailing evidence to the dominant contemporary narrative that frequently blamed what was characterized as ill-informed and inattentive care provided by poor and immigrant mothers for the alarmingly high infant mortality rates in many nineteenth-century cities. Similarly, maternal malnutrition and poor health undoubtedly contributed to the alarmingly high rates of infant mortality among the enslaved population in the southern United States under conditions in which most expectant women received inadequate rations and insufficient relief from hard labour, particularly in the early stages of their pregnancies. Problems of infant weight thus often preceded birth and were due to factors beyond the control of individual mothers. Yet the blame placed on these mothers (and indeed all mothers) for either overfeeding, underfeeding, or wrongly feeding their infants would become a persistent theme in the late nineteenth and early twentieth century.[30]

By the late nineteenth and early twentieth centuries, medical and child-care experts argued that the best way to ensure the healthfulness of these infants and young children was to carefully monitor their growth and weight gain. T.C. Duncan's *The Feeding and Management of Infants and Children* (1880) included a list outlining the expected monthly weight gain from birth. He also referenced the increasing expectation that babies should be weighed regularly, with a preface picture entitled "Weighing the Baby," accompanied by a truly terrible poem that read in part: "How many pounds does the baby weigh,/ Baby, who came but a month ago;/ How many pounds, from the crowning curls/ To the rosy point of the restless toe?"[31] Such verse, regardless of its quality, normalized the weighing of the young child as something that careful parents would do. Popular culture, of significantly higher quality than Duncan's poem, would also increasingly reinforce this message by celebrating the image of the fat baby.

Dr Thomas Sozinskey's *The Care and Culture of Children,* also published in 1880, avoided Duncan's doggerel but did similarly emphasize the importance of weighing and measuring young children, outlining the expected weights as they developed:

> The weight of Anglo-Saxon children, at birth, averages about seven and a half pounds. At the end of the first six months it is about 15 pounds; at the end of the first year, twenty; at the end of the second, twenty-six; at the end of the 5th, thirty-nine. At each of these periods males are about a pound heavier than females.[32]

By 1903, J.P. Crozer Griffith's *The Care of the Baby,* would insist that "the baby *should* weigh anywhere from 6½ to 10 pounds, the average being 7½ pounds," adding that "any child which comes within these limits of weight and length is to be called normal. Occasionally, these figures are much exceeded, but not often." The precise measurements still faced some debate. Even Griffith himself sounded a cautionary note, remarking: "There have been very many estimates made of the average height and weight of children at different ages, and there have even been constructed an elaborate algebraic formula for calculating what these should be," but he warned "the truth of the matter is that the variation is too considerable to allow of any iron-bound statements regarding it." Nonetheless, he did provide his readers with a pull-out chart on which they could record their children's weekly weight gain, and he even recommended the specific scales that new parents should purchase to take these weights, asserting that the scale "must show variations in weight down to one ounce. Those with markings of only a quarter of a pound or more are useless for our purpose." Yet Griffith also continued to insist that "all the figures in the table are, of course only average ones, and a child may measure or weigh somewhat less without there being any occasion for anxiety if it is perfectly healthy; while it may decidedly exceed the figures without being phenomenal." Clearly, there were debates about how much a baby ought to weigh not only within the medical community, but within the minds of individual practitioners. Still, by the last decades of the nineteenth century, the general public seemed to have been largely convinced that all responsible parents should regularly weigh their baby from birth until well into childhood.[33]

Dr Louis Starr's 1894 guide also took a scientific approach to the subject, arguing that "from the first day, growth or increase in length and weight steadily progress, according to certain definitely fixed rules." To monitor this progress, Starr recommended frequent weighing and measurement of the child's chest girth. To help parents track their child's conformity to the "fixed rules," Starr, like Griffith, included a detailed chart of average weights, and information on expected weight gain extending into the sixteenth year. In a copy of the book available on archive.org, the former owner has carefully recorded the weights of Morris (1894), Hamilton (1896), and Laura (1899) on the printed chart, as well as noting that they were weighed naked as recommended by the author. Clearly, readers were taking this advice seriously.[34]

Such charts had, by the late nineteenth century, become increasingly available to parents, aiding in the adoption of quantitative assessments of their child's development. They were found not only in medical and parenting guides, but in "Baby Books" used to record developmental milestones from first steps to first words, and distributed by health departments, baby food manufacturers, and insurance companies. Fancier, bound versions of these books were also available for purchase, becoming popular gifts for new parents. But whether an expensive volume, a mass-produced pamphlet, or a medical guidebook, all sought to normalize the close monitoring and recording of a baby's weight gain as a key duty of parents in ensuring the proper, healthy development of their infants and young children.[35]

This ideal was taken even further in the increasing popularity of "baby shows" that began at county and state fairs, but soon became a national sensation under the sponsorship of the *Woman's Home Companion*. Local versions of these shows, besides looking for the overall "finest" baby, also often had a category specifically for the "fattest baby," and commentators were prone to rhapsodize, as one Ohio newspaper did: "Who is there that does not like to see a plump rosy-cheeked infant." It is not entirely clear if the young contestants were weighed as part of these competitions, but in a context in which prized pumpkins and piglets were put on a scale, the possibility certainly existed. Historian Richard Meckel has noted that in these competitions "the scoring criteria were rather vague and the baby who won was usually the plumpest, fairest, and most blue-eyed." Besides the obvious racial elements of such judgments, fat was clearly considered a key element of the attractive and healthy babies put up for judgment in these shows.[36]

The popular culture understanding of fat babies as healthy babies was also apparent in the photographs that many well-off parents had taken of their young children in the latter decades of the nineteenth century. While photographic images, of necessity, reflected the shape and size of the infant in the lens, an effort seemed to be made to emphasize the chubbiness of a child – ample bellies, pudgy limbs, and rolls of fat at the neck and ankles – suggesting the positive valuation of the fat baby as signifying health and well-being (Figures 3.2 and 3.3). Similar

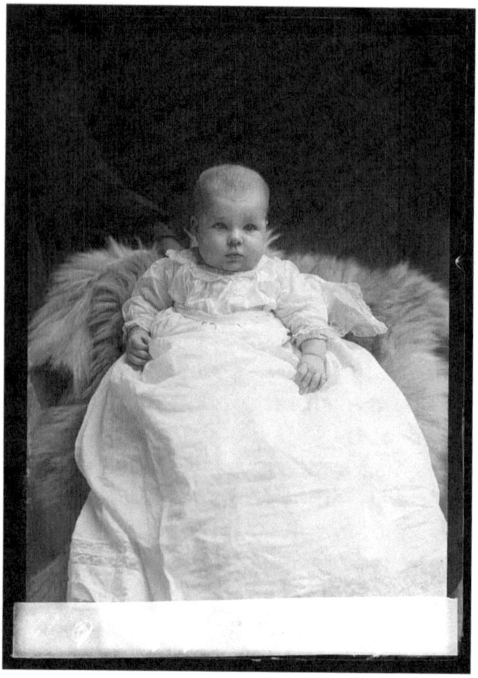

Figure 3.2. Bland Baby, Library of Congress, Prints & Photographs Division, C.M. Bell Studio Collection, LC-DIG-bellcm-04263 (digital file from original).

aesthetic values were reflected in both high art and commercial advertising during this era. Images of loving mothers and angelic infants became common cultural tropes. American artist Aaron Draper Shattuck, for example, portrayed his own family in an 1865 painting centred on his chubby-cheeked infant William surrounded by both his mother and grandmother, suggesting the intergenerational caregiving necessary to tend this fat, healthy baby (Figure 3.4).[37] Artist Arthur John Elsley fully embraced the trope of the fat, healthy child in his work titled "This Little Piggy Went to Market," which shows a naked infant with a prominent potbelly posed on his mother's lap while a doting sister plays with his toes. Elsley's paintings had broad appeal and a number were adapted for use in the rapidly expanding advertising industry. Infant-food manufacturers, not surprisingly, adopted chubby babies to their cause. Soap advertisements also frequently made use of plump infants. An 1886 ad for Pear's Soap, for example, featured a chubby naked infant laying across his mother's lap as she bathes him, his fat

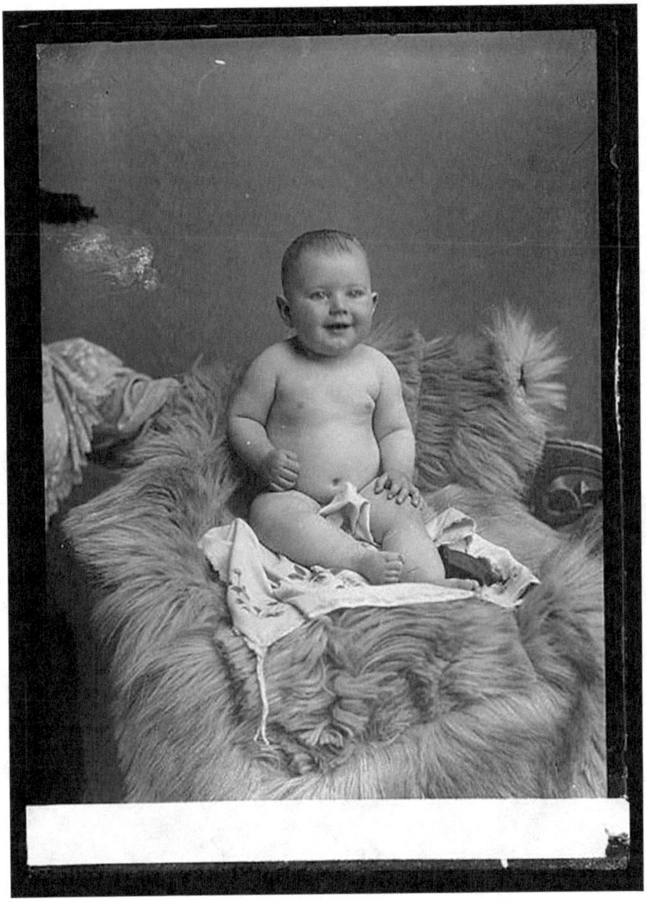

Figure 3.3. Fitzsimmons Baby, Library of Congress, Prints & Photographs Division, C.M. Bell Studio Collection, LC-DIG-bellcm-05978 (digital file from original).

little arms reaching out to pet a kitten. In another ad, a rotund baby in a tub is apparently made ecstatic by gaining hold of the bar of Pear's soap. The fat baby as a model of health and happiness thus became a cultural touchstone, a shorthand that advertisers could use to create positive associations with their products.

The dominant messaging about the correlation between fatness and health in both popular culture and medical literature might appear to provide a clear understanding of fat babies, with an assumption that a mother with such a child should be deemed a success, fulfilling her role

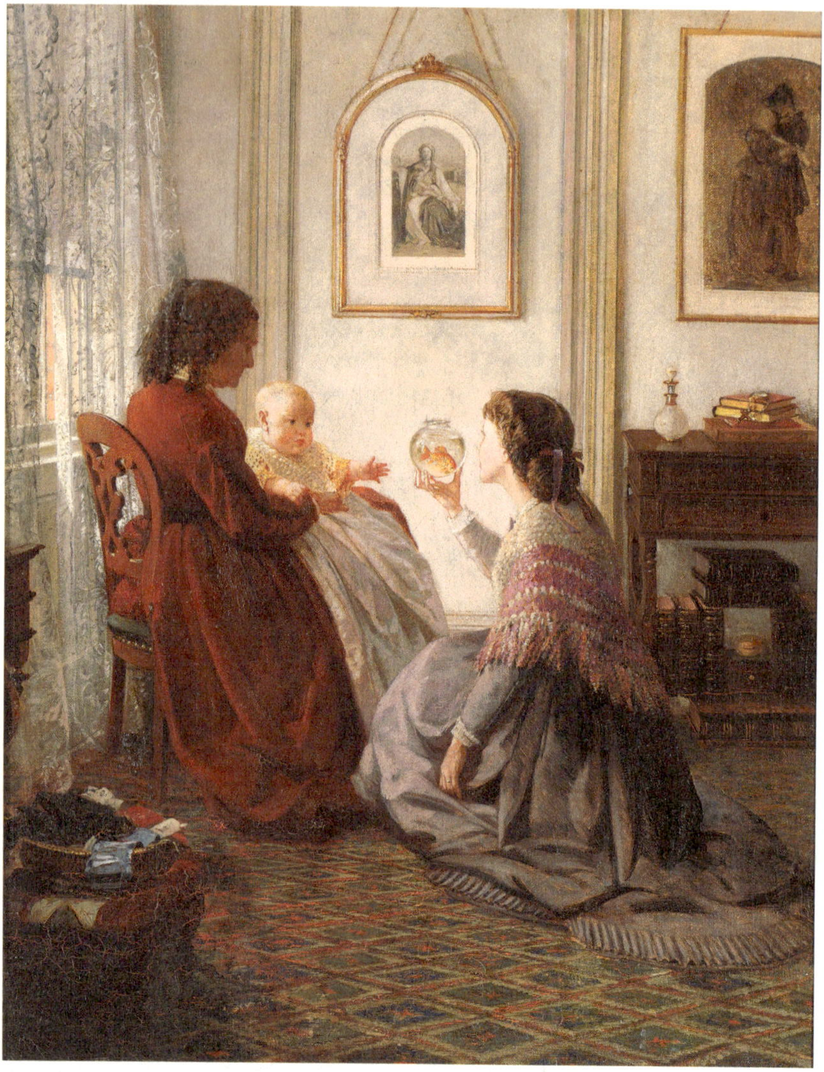

Figure 3.4. Aaron Draper Shattuck (American, 1832–1928). *The Shattuck Family, with Grandmother, Mother and Baby William*, 1865. Oil on canvas, 20 x 15⅞ in. (50.8 x 40.3 cm). Brooklyn Museum, Given in memory of Mary and John D. Nodine, by Judith and Wilbur Ross, 80.192.

in raising a healthy infant. And yet, the message to mothers was never quite that simple or straightforward; a counter-narrative also existed that not all fat was good, and indeed caregivers might be being lulled into a false sense of security by a chubby child. T.C. Duncan, who had lauded the fat baby as possessing superior health, subsequently wrote a book entitled *The Feeding and Management of Infants* in which he at first seemed to sound a similar note, remarking that "A healthy child should be large and plump," but then cautioned that the child "should not be too large nor too fleshy[.]"[38] This mixed messaging meant that caregivers walked a fine line, subject to blame almost regardless of what they did, for while celebration of the fat baby persisted into the twentieth century and beyond, a *too* fat baby could be just as problematic as one who was too thin.

Conclusion

As thinness became increasingly celebrated in the twentieth century as a marker of both health and aesthetic beauty, infants were seemingly the last group in which fatness remained apparently desirable. From the announcement of a newborn's weight to the chubby-cheeked Gerber babies, this plumpness came with the tacit assumption of health and well-being, even as the opposite assumption has come to dominate the discourse not only of adults, but increasingly of overweight children and teenagers.[39] But on the fat infant, experts, parents, and popular culture seemed to agree. Or at least they did until the mid-twentieth century when the foremost expert of that era changed the expectations yet again. While parents had been convinced over the course of the late nineteenth and early twentieth centuries to carefully weigh and measure their infants, the 1946 version of Dr Benjamin's Spock's *Baby and Child Care* counselled new parents: "If you have scales, don't weigh more often than once a week. Once in 2 weeks is even better. If you weigh your baby every day, you encourage yourself to get too wrapped up in the weight." Yet significantly, in the same pages he warned about the future dangers of the fat infant, warning that "fatness in infancy tends to foster fatness for the rest of life." Concluding: "So it is not a kindness to babies to get them fattened up, it's almost a curse in a society that dislikes and ridicules fatness." Experts once again shifted the narrative, reflecting contemporary social views about fatness and health – although how closely parents adhered to these new recommendations is not yet entirely clear.[40]

Fat babies continue to be celebrated in popular culture even as the so-called obesity epidemic has raised alarms about virtually all other demographic groups. But this ongoing acceptance should not obscure the shifting and complicated ideas underlying the discussion of fat infants as an expression of the authority by physicians and other experts in child care in the nineteenth century, nor the judgments they made on the parents, particularly mothers, of these infants. Early in the nineteenth century, parenting manuals rarely mentioned weight, and parents generally assessed their infants in qualitative terms praising fat, fine, and healthy babies, but also painfully aware that even such robustness offered no real guarantee of survival when infant mortality rates were so disturbingly high. As the medical community became increasingly involved in delivering, treating, and feeding infants, and as statistical measures of the human body in all its forms became more common, qualitative assessments were increasingly displaced by quantitative measurements. Mothers were encouraged not only to weigh their babies at more frequent intervals, but to plot that weight against statistical norms to see how their infant, and by inference, they as mothers, measured up. This chapter has shown not only how measuring became standard practice in infant care, but how this practice was used to create precise expectations and standards that were then used to both sanctify the authority of "experts" and to judge mothers whose infants failed to live up to these newly established markers of proper development. Such shifts in how weight should be monitored and understood suggest that the health of the infant was only one concern. Lurking just beneath the surface of the celebrated imagery of the fat baby was a complicated narrative that laid the foundation for the authority of experts and the increasingly contested meanings of fat that embodied not only the physical body and health of the infant, but the care of the mother.

NOTES

1 Henry Chavasse Pye, *Advice to a Mother on the Management of Her Children, and on the Treatment on the Moment of Some of Their More Pressing Illnesses and Accidents*, 9th ed., (London: John Churchill & Sons, 1868), 99.

2 Julia Clark Hallam, *Studies in Child Development: A Manual for Mothers and Mothers' Clubs* (Chicago: Row, Peterson & Co., 1913), 29. For biographical details on Hallam, see Pat Schultz, "Julia Clark Hallam," in *Biographical Database of NAWSA Suffragists, 1890–1920*, alexanderstreet.com.

3 Sander L. Gilman, *Obesity: The Biography* (Oxford University Press, 2010), 45–112, traces the writings of various self-proclaimed experts often writing from their own personal bodily struggle offering diverse solutions to

weight gain and dieting, including Benjamin Franklin, George Cheyne, and William Banting.

4 Julia Grant, *Raising Baby by the Book: The Education of American Mothers* (Yale University Press, 1998), esp. chapter 1.

5 Kathleen W. Jones, "Sentiment and Science: The Late Nineteenth Century Pediatrician as Mother's Advisor," *Journal of Social History* 17 (Autumn 1983): 79–96.

6 This blaming of the mother for all difficulties suffered by her children is a paradigm that continued to exist into the twentieth century and beyond. See for example, Wendy Mitchinson, "Mother Blaming and Obesity: An Alternative Perspective," 187–217, in *Obesity in Canada: Critical Perspectives*, ed. Jenny Ellison, Deborah McPhail, and Wendy Mitchinson (University of Toronto Press, 2016); and Molly Ladd-Taylor and Lauri Umansky, eds., *"Bad" Mothers: The Politics of Blame in Twentieth-Century America* (New York University Press, 1998).

7 L.H. Sigourney, *Letters to Mothers*, 2nd ed. (New York: Harper & Bros, 1839), 29; Nancy Schrom Dye & Daniel Blake Smith, "Mother Love and Infant Death, 1750–1920," *Journal of American History* 73 (Sept., 1986): 329–53. Sentimental motherhood began with a focus on the moral and religious training of the children, but soon took on a more expansive understanding of the well-being of the child.

8 Hugh Smith, *The Female Monitor, Consisting of a Series of Letters to Married women on Nursing and the Management of Children* (Wilmington, Peter Brynberg, 1801); An American Matron, *The Maternal Physician: A Treatise on the Nurture and Management of Infants, from the birth until two years old* (Philadelphia: Lewis Adams, Clark & Raser, 1818); William P. Dewees' *Treatise on the Physical and Medical Treatment of Children*, 3rd ed. (Philadelphia: Carey, Lea & Carey, 1829). A keyword search for words such as weigh, weight, pounds, fat, thin, plump, and puny was conducted in all of the manuals used in this study through archive.org.

9 The shift toward doctor-attended births and then hospital deliveries occurred gradually and only became common in the twentieth century. Judy Barrett Litoff, *American Midwives, 1860 to the Present* (Westport, CT: Greenwood Press, 1978), ix; and Richard Wertz and Dorothy Wertz, *Lying-In: A History of Childbirth in America* (New Haven, CT: Yale University Press, 1989), 211. On the shifting availability of scales available to weigh infants, see Deborah Warner, "Weighing the Baby," National Museum of American History, 10 July 2017. americanhistory.si.edu/blog/weighing-baby.

10 Margaret Law Callcott, ed., *Mistress of Riversdale: The Plantation Letters of Rosalie Stier Calvert, 1795–1821* (Baltimore: Johns Hopkins University Press, 1991), 150, 154, and 192.

11 William Pollock to Elizabeth Pollock, 25 May 1839, Folder 9, Pollock Family Papers, Tulane; Betty Cole to Marion Singleton, 20 Jan. 1831, Singleton Family Papers, LC; William F Colcock to Charles J. Colcock, 9 June 1834, Folder 5, Colcock Family Papers, Tulane.

12 Callcott, ed., *Mistress of Riversdale*, 176.

13 Smith, *The Female Monitor*, 90.

14 Charles D. Meigs, *An Introductory Lecture, Delivered to the Class of Midwifery and Diseases of Women and Children, in Jefferson Medical College, Oct. 18th, 1848, Published by the Class* (Philadelphia: C. Sherman Printer, 1848), 12. On the professionalization of the medical profession, see Steven M. Stowe, "Seeing Themselves at Work: Physicians and the Case Narrative in the Mid-Nineteenth-Century American South," *American Historical Review* 101 (Feb., 1996): 41–79.

15 Stephen Tracy, MD, *The Mother and Her Offspring* (New York: Harper & Bros., Pub., 1853), 117. For a discussion of the development statistic keeping about average baby weights see Lawrence T. Weaver, "In the Balance: Weighing Babies and the Birth of the Infant Welfare Clinic," *Bulletin of the History of Medicine* 84 (Spring 2010): esp. 34–5. More generally on biometrics, see Jeffrey P. Brosco, "Weight Charts and Well Child Care: When the Pediatrician Became the Expert in Child Health," in *Formative Years: Children's Health in the United States, 1880–2000*, ed. A.M. Stern & H. Markel (Ann Arbor, MI: University of Michigan Press, 2002), 91–2; Amanda M. Czerniawski, "From Average to Ideal: The Evolution of the Height and Weight Table in the United States, 1836–1943," *Social Science History* 31, no. 2 (Summer, 2007): 273–96; and Michael Shimkin, "The Numerical Method in Therapeutic Medicine," *Public Health Reports*, 79 (Jan 1964): 2.

16 Pye, *Advice to a Mother on the Management of Her Children*, 55. Patricia Vertinsky, "'Weighs and Means': Examining the Surveillance of Fat Bodies Through Physical Education Practices in North America in the Late Nineteenth and Early Twentieth Centuries," *Journal of Sports History* 35 (Fall 2008): 449–68, discusses the move from averages to norms in the field of physical education, and how moral judgments eventually became attached to these norms.

17 Arthur Ritchie to the Murdock sisters, 28 July 1843, Murdock-Wright Papers, Southern Historical Collection, UNC; Henry Lesesne to Adèle Allston, 19 Dec. 1842, Allston Family Papers, South Carolina Historical Association.

18 Mary Lowndes to "Mama," 15 Sept. 1850, Middleton Family Papers, South Carolina Historical Society; Eliza Fisher to Mary Middleton, 17 Dec. 1840, & 10 Jan. 1842, in *Best Companions: Letters of Eliza Middleton Fisher and Her Mother, Mary Hering Middleton, from Charleston, Philadelphia, and*

Newport, 1839–1846, ed. Eliza Cope Harrison (Columbia: University of South Carolina Press, 2001), 160 and 234; Tryphena Fox to her Sister, 7 Feb., 1867, and to her Brother, 6 Apr. 1875, in *A Northern Woman in the Plantation South: Letters of Tryphena Blanche Holder Fox, 1856–1876*, ed. Wilma King (Columbia: University of South Carolina Press, 1993), 207 & 258. H.L. [likely Harriet Lesesne] to Adèle Allston, 8 June 1854, Allston Family Papers, South Carolina Historical Society. Another of Carey Pettigrew's aunts, Louise Porcher, also wrote to Allston commenting that the infant "is a very delicate little child – very small & suffering with cholic incessantly. I feel very anxious about it." – Louise Porcher to Adèle Allston, 9 June 1854, Allston Family Papers, SCHS. Despite the concern that his puniness generated, the child, Charles Louis Pettigrew, survived into his 70s.

19 Mahala Roach Diary, 3 July 1856, 2 May 1859, 9 June 1860, and 27 Nov. 1860, on birth weights, and 4 Dec. 1860 and 13 Sept 1866, for incidents of weighing herself, Southern Historical Collection, UNC.

20 Dewees, *Treatise on the Physical and Medical Treatment*, 81.

21 Sigourney, Letters to Mothers, 29; Thomas Ewell, MD, *Letters to Ladies, Detailing Important Information Concerning Themselves and Infants* (Philadelphia: W. Brown, 1817), 255; Louis Starr, MD, *Hygiene of the Nursery*, 156–7. See also Sally McMillen, "Mothers' Sacred Duty: Breast-Feeding Patterns among Middle- and Upper-Class Women in the Antebellum South," *Journal of Southern History* 51 (Aug., 1985): 333–56; and Marylynn Salmon, "The Cultural Significance of Breastfeeding and Infant Care in Early Modern England and America," *Journal of Social History* 28 (1994): 247–69. Currently, the World Health Organization recommends infants should be exclusively fed breastmilk for the first six months, with weaning occurring, discretionally, up to the second year; who.int/topics/breastfeeding/en/.

22 H. Lesesne to Adèle Allston, 22 Jul. 1856, Allston Family Papers, SCHS. See also E. West and R.J. Knight, "Mother's Milk: Slavery, Wetnursing, and Black and White Women in the Antebellum South," *Journal of Southern History* 83 (2017): 37–68; Janet Golden, *A Social History of Wet Nursing in America: From Breast to Bottle* (Cambridge: Cambridge University Press, 1996); Valerie A. Fildes, *Breasts, Bottles and Babies: A History of Infant Feeding* (Edinburgh: Edinburgh University Press, 1986), esp. chs. 6 and 7.

23 Harrison, ed., *Best Companion*, 416, 263, 244.

24 Anne Webb to Ann Moore, 9 Apr. 1840, Webb Family Papers, Southern Historical Collection, UNC; Jaqueline H. Wolf, *Don't Kill Your Baby: Public Health and the Decline of Breastfeeding in the Nineteenth and Twentieth Centuries* (Columbus: Ohio State University Press, 2001), 74; Dewees, *Treatise*, 82.

25 Rima D. Apple, "'To Be Used Only Under the Direction of a Physician': Commercial Infant Feeding and Medical Practice, 1870–1940," *Bulletin of*

the History of Medicine 54 (Fall 1980): 402–17; Rima D. Apple, "'Advertised by our Loving Friends': The Infant Formula Industry and the Creation of New Pharmaceutical Markets, 1870–1910," *Journal of the History of Medicine and Allied Sciences* 41 (Jan. 1986): 3–23; Starr, *Hygiene*, 175; Wolf, *Don't Kill Your Baby*, 77.

26 Griffith, *The Care of the Baby*, 34; T.C. Duncan, *How to be Plump: or Talks on Physiological Feeding* (Chicago: Duncan Bros. Pub., 1878), 44.

27 Aunt A.M.F. to Miss Mary Custis, 4 Jan. N.Y., Lee-Mason Papers, Library of Virginia; Elizabeth Perry Diary, 6 Apr. 1843, Southern Historical Collection, UNC.

28 For one such study see M.C. McCormick, "The Contribution of Low Birth Weight to Infant Mortality and Childhood Morbidity," *New England Journal of Medicine* 312 no. 2 (10 Jan. 1985): 82–90.

29 George Newman quoted in Weaver, "In the Balance," 30; Louis Starr, *Hygiene of the Nursery*, 23.

30 W. Peter Ward & Patricia C. Ward, "Infant Birth Weight and Nutrition in Industrializing Montreal," *American Historical Review* 89 (Apr. 1984): 324–45; Robert Millward & Frances Bell, "Infant Mortality in Victorian Britain: The Mother as Medium," *Economic History Review* 54 (Nov. 2001): 699–733; Richard A. Meckel, *Save the Babies: American Public Health Reform and the Prevention of Infant Mortality, 1850–1929* (Baltimore: Johns Hopkins University Press, 1990), 24. Mortality rates for enslaved infants has been estimated to be as high as 30 to 35 percent, in part due to the harsh labour regimes and poor nutrition endured by their mothers. Richard H. Steckel, "Birth Weights and Infant Mortality among American Slaves," *Explorations in Economic History* 23 (Apr. 1986): 173–98; and John Campbell, "Work, Pregnancy, and Infant Mortality among Southern Slaves," *Journal of Interdisciplinary History* 14 (Spring 1984): 793–813.

31 T.C. Duncan, *The Feeding and Management of Infants and Children, and the Home Treatment of the Diseases* (Chicago: Duncan Bros., 1880), 6.

32 Thomas Sozinskey, *The Care and Culture of Children: A Practical Treatise for the Use of Parents* (Philadelphia: H.C. Watts Co, 1880), 317. The use of "Anglo Saxon" was not coincidental here; according to Sabrina Strings, *Fearing the Black Body: The Racial Origins of Fat Phobia* (New York: New York University Press, 2019), esp. ch. 5, ideas about weight and an Anglo-Saxon heritage were increasingly being tied together to define the American identity during this period.

33 J.P. Crozier Griffith, *The Care of the Baby: A Manual for Mothers and Nurses*, 3rd ed. (Philadelphia: W.B. Saunders & Co., 1903), 53–7, 34–5 (emphasis added). For a discussion of the broader debates over infant weight charts, see Jeffrey P. Brosco, "Weight Charts and Well Child Care," 91–120.

34 Louis Starr, MD, *Hygiene of the Nursery,* 4th ed. (Philadelphia: P. Blakiston, Son & Co., 1894), 23, 26.

35 Janet Golden & Lynn Weiner, "Reading Baby Books: Medicine, Marketing, Money and the Lives of American Infants," *Journal of Social History* 44 (Spring 2011): 667–87.

36 The Ohio newspaper is quoted in Susan J. Pearson, "'Infantile Specimens': Showing Babies in Nineteenth-Century America," *Journal of Social History* 42 (Winter 2008): 346–7 and also 343–4; Meckel, *Save the Babies,* 151. There is some disagreement between Meckel and Pearson. Meckel identifies the baby show as a phenomenon that emerged only in the early twentieth century, whereas Pearson identifies a much longer history for the exhibition of babies on both the local and national level. On the representation of children in photography, see Josephine Gear, "The Baby's Picture: Woman as Image Maker in Small Town America," *Feminist Studies* 13 (Summer 1987): 419–42.

37 Gallati, Barbara Dayer, "The Shattuck Family: Aaron Draper Shattuck's Experiment in Narrative Content," *The American Art Journal* 20, no. 3 (1988): 36–47. A reproduction of the painting appears in this article. Mann's "The New Baby" is reproduced at victorianweb.org/painting/mann/1.htm. Both of these paintings have been compared to the Madonna and child in their composition.

38 Duncan, *The Feeding & Management of Infants,* 26.

39 It is not entirely clear at what age the delightfully fat baby transforms into the problematically overweight child or if this shift has altered over the course of the twentieth century; current discussions seem to frequently begin their statistical evidence at age two and caloric reductions are not generally recommended before then. After age two, however, there seems to be a radical shift in perspective with an almost alarmist tone of this discussion of childhood weight gain, noting the global dimensions of this "epidemic" citing a doubling, or more, in children deemed obese and linking these statistics to long term health problems such as diabetes and heart disease. See, for example, Krushnapriya Sahoo et al., "Childhood Obesity: Causes and Consequences," *Journal of Family Medicine and Primary Care* (India) 4, no. 2 (2015): 187–92. Similar messages are conveyed on the websites of the National Institutes of Health and the Childhood Obesity Foundation of Canada. Wendy Mitchinson, *Fighting Fat: Canada, 1920–1980* (Toronto: University of Toronto Press 2018), 180–1, traces the efforts to prevent or treat obesity in the twentieth century, and suggests that by the 1960s even fat infants were beginning to be seen as suspect.

40 Dr Benjamin Spock, *Baby and Child Care* (New York: Pocket Books, 1946), 91. archives.org.

4 Physical Culture and the Denial of Fat in fin de siècle America

CONOR HEFFERNAN

In 1893, Eugen Sandow, a Prussian strongman soon to be declared the world's "most perfectly" developed specimen, debuted to an American audience at the Chicago World's Fair. Still in the infancy of his fame, Sandow would, in time, be known as the first modern bodybuilding celebrity, and the man who helped initiate a growing leisure interest in gym cultures across the western world. This did not, however, immediately endear him to audiences. Sandow's biographer, David Chapman, has highlighted the muted reception to Sandow, who many labelled an oddity.[1] His 1893 tour of America was not, however, a waste. Within months of his World Fair debut, Sandow was attracting thousands of Americans to the cause of "physical culture." Broadly described as a late-nineteenth and early-twentieth-century concern with the ideological and commercial cultivation of the body, physical culture has been described by scholars as a precursor to the modern interest in fitness or gym culture.[2] In the case of Sandow and others, physical culture became an all-encompassing term used to describe highly specified forms of weight training, calisthenics, and dieting. While calisthenics and weight training had existed in America before this time, the resultant physical culture craze that emerged in the late nineteenth and early twentieth century was unprecedented.[3] Inspired by Sandow's physique at the 1893 World Fair, Bernarr Macfadden, a Missouri-born entrepreneur, established his own *Physical Culture* magazine in 1899, which soon claimed thousands of readers across the United States.[4] Many Americans bought Sandow's monographs, workout devices, or health supplements, or turned to the emerging number of physical culture experts whose gymnasiums promised strength, health, and beauty. Although physical culture was primarily aimed at a young male audience, American physical culturists were equally comfortable speaking about female exercise. All bodies were now subject to measurement, evaluation, and the possibilities of improvement.

Importantly for the present collection, the bodies most praised and coveted by the physical culture community were lean, muscular, and strong. For men, entrepreneurs like Sandow and Macfadden used Greco-Roman art and anthropometric charts to highlight the "ideal" male body. The same was done for women who, although discouraged from building excessive muscle, were faced with the same pressure to exercise. The physical culturist's body was taken to represent vibrant health, strength, and the absence of disease. Furthermore, the muscular and athletic body became linked to one's success in life. It was advertised as a form of physical capital that would allow practitioners to progress in their career, relationships, and hobbies. In short, the muscular physical culture body, which grew in importance during the early 1900s, was promoted and desired by countless Americans. Physical culture represented a rejection of the rotund bodies previously deemed desirable by many in the United States, and a glimpse into the new obsession with thinness that would dominate most of the twentieth century.

In highlighting this new rejection of the fat body in favour of a muscular ideal, this chapter examines the creation of a definitive physical culture body and explores its subsequent promotion in the United States, tracing the rise of the muscular body as a desirable form among middle- and upper-class Americans. This, as will be shown, was a slow process which began to reach a crescendo by the late 1800s. Physical culture was a pivotal step in the transition toward the muscular body as an ideal. Emerging in the late 1800s, physical culture materials and marketers reinforced the idea that fat was abject and muscularity desirable. Tracing this shift requires us to explore fit and fat bodies in the context of physical culture diets and advertisements. Physical culture did not lead the charge against fat bodies, but it did play a substantial role in public perceptions of the healthy and desirable body. In this way, physical culture was part of a gradual transition from a greater variety of acceptable bodies to a new hegemonic narrative of thinness that came to dominate the twentieth century and beyond.

Desirable Bodies in Nineteenth-Century America

In *Fat Shame: Stigma and the Fat Body in American Culture*, Amy Farrell argues that body size has long been related to issues of status and social belonging in American thought especially with regard to race, gender and class.[5] In discussing fat bodies in nineteenth-century America, Farrell, like Hillel Schwartz and Peter Stearns, highlighted a dichotomy between middle- and upper-class physiques.[6] Earlier in the nineteenth century, the rotund physique was taken by many as an indicator of one's success, evidence of access to vast quantities of food and a lifestyle free from manual labour. The fat body was a visual signifier of wealth at a time of scarce resources and labour-intensive employment. Some critics derided the "fat cats," whose corpulence stemmed from their privileged lifestyles,[7] deeming the fat body undesirable not because of its aesthetics but rather because it was associated with a capitalist greed said to be damaging American society. Despite this negative view of the fat body as evidence of a lack of moral scruples, advertisements from the mid to late nineteenth century were much more likely to highlight the virtues associated with fat bodies as a sign of mental and sexual strength.[8]

Illustrative of this approbation was "Fat-Ten-U," a late-nineteenth-century product whose sole purpose was to increase the consumer's weight. Advertised in the *Boston Daily Globe* in 1895, "Fat-Ten-U," promised users as much as a one-pound weight gain a day.[9] This, potential customers were assured, would produce in them a healthy glow, a sound constitution, and give them the energy they needed to progress through life. Other advertisements for this product made similar promises, with some explicitly linking weight gain to greater financial health.[10] One of the more popular weight gain products of the age, "Fat-Ten-U" and its accompanying rhetoric was replicated by a series of other products. That individuals paid money for products to increase their weight was testament to their popularity. Corpulence was also at times attractive because it was linked to intelligence. Sander Gilman's study of crime novels in the late nineteenth and early twentieth century found that turn of the century detectives' excess fat was seen as corporeal proof of their intelligence.[11] The detective's thinking and judging body was fuelled by their fat. Accordingly, Gilman argued that "the male body thinks with its visible fat. It is empathetic and responsive. His body is a healthy body because of its fat."[12] The discourses surrounding the fat body in some quarters viewed it as a signifier of one's wealth, health, and intelligence. All of this pointed to the fact that fat bodies were not only permissible for many in the United States, but even celebrated.

Existing concurrently with the promotion of the fat body in nineteenth-century America was a growing idealization of lean and muscular bodies. There were several reasons for this development. One of these, according to Georges Vigarello, was medical changes that meant that the body was no longer understood through nerves and humours but rather as a physiological entity akin to a machine.[13] Under this new model, the body's health and weight were determined by inputs and outputs like diet, exercise, and medicine. This new medical model, which began in the early nineteenth century, later encouraged the rise of a sports-focused medicine which sought to understand the limits of the human "machine." Academic developments regarding the body and its functioning coincided with a growing leisure culture in the United States that permitted more and more individuals spare time to exercise.[14] Typically, economic developments in the nineteenth century, which created a growing middle class with time for exercise, have been cited as a key component in the rise of American sport. Increases in leisure time and more disposable income also precipitated the physical culture phenomenon of the late nineteenth century, and a changing assessment of fat and thin bodies.

Many have cited the mid-nineteenth century as a pivotal moment in the rise of an American fitness industry.[15] Katharina Vester has previously problematized claims that dieting first emerged in 1920s America with a thorough examination of mid-nineteenth century literature which explicitly targeted white men and women interested in losing weight.[16] By 1860, American society, predominantly white, middle-class American society, was beginning to take a clear interest in health and fitness. Amy Farrell explains that the idea that "lower races and ethnicities" tended toward obesity took a remarkable cultural hold in the mid to late nineteenth century.[17] Thus the ability to remain svelte, or athletic, told much about one's social standing. More recent work by Sabrina Strings has demonstrated that fatness became linked first to immorality during this period and then to "otherness."[18] In the case of the United States, the other was predominantly Black and non-white groups. That physical culturists often attempted to link their heritage to Ancient Greece and Rome demonstrated an anxiety about maintaining strict racial and ethnic divisions.

In time, the aversion to fat manifested for some into an interest in strong and muscular physiques that were linked to middle-class ideals of rationality and self-discipline. A clear instance of this was William Blaikie's 1879 monograph *How to Get Strong and Stay So*.[19] An athlete, lawyer, and one of the first American evangelists of physical fitness, Blaikie wrote two influential books on health and fitness in the late nineteenth century.[20] Inspired by the anthropometric fitness studies conducted in Great Britain by Archibald MacLaren in the 1860s, as well as the growing American concern with phrenology, Blaikie presented clear guidelines as to the ideal body type for men and women.[21] Much

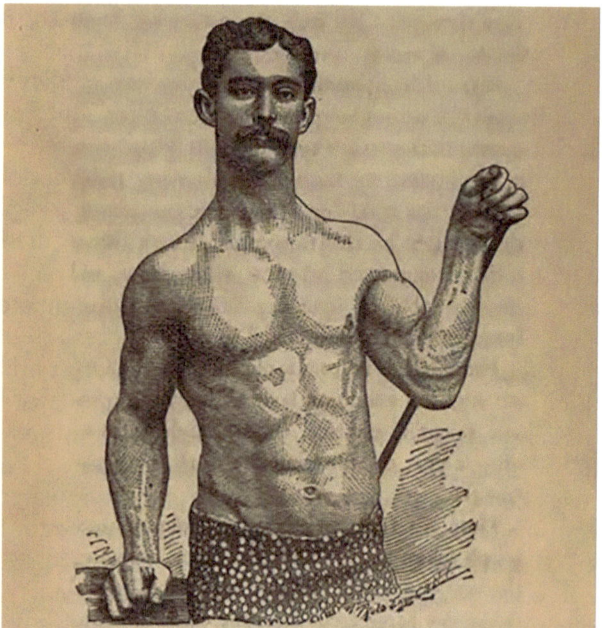

Plate No. II.—The Author, 1882.

Figure 4.1. Dowd after a course of weight training in 1882 (D.L. Dowd, *Physical Culture for Home and School, Scientific and Practical* (New York: D.L. Dowd, 1895).

like MacLaren, a Scottish-born physical educationist who helped create the first system of physical training for the British military, Blaikie saw health as both a personal and national concern.[22] Importantly, Blaikie linked muscular bodies to rationality, discipline, and restraint. In this regard, he was followed by Professor Dowd, whose works in the 1880s were among the first to clearly promote the ideal, fitness-built physique (Figure 4.1).

Where Blaikie and Dowd promoted lean and muscular physiques as precursors to sporting, sexual, or entrepreneurial success, others in the United States, notably Dr John Harvey Kellogg, and before him, Sylvester Graham, linked dietary restraint to forms of godliness and spiritual purity.[23] Kellogg and Graham, as retold by Adam Shprintzen, were part of a growing movement in the United States that linked religious piety and dietary restraint.[24] These two paths, which both stressed the importance of the slender or lean body over the corpulent one, eventually merged in the late nineteenth-century fascination with physical culture. Sections of

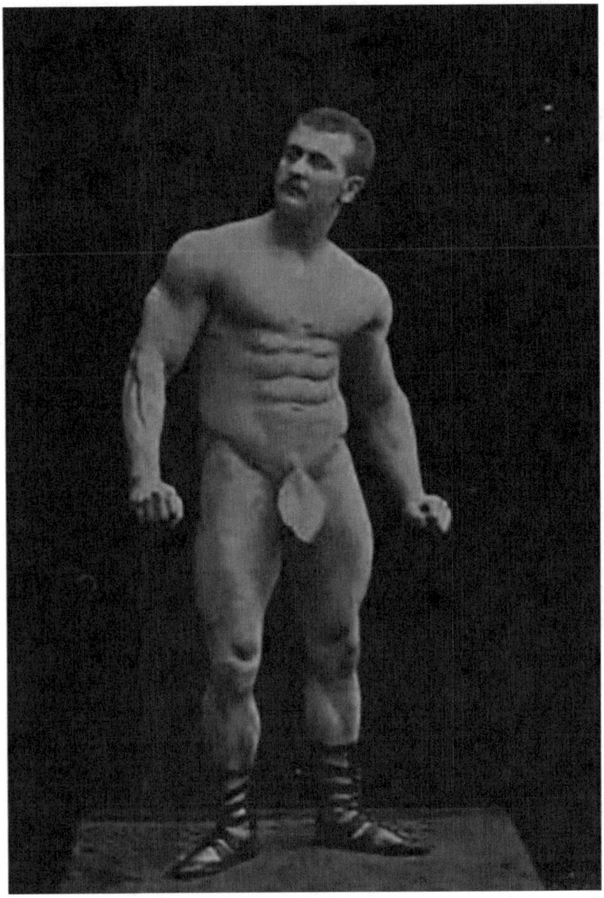

Figure 4.2. Eugen Sandow c. 1890. (Eugen Sandow, *Strength and How to Obtain It* (London: Gale & Polden, 1897).

American society, predominately middle-class white men, had begun to rebel against the celebration of excess and instead privileged discipline over all else. Through diet and exercise, one could embody these values. Thomas Murray's examination of the language of bodybuilding has cited the late 1860s as the period in which the term "physical culture" first came into common use although its first use can be traced to the late eighteenth century.[25] A continuation of previous health trends, physical culture was nevertheless presented by many as new, scientific, and inherently advantageous. Eugen Sandow is widely regarded as the individual who popularized the term physical culture (Figure 4.2).[26]

Following victory in a weightlifting contest over a fellow strongman, Charles A. Sampson, or "Sampson," in London in 1889, Sandow toured Great Britain, promoting physical culture. Seen by his biographers as one of the most influential men of the fin de siècle period, Sandow's physical culture interests would, by the end of the century, include a magazine series, a range of nutritional supplements and workout devices, alternative medical institutes, and a series of monographs.[27] Following Sandow's rise to prominence, numerous other strongmen and in some cases, strongwomen, began to promote themselves as physical culturists. This situation was echoed in the United States both before and after Sandow's 1893 to 1895 tour.[28] Previous health trends coincided with increases in leisure time as well as with the dietary purity campaigns headed by individuals like Kellogg. Gail Bederman has also cited a destabilization of white middle-class masculinity in this era owing to economic changes, the growth in the numbers of working women, and an influx of foreign labour.[29] Reacting to these threats, middle-class American men in particular, turned to physical culture exercises as a means of re-establishing a masculine dominance over other groups. For the historian John Kassan, the body of the male or female physical culturist became a symbol of traditional white America during this time.[30] Stemming from this, physical culturists, like Eugen Sandow, often promoted exercise to demonstrate the white race's racial superiority. Where the corpulent body had been associated with wealth, health and, at times, intelligence, a new ideal began to form around the physical culturist's body. The excess that had previously been celebrated was now being challenged by a white, middle-class privileging of discipline, work ethic, and self-restraint. As the physical culturist's body required steadfast attention to build, this physique became an embodiment of these ideals. This celebration of discipline was clear in physical culture advertising, body prescriptions, and diet monographs.

Measuring Fat and Fit Bodies

Dedicating his monograph to Archibald MacLaren, the English physical educationist, William Blaikie's 1879 health tract, *How to Get Strong and Stay So*, marked a turn in American health writing.[31] Inspired by MacLaren's extensive measuring of soldiers' bodies, Blaikie encouraged parents to measure their boys' limbs, weight, and height. Like MacLaren, Blaikie did so in the belief that one's outer measurements were an indication of health and strength.[32] When MacLaren measured soldiers' bodies, he did so to prove the efficacy of his training system.[33] Blaikie helped bring this measuring to the American public in the form of fitness manuals, although American phrenologists had already popularized the practice. At the same time that Blaikie's book reached the presses, Harvard had just hired a new director for its Hemenway gymnasium. Inspired by the growth of phrenology as a recognized discipline in the United States and also concerned with perfecting human health, the new director, Dudley Allan Sargent, began to measure every student who entered his gym.[34] Later, when the opportunity arose, Sargent sought famous athletes and sportsmen to take their measurements, thereby allowing him to compare the public to the perceived healthiest groups in America.[35]

Taken together, Blaikie and Sargent represented a growing trend in American health and education, the quantification of health. Shannon Walsh's work on physical culture and whiteness stresses the multiple ways in which Sargent's measurements were part of a broader project related to whiteness. Physical activity, in Sargent's lectures and writings, would help white bodies return to nature, build balance and perfection, and nurture future generations. This was no trivial matter as Sargent was often keen to link his system of physical culture to the survival of the white race. In pointed comments toward educated women, Sargent warned of race deterioration should they ignore their physical health. The need to measure, to monitor, and above all else, control the white body, and discipline it through exercise was deemed essential to maintain the presumed rationality and scientific discipline exhibited by western civilization.[36]

Georges Vigarello cited the late nineteenth and early twentieth century as a time when new measuring techniques for the body were created and used to distinguish healthy bodies from fat bodies.[37] Tapping into a longer-held acceptance of phrenology in the United States, a practice that linked cranial and body size to behavioural characteristics, men's bodily measurements, typically the size of the waist, chest, and biceps, began to be linked to broader societal messages.[38] And, as Lynn Kennedy suggests in chapter 3 of this collection, such practices were not restricted to adults but began with weighing and measuring babies. In adulthood, the man who was slim-waisted, broad-chested, and in possession of large bicep muscles was often depicted as hard-working, attractive, successful, and brave in both the United States and parts of Western Europe.[39] Body measurements were not only accepted, but encouraged by politicians, public health officials and, in time, physical culturists. A further important development was the creation of insurance tables at the end of the nineteenth century in America, which linked weight to mortality.[40] A higher weight meant a higher insurance premium, furthering the importance of measuring one's body. When physical culturists began to publish their own health monographs en masse at the end of the nineteenth century, it is not surprising that so many included measurements and anthropometric charts depicting the ideal body.

One of the first to initiate this trend was Eugen Sandow. Sandow, who was measured by Dudley Allen Sargent in 1893, included anatomical charts in the first of his training manuals, *Sandow on Physical Training*, published in 1894.[41] Capitalizing on his meeting with Sargent, Sandow published his measurements before imploring his new followers to similarly measure their own physiques.[42] To increase their motivation, Sandow even promised medals to students who improved their physical measurements using his system.[43] This tactic, which Sandow perfected over the following decade, was furthered in 1897, when Sandow's second monograph, *Strength and How To Obtain It*, included anthropometric charts for his "pupils" to complete, preferably under the guidance of a physician (Figure 4.3).[44]

Men, and it was predominantly men who Sandow targeted, were told that the closer they could bring their body into alignment to Sandow's measurements, the greater their vitality, health, work rate, and control would be.[45] Whereas the rotund figure was often a sign of wealth in much of the nineteenth century, the end of the century saw a muscular body become the ideal. Originally published in London, Sandow's work quickly made its way to the United States and even South America, where it became a best seller, being published in several editions before Sandow's death in the 1920s.[46]

But the vogue for quantification was not all-encompassing. Although his work sold widely in the United States, Sandow's influence paled in comparison to Bernarr Macfadden's. Where Sandow gave definitive measurements for male bodies, which explicitly rejected the fat body, Macfadden's prescriptions were often more confused. In works such as *Macfadden's Physical Training*, published in 1900, he decried the use of anthropometric charts and body measurements, claiming that efforts to homogenize the human body were problematic owing to individual variance.[47] Macfadden's unease with body measurements, at least within this work, did not, however, prevent him from commenting on the ideal human form. Though its appropriate extent was different for men, women, and children, Macfadden cited a common goal across age and sex: slenderness. This was made clear in his claim that "A thorough development of all parts of the muscular system tends to drive away surplus accumulations of flesh."[48]

Rather than anatomical charts, the ideal male and female forms for Macfadden were rooted in Greco-Roman art, which, again, was a signifier of the long lineage of western health. Men were to model themselves on the sculptures of Apollo, Hercules, or Adonis. Women were

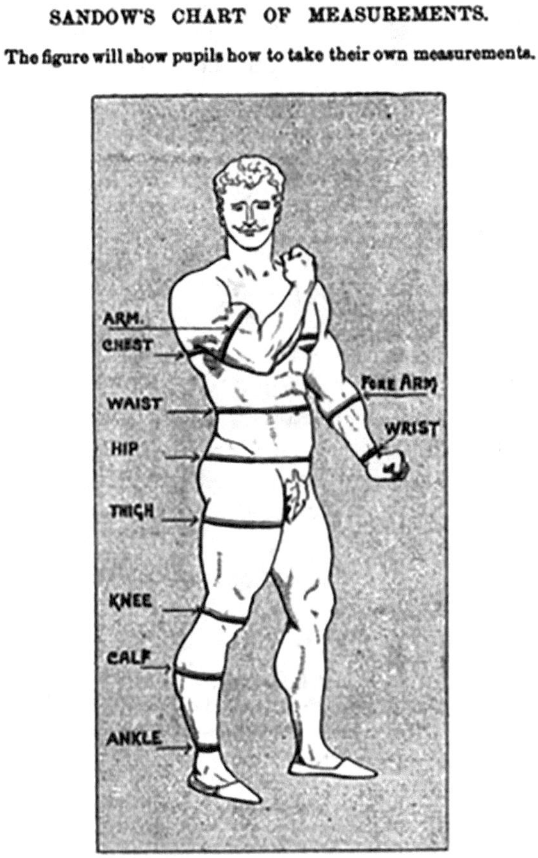

Figure 4.3. Sandow's Chart of Measurements. (Eugen Sandow, *Strength and How to Obtain It* (London: Gale & Polden, 1897).

instructed to use the Venus de Milo as inspiration.[49] Underpinning these instructions was Macfadden's steadfast belief that strong, muscular bodies reflected robust health. In *Macfadden's Physical Training*, the author claimed that

> [i]f physical training always tends towards the development of the highest degree of health and strength, if under its influence every function performs its office more thoroughly, and every organ is accelerated in its efforts to produce the purest, strongest, bodily conditions – is not the riddle, how can it deposit flesh on a thin person and lessen the weight of an obese one, fully solved.[50]

In this instance, Macfadden rejected bodies that were overly thin or overly fat in favour of a body developed through physical training and dietary restraint. Such a frame, modelled on Greco-Roman principles, was linked to the perfect functioning of the body.

However, Macfadden's disapproval of quantified measuring of the body did not last long. In 1901 he published *The Power and Beauty of Superb Motherhood*, in which he urged female readers to measure the size of their bust, waist, and arms before and after a course of training.[51] For the stout, he promised a return to perfect health, as epitomized by the Venus de Milo, whose measurements Macfadden promoted as the ideal form. For men, Macfadden's *Physical Culture* magazine began to include measurements of athletes and well-known physical culturists, as a means of encouraging readers to emulate their physiques.[52] The ideal body, for Macfadden and those who supported him, was linked to a higher vision of humanity. Two of Macfadden's business slogans, used throughout his several-decade career, were "weakness is a crime, don't be a criminal" and "sickness is a sin, don't be a sinner."[53] Like Sandow, who envisioned muscularity and strength as precursors for a man's work ethic, character, and gentlemanly bearing, Macfadden depicted strong, muscular bodies as expressions of a desirable personality. The quantified human body, which rejected both thinness and fatness, became linked to broader personality traits deemed important in turn of the century America.

Fat Bodies and Diet

Exercise was key to the new ideal body, with its associations of discipline and control, but regulating one's diet was equally important. Writing in 1895, one American physical culturist, Edwin Checkley, claimed that "with all the hurrying and scurrying brought by the Nineteenth Century method of living, a large number of people suffer from an accumulation of fat."[54] In doing so, Checkley highlighted a growing physical culture industry concerned with fat and weight loss. Newspaper advertisements decried the fat body, physical culturists promoted ideal human forms, and a host of Americans turned toward new foodstuffs and devices to improve their health. This included, as noted by Carolyn Thomas de la Peña, fantastical sounding devices like magnetic belts, whose electrical vibrations were thought to decrease fat, increase vitality, and improve one's health.[55] Some physical culturists attached their names to health devices but were far more focused on diet and exercise, with physical culturists like Sandow or Macfadden stressing the importance of moderation in one's diet.

Interviewed during his first tour of the United States, Sandow told reporters in 1894 that his own diet, which included cigar smoking and alcohol, was centred on moderation.[56] This, as retold by Sandow's biographer David Chapman, further endeared Sandow to the American public.[57] Sandow's promotion of moderation in everything and excess in nothing further substantiated his attempt to link the physical culturist's body to ideals of restraint and self-discipline. The antithesis to this was of course the fat body, often reviled by Sandow and other physical culturists. In an age of abundance, as fin de siècle America was often depicted, one's inability to control appetite, and thus to carry excess weight, was a cause for concern.[58] Whereas fat bodies may have represented success in times of scarcity, the inverse became true during a time of perceived plenty.

The cookbooks and diets Macfadden produced during this time similarly stressed the importance of the disciplined, healthy body. In his 1900 *Physical Culture Cookbook*, Macfadden criticized the general public's eating patterns which, he claimed, resulted from a complete ignorance of wholesome food.[59] His recipes, he assured readers, would bring them closer to a state of vibrant health. They would nourish body and brain, strip excess flesh, and build strength.[60] This narrow understanding of health deliberately excluded the fat or obese body, which was, oftentimes explicitly, linked with ill health. Macfadden even rejected the very idea of gaining weight for the sake of health, as was often recommended for convalescents.[61] Eschewing this advice, which often brought him into conflict with American physicians, whom he labelled misguided, Macfadden instead promoted a small amount of nourishing food rather than "eating heartily" without discipline.[62] Like Sandow, Macfadden, too, promoted moderation in eating. This point was reiterated in 1902 when Macfadden opened his own restaurant in New York. Selling one-cent meals, Macfadden's restaurant sold only "wholesome" food, thought to enhance New Yorkers' health and vitality.[63] Later criticized for its bland fare, consisting of unsweetened bread, barely boiled vegetables, and nut loaves, the restaurant highlighted Macfadden's commitment to an ascetic style of eating.[64]

On the rare occasions when Macfadden allowed for weight gain, he was quick to stipulate what kind. In his *Miracle of Milk* monograph, in which he promoted the health-giving properties of an all-milk diet, he distinguished between good and bad forms of weight:

> Milk does not create flabby fat. It is a corrective diet for tissues below par, and it aids these tissues and the entire body to approach normality. This means that an improvement is established in the "selective action" of

> the cells, by which action they are enabled to discard elements not necessary for natural growth, repair and bodily functions. Worthless, unsightly, cumbersome or burdensome fat is therefore never developed or deposited from a milk diet[.][65]

Again, the emphasis was on controlling and containing the body through science and assessment.

Sandow and Macfadden were more vocal, and more publicized, than other American-based physical culturists on the matter of diet but they were not alone. In 1899, the unnamed author of the *Philadelphia Inquirer*'s "Womanly Wisdom" column responded to one reader's question on how best to lose weight in officious tones: "There is no simple home remedy for getting thinner. Reducing weight requires the most thorough treatment from physical culture to diet. Few women are persistent enough to pursue an anti-flesh reform, vigorously."[66] The author later linked slender female physiques, as forged through physical culture exercises and eating habits, to healthy motherhood and vibrancy.[67] The woman's body thus held a dual importance – her health was both a personal matter and a concern for the human race. Such dietary advice became a means of asserting the broader importance of slender bodies. In Iowa, a lesson on "physical culture diets" was added to a charitable Chautauqua assembly, which aimed to increase the health, strength, and nerve of the rural American man or woman.[68] Once described as "the most American thing in America," by President Theodore Roosevelt, Chautauqua assemblies were romanticized as part of a white, rural, American identity.[69] The fat body explicitly was no longer part of this American project.

Physical Culture Advertisements and the Fat Body

The late nineteenth and early twentieth century witnessed a vast array of workout devices, fitness manuals, and dietary supplements. Entrepreneurs preyed upon male and female anxieties about their bodies to turn a profit.[70] Sandow, like later popular strongmen such as Earle Lierderman and Charles Atlas (who operated in the 1920s and 1930s), used his own physique to sell products.[71] These products were marketed in a highly gendered way, particularly for men, and promoted as patriotic, modern, and scientifically advanced. This is explored in Lesley Steinitz's study of early food supplements. Bernarr Macfadden's many biographers have also noted his use of powerful masculinities and domestic femininities to market his goods.[72] The social, sexual, and entrepreneurial importance of the physical body during this time was clearly key.

At the core of the physical culture enterprise was the white body. Marketing discourses in Great Britain and the United States targeted a growing middle-class consumer base, typically employed in sedentary positions, who were dissatisfied with their bodies.[73] This explains why Irish author James Joyce made his protagonist in *Ulysses*, Leopold Bloom, a devoted "Sandow-ite." Counted among Bloom's possessions were "The indoor exercises, formerly intermittently practised, subsequently abandoned, prescribed in Eugen Sandow's *Physical Strength and How to Obtain It* ... designed particularly for commercial men engaged in sedentary occupations."[74] For men, the muscular body became something they could purchase through the latest equipment, course, or supplement. Whereas previously a corpulent frame was a social signifier of one's wealth, now the physical culturist's body was taken to represent both wealth and, significantly, a high work ethic. The physical culture body became the antithesis to the fat body.

Despite the efforts of some marketers to sell a "corset for fat men," the majority of physical culture advertisements in American newspapers promised to reduce fat through some form of physical culture intervention.[75] What was remarkable about such advertisements was not the targeting of fat, but rather the implicit and often undefined assertion that excess fat was undesirable and made one lesser. Julian R. Brandon, an American physical culturist, of whom little else is known, made this point apparent to audiences in Iowa in 1901. Lecturing both male and female consumers, whom he wished to convert to his patented exercise system, Brandon decried the overeating, physical sluggishness, and inactivity he saw plaguing America.[76] Such behaviour, he argued, was leading to fatter bodies, thereby depriving Americans – and by that white Americans were meant – of their vitality. To recover their health and build bodies akin to the slender and muscular white bodies shown in Brandon's subsequent articles, a course of physical culture was needed.[77]

After publishing his book, *Physical Culture for Fat People*, in 1903, Anthony Barker went on a prolonged media campaign, which included interviews, articles, and a series of photographs.[78] In these works, and his larger monograph, Barker cited the "fat, clumsy body" as the prime threat facing American men.[79] This threat, often undefined, was linked, among white Americans, to physical degeneracy, financial instability, and a lack of vigour in one's love life. Barker's solution was set out in his new physical culture monograph, a program through which he promised that men would build muscle and nerve in equal measure.[80] In Barker's thinking, strong and muscular bodies, similar to Eugen Sandow's, revealed mental as well as physical strength. The inverse of this was the fat or obese body which Barker depicted as gluttonous, comical, and deserving of pity. What is important to state about these campaigns is the absence of African-American or Asian bodies. Were one to encounter these advertisements without knowing the composite of American society, the assumption would be that only white bodies existed.[81]

Messages aimed at women likewise critiqued and rejected the fat body. An advertisement in the *Boston Daily Globe* targeted "women who are eager to reduce their avoirdupois" and encouraged them to hire physical culture teachers.[82] Using terms like "heavyweights" to describe former clients, the paper spoke of women whose "adipose tissue" had become problematic.[83] It was for this reason that a Boston teacher of physical culture boasted a "large and flourishing fat ladies class."[84] One of Bernarr Macfadden's many advertisements for female physical culture at this time promised that fat would "vanish" from the stout through his brand of physical exercise.[85] The advertisements encouraged the message that the ideal female physique was slender, poised, and dainty.

That the perceptions of female beauty had changed with the advent of physical culture was clear to many of Macfadden's contemporaries. One writer for the *Seymour Daily Republican* claimed that desired body types had so altered that

> With regard to figures, it is amusing to note that the ideal forms for woman varies from decade to decade. The straight-fronted effect has become outmoded, and we now go in strong for small waists, big hips and broader shoulders, and – most serious of all – we make a dead set against obesity.[86]

Big hips and broad shoulders, as built by physical culture, represented healthy women and, by virtue of that, healthy mothers. The obese body, in this understanding, was linked with large stomachs, stooped shoulders, and energy deficits. Physical culture's rising popularity facilitated a shift away from fat bodies as an indicator of wealth and desirability toward slender and muscular bodies. Bernarr Macfadden's *Physical Culture* magazine, the most popular American magazine of its kind, regularly featured articles on the dangers of fat bodies.[87] For Macfadden and other physical culturists, the fat body, for men and women, signified a body in need of reform. The answer, typically, lay in the latest Macfadden book or exercise device. That a physical culture magazine would promote physical culture products is not surprising; after all, it fuelled the industry. Importantly, newspaper advertisements also published messages decrying fat bodies by promoting physical culture.

The fat body was still critiqued while muscular or slender bodies were praised.

Lectures and advertisements for physical culture diets prove equally illustrative. Promoting his "Barton Method," one lesser-known physical culturist, John Barton, claimed that his diet alone could strengthen the body, calm nerves, and treat a variety of illnesses.[88] Unlike the "weakened body" or the body deprived of vitality, the Barton Method promised a body quickly toned through physical exercise and nourished through food.[89] Discipline and an ascetic lifestyle were linked to a toned, strong, and muscular body. This body, unlike the fat body, was assumed to be impervious to illness or "excited nerves."[90] The strong body was seen as reflecting a strong will and a strong will was deemed necessary to build the physical culture body. There was no room for other shapes or sizes.

Conclusion

After the Great War, large numbers of Americans took part in the "reducing craze" of the 1920s. Commonly identified with the growing influence of Hollywood filmdom and print media more generally, the "craze" has often, incorrectly, been cited as the first major weight loss movement in the United States.[91] Physical culture in the fin de siècle period was clearly one precursor to this trend. Spurred on by the muscular bodies of men like Eugen Sandow and Bernarr Macfadden, physical culture promoted a total lifestyle that influenced eating and exercising behaviours and was intensely focused on the corporal frame.

Muscular, lean, and strong bodies were promoted as the ideal male form. Often comparing themselves to the statues of antiquity, physical culturists, like Sandow, linked the muscular body to behavioural and personality traits. The muscular body was not a neutral thing. It was advertised to represent strong-willed, hard-working individuals brimming with vitality. To build this body, individuals were required to spend time exercising in the gymnasium or their home. They were instructed to watch their diets, to refuse certain foodstuffs, and to concentrate on nourishment above all else. It is difficult to know how many men fully subscribed to such ascetic lifestyles, but the continued popularity of Bernarr Macfadden's *Physical Culture* magazine demonstrates some form of market. Within these discourses, little room, if any, existed for the fat or corpulent body. This body was a project, something that required steady attention and, at times, drastic action. The fat body lacked the aesthetics coveted by physical culturists. It also represented a body deprived of vitality and was seen as a sort of embodied gluttony. The physical culturist's body was a complete rejection of the corpulent one.

The situation was much the same for women. Here slender and petite bodies became the ideal. Female strength was encouraged among physical culturists, but far less emphasis was placed on muscularity. Where men were encouraged to build muscle and, in doing so, become conquerors of their social or sexual worlds, women were implored to exercise for the sake of future races or the nation-state. For women, just as for men, the physical culturist's body became an embodiment of discipline and hard work. It was a symbol of strength and racial superiority for others. Yet again the fat body was reviled in discourses on female physical culture. Not only was it seen as undesirable but ill-suited to the demands of modern life. Taken together, physical culture in fin de siècle America privileged muscular, slender, and strong bodies over fat ones. In the early nineteenth century, the fat body was a symbol of health and wealth and was seen as desirable. By the end of the century, embodied forms of excess were no longer permissible for the middle class in America. Hard work, discipline, rationality, and a certain kind of ascetism became socially important values. Physical culturists not only promoted these values, they inscribed them on their flesh.

NOTES

1 David L. Chapman, *Sandow the Magnificent: Eugen Sandow and the Beginnings of Bodybuilding* (Chicago: University of Illinois Press, 1994), 56–68.
2 Michael Anton Budd, *The Sculpture Machine: Physical Culture and Body Politics in the Age of Empire* (New York: NYU Press, 1997), xi.
3 Elizabeth A. Gagen, "Making America Flesh: Physicality and Nationhood in Early Twentieth-Century Physical Education Reform," *Cultural Geographies* 11, no. 4 (2004): 417–42.
4 William R. Hunt, *Body Love: The Amazing Career of Bernarr Macfadden* (Wisconsin: Popular Press, 1989), 1–15.
5 Amy Erdman Farrell, *Fat Shame: Stigma and the Fat Body in American Culture* (New York: NYU Press, 2011), 3–21.
6 Hillel Schwartz, *Never Satisfied: A Cultural History of Diets, Fantasies, and Fat* (New York: Doubleday, 1986), 120; Peter N. Stearns, *Fat History: Bodies and Beauty in the Modern West* (New York: New York University Press, 1997), 58–60.
7 Debbie Rodan and Katie Ellis, *Disability, Obesity and Ageing: Popular Media Identifications* (New York: Routledge, 2016), 25.

8 Juliann Sivulka, *Soap, Sex, and Cigarettes: A Cultural History of American Advertising* (Boston: Cengage Learning, 2011), 43.
9 "Fat-Making Foods," *Boston Daily Globe*, 25 May 1895, 6.
10 "Fat-Making Foods," *Indianapolis News*, 21 April 1897, 6.
11 Sander L. Gilman, "How Fat Detectives Think," in *Cultures of the Abdomen*, ed. Christopher Forth and Ana Carden-Coyne (Palgrave Macmillan, New York, 2005), 221–37.
12 Gilman, "How Fat Detectives Think," 226.
13 Georges Vigarello, *The Metamorphoses of Fat: A History of Obesity* (Columbia: Columbia University Press, 2013), 141–5.
14 Steven A. Riess, *Sport in Industrial America, 1850–1920* (New York: John Wiley & Sons, 2012), 2–12.
15 Jan Todd, "The Strength Builders: A History of Barbells, Dumbbells and Indian Clubs," *The International Journal of the History of Sport*, 20, no. 1 (2003): 73–5.
16 Katharina Vester, "Regime Change: Gender, Class, and the Invention of Dieting in Post-Bellum America," *Journal of Social History*, 44, no. 1 (2010): 39–70.
17 Farrell, *Fat Shame: Stigma and the Fat Body*, 80.
18 Sabrina Strings, *Fearing the Black Body: The Racial Origins of Fat Phobia* (New York: New York University Press, 2019), 1–9.
19 William Blaikie, *How to Get Strong and Stay So* (New York: Harper & Brothers, 1879).
20 "Author Athlete Dies Suddenly. William Blaikie, Well-Known Lawyer, Pioneer Advocate of Physical Culture, Stricken with Apoplexy While Asleep," *The Evening World*, 6 December 1904, 6.
21 "Author Athlete Dies Suddenly. William Blaikie, Well-Known Lawyer, Pioneer Advocate of Physical Culture, Stricken with Apoplexy While Asleep," *The Evening World*, 6 December 1904, 1–20; Susan Branson, "Phrenology and the Science of Race in Antebellum America," *Early American Studies: An Interdisciplinary Journal*, 15, no. 1 (2017): 164–93.
22 Archibald Maclaren, "Military Gymnasia," *Royal United Services Institution*, 8, no. 31 (1864): 217–30.
23 James C. Whorton, "Historical Development of Vegetarianism," *The American Journal of Clinical Nutrition*, 59, no. 5 (1994): 1103S–1109S.
24 Adam D. Shprintzen, *The Vegetarian Crusade: The Rise of an American Reform Movement, 1817–1921* (North Carolina: UNC Press Books, 2013), 120–45.
25 Thomas E. Murray, "The Language of Bodybuilding," *American Speech*, 59, no. 3 (1984): 195–206.
26 Chapman, *Sandow the Magnificent*, 1–12; David Waller, *The Perfect Man: The Muscular Life and Times of Eugen Sandow, Victorian Strongman* (London: Victorian Secrets, 2011), 1–12.

27 Dominic G. Morais, "Branding Iron: Eugen Sandow's "Modern" Marketing Strategies, 1887–1925," *Journal of Sport History*, 40, no. 2 (2013): 193–214.
28 John F. Kassan, *Houdini, Tarzan and the Perfect Man: The White Male Body and the Challenge of Modernity in America* (New York: Hill and Wang, 2001), 28–60.
29 Gail Bederman, *Manliness and Civilization: A Cultural History of Gender and Race in the United States, 1880–1917* (Chicago: University of Chicago Press, 1995), 5–12.
30 Kassan, *Houdini, Tarzan and the Perfect Man*, 8.
31 Blaikie, *How to Get Strong and Stay So.*
32 Blaikie, *How to Get Strong and Stay So*, 1–10.
33 Archibald Maclaren, *A Military System of Gymnastic Exercises for the Use of Instructors* (London: Her Majesty's Stationery Office, 1862).
34 E. Melanie DuPuis, *Dangerous Digestion: The Politics of American Dietary Advice* (California: University of California Press, 2015), 79.
35 Carolyn De la Peña, "Dudley Allen Sargent: Health Machines and the Energized Male Body," *Iron Game History*, 8, no. 2 (2003): 3–19.
36 Shannon L. Walsh, *Eugenics and Physical Culture Performance in the Progressive Era: Watch Whiteness Workout* (New York: Springer, 2020), 55–83.
37 Vigarello, *The Metamorphoses of Fat*, 141–5.
38 De la Pena, "Dudley Allen Sargent"; Jan Todd, *Physical Culture and the Body Beautiful: Purposive Exercise in the Lives of American Women, 1800–1870* (Macon: Mercer University Press, 1999), 250–60.
39 J. Reich, "The World's Most Perfectly Developed Man: Charles Atlas, Physical Culture, and the Inscription of American Masculinity," *Men and Masculinities*, 12, no. 4 (2010): 444–61.
40 Amanda M. Czerniawski, "From Average to Ideal: The Evolution of the Height and Weight Table in the United States, 1836–1943," *Social Science History*, 31, no. 2 (2007): 273–96.
41 Eugen Sandow, *Sandow on Physical Training: A Study in the Perfect Type of the Human Form* (London: JS Tait & Sons, 1894), 171.
42 Sandow, *Sandow on Physical Training*, 171–4.
43 Sandow, *Sandow on Physical Training*, 171–4.
44 Sandow, *Strength and How to Obtain It*, 26–7.
45 Sandow, *Strength and How to Obtain It*, 27–34.
46 Morais, "Branding Iron"; Andrés Horacio Reggiani, "Physical Culture, Athletic Performance and Hygiene of the Nation: The Rise of Sports Medicine in Argentina (1930–1940)," *Historia Crítica*, 61 (2016): 65–84.
47 Bernarr Macfadden, *Macfadden's Physical Training* (New York: The Macfadden Company, 1900), 37–8.
48 Macfadden, *Macfadden's Physical Training*, 106.

49 Bernarr Macfadden, *The Power and Beauty of Superb Motherhood* (New York: The Macfadden Company, 1901), 31.
50 MacFadden, *Macfadden's Physical Training*, 23–4.
51 Macfadden, *The Power and Beauty of Superb Motherhood*, 1–12.
52 "Our Premium Instruction Course," *Physical Culture*, 2, no. 5 (1900): 4.
53 Mary Williamson Macfadden and Emile Gauvreau, *Dumbbells and Carrot Strips: The Story of Bernarr Macfadden* (New York: Holt, 1953), 71.
54 Edwin Checkley, *A Natural Method of Physical Training* (New York: William C. Bryant, 1895), 85.
55 Carolyn Thomas De La Peña, *The Body Electric: How Strange Machines Built the Modern American* (New York: NYU Press, 2003).
56 "To Get Strong," *Newark Daily Advocate*, 27 April 1894, 3.
57 Chapman, *Sandow the Magnificent*, 93.
58 See for example, Eric C. Schneider, *In the Web of Class: Delinquents and Reformers in Boston, 1810s–1930s* (New York: NYU Press, 1993), 105.
59 Bernarr Macfadden, *Physical Culture Cookbook* (New York: The Macfadden Company, 1901), 1–10.
60 Macfadden, *Physical Culture Cookbook*, 12–14.
61 Macfadden, *Physical Culture Cookbook*, 215.
62 Macfadden, *Physical Culture Cookbook*, 215.
63 "The One-Cent Meal Restaurant," *Physical Culture*, 7, no. 2 (1902): 102.
64 Andrew F. Smith, *New York City: A Food Biography* (Lanham: Rowman & Littlefield, 2013), 140–1.
65 Bernarr Macfadden, *The Miracle of Milk: How To Use The Milk Diet Scientifically at Home* (New York: The Macfadden Company, 1923), 7–8.
66 "Womanly Wisdom," *The Philadelphia Inquirer*, 27 March 1899, 7.
67 "Womanly Wisdom," *The Philadelphia Inquirer*, 27 March 1899, 7.
68 "Treats in Store," *Des Moines Daily News*, 3 May 1899, 4.
69 Charlotte Canning, *The Most American Thing in America: Circuit Chautauqua as Performance* (Iowa: University of Iowa Press, 2005), 227.
70 Conor Heffernan, "Strength Peddlers: Eddie O'Callaghan and the Selling of Irish Strength," *Sport in History*, 38, no. 1 (2018): 23–45.
71 Heffernan, "Strength Peddlers; Morais, "Branding Iron."
72 Benjamin Pollack and Janice Todd, "Before Charles Atlas: Earle Liederman, the 1920s King of Mail-Order Muscle," *Journal of Sport History* 44, no. 3 (2017): 399–420; Lesley Steinitz, "The Language of Advertising: Fashioning Health Food Consumers at the Fin de Siècle," in *Food, Drink, and the Written Word in Britain, 1820–1945*, eds. Mary Addyman, Laura Wood, Christopher Yiannitsaros (London: Routledge, 2017), 135–63; Jan Todd, "Bernarr Macfadden: Reformer of Feminine Form," *Journal of Sport History* 14, no. 1 (1987): 61–75.

73 Shelly McKenzie, *Getting Physical: The Rise of Fitness Culture in America* (Lawrence: University Press of Kansas, 2013), 3–12.
74 James Joyce, *Ulysses* (London: Bodley Head 1960), 17. 509.
75 "New Corsets for Fat Men," *The Biloxi Daily Herald*, 13 September 1901, 1.
76 "Dignity is Killing Four-Fifths of the World," *Daily Times*, 17 November 1901, 15.
77 "A Beautiful Pair of Shoulders," *San Francisco Call*, 23 June 1901, 10.
78 Anthony Barker, *Physical Culture for Fat People* (Anthony Barker: New York, 1903); "Physical Culture for the Lean," *The Leader*, 4 March 1903, 3; "Physical Culture for Men Who Are Busy," *Atlanta Constitution*, 2 November 1902, 6; "Real Physical Culture And Corrective Exercises." 2545, Ottley Coulter Clippings, Stark Center, University of Texas at Austin.
79 Anthony Barker, "Physical Culture for Busy People," *The Sunday Oregonian*, 2 November 1902, 10.
80 Barker, *Physical Culture for Fat People*.
81 While physical culture historians have also been guilty of this, existing work by Shannon Walsh (cited above) and other forthcoming work is helping to address it. Ava Purkiss, *Fit Citizens: A History of Black Women's Exercise, 1900–1960* (Chapel Hill, forthcoming). See also Louis Moore, "Fit for Citizenship: Black Sparring Masters, Gymnasium Owners, and the White Body, 1825–1886," *The Journal of African American History* 96, no. 4 (2011): 448–73.
82 "Physical Culture Lessons, Daily," *The Boston Globe*, 21 April 1904, 17.
83 "Physical Culture Lessons, Daily," *The Boston Globe*, 21 April 1904, 17.
84 "Physical Culture Lessons, Daily," *The Boston Globe*, 21 April 1904, 17.
85 "Physical Culture for Boys and Girls," *Anaconda Standard*, 3 November 1902, 4.
86 "For the Ladies," *Seymour Daily Republican*, 22 June 1908, 7.
87 Greg Mullins, "Nudes, Prudes, and Pigmies: The Desirability of Disavowal in Physical Culture," *Discourse*, 15, no. 1 (1992): 27–48. "How to Remedy Obesity," *Physical Culture*, 2, no. 6 (1900): 259; W.M.J. Cromie, "Why Should we Exercise?," *Physical Culture*, 3, no. 2 (1900): 77–8; W.M.J. Cromie, "Inactivity Means Death," *Physical Culture*, 4, no. 2 (1900): 80–1.
88 "Advertisement," *Hamilton Evening Democrat*, 16 October 1903, 4.
89 "Advertisement," *Hamilton Evening Democrat*, 16 October 1903, 4.
90 "Advertisement," *Hamilton Evening Democrat*, 16 October 1903, 4.
91 Heather Addison, *Hollywood and the Rise of Physical Culture* (New York: Routledge, 2003), 32–40.

5 Prison Bodies: The Height and Weight of Men in Canadian Prisons, 1874–1935[1]

LUIZA ANTONIE, KRIS INWOOD, AND HAMISH MAXWELL-STEWART

Humans have long been fascinated by body size. As the Canadian economist John Kenneth Galbraith once put it, the favouritism bestowed on the tall is one of society's "most blatant and forgiven prejudices."[2] While the tall, particularly tall men, are today paid more and often favoured socially, the overweight in the twentieth century have frequently been discriminated against. In Margaret Atwood's novel *Lady Oracle*, Joan Foster reveals that she was able to see "*Adult* pictures" long before she came of age as she was "fat" and therefore less noticeable, the ushers and ticket sellers merely seeing her "as a huge featureless blur."[3] Fat people in contemporary society are seen differently, when they are seen at all.

There is some evidence, however, that perceptions of what might constitute tall or overweight, and the desirability or attractiveness of various body types, have changed from one generation to another. Deborah McPhail and Wendy Mitchinson, for example, have both analysed changes during the twentieth century in the ideal size and shape of Canadians.[4] This collection extends such work back to the nineteenth century when body size and shape were contested terrain. Our focus in this chapter is not the construction of cultural values or the health consequences of excess weight – both important topics that are addressed in other chapters. Rather, we consider a simpler question: how tall were Canadians and how much did they weigh in the past? Measures of height and weight do not speak directly to "fat" or perceptions of fatness, at least not in a simple way, but they do suggest the methodological possibilities and issues for historians considering the empirical realities underlying the increasing emphasis on measurement and body size in the nineteenth century. These anthropometric characteristics are well documented, as early as the 1950s, thanks to a representative national survey taken in 1953.[5] Since that date, a long series of nutrition, fitness, and health surveys have confirmed that Canadian average height, weight and, importantly, weight adjusted for height, have increased steadily from the 1950s to the present day.[6]

But what about earlier generations? In this paper, we introduce new evidence about the height and weight of Canadians who were incarcerated during the later nineteenth and early twentieth centuries. Our goal is to provide a first glimpse of the prison bodies, rather than to undertake a detailed quantitative analysis. The historical prison records reveal marked differences in the size of French Canadians, Indigenous peoples, African-descended individuals, and immigrants from both Europe and East Asia. Unexpectedly, there was no evidence of systematic change over time in the height or weight of prisoners during the long nineteenth century (despite the increasing emphasis on issues of weight medically, culturally, and politically described elsewhere in this volume). We speculate briefly about the historical significance of the new evidence, but our primary goal is simply to describe the size of prison bodies in the past, and to suggest methodologies for ascertaining these figures. To anticipate our findings, in this case the present does *not* resemble the past, at least not insofar as the bodies of prisoners were representative of other Canadians.

Sources for Body Size and Weight in the Canadian Past

Medical and insurance professionals in the twentieth century came to identify overeating and excess body mass as a health risk, although by itself this does not tell us how tall or heavy Canadians were in general, or the extent to which height and weight varied across different subsections of the population.[7] During the 1920s, there were occasional remarks in the medical literature, and some stigmatization of overweight people in the popular press, although it appears to have been more common to highlight undernutrition among the poor.[8] By the 1940s, public health and nutrition professionals were beginning to suggest that occasional undernutrition might mask a broader and potentially more serious problem of overnutrition and excess body mass. The 1953 survey mentioned earlier did not reveal a particularly wide pattern of excess weight, although soon afterward expressions of alarm about the "obesity epidemic" became common.[9]

Continuous change in body size since the mid-twentieth century might lead us to think that the increase of obesity is a natural and irrepressible characteristic of modern societies, and that earlier generations shared a similar experience even if change might have been slower. In fact, the first historical research suggests otherwise. Evidence drawn from Canadian military personnel records, one of the few systematic sources of information about the human body before the emergence of national health surveys, found no tendency before 1900 for adult height to increase.[10] The first half of the twentieth century saw the beginning of a secular (long-term) increase of stature but not of weight. After taking account of height and age, the weight of soldiers enlisting in the Second World War appears to have been *less* than that for First World War soldiers.[11] But these studies are based on soldiers – reasonably fit young men – whose experience may have been atypical. Moreover, the timing of the Great Depression complicates any inference about longer-run trends, since widespread unemployment during the 1930s likely impaired nutrition in the years leading to men enlisting for the Second World War.

What other sources are available? The routine measuring and weighing of people did become increasingly common during the nineteenth century, as part of a broader movement to accumulate social data.[12] High levels of numeracy in North America and Europe facilitated the emergence of an "information state" and new forms of governance that used knowledge to normalize and discipline individuals.[13] Some contemporaries associated physical robustness with broader notions of national and racial superiority. Mathematicians used the same information to develop and demonstrate innovative statistical tools.[14] Evidence of body size also informed social reformers concerned about the health consequences of early industrialization.[15] Life insurance companies managed risk by assessing individual characteristics in relation to those of a broader population.[16] Military planners sought reassurance about the physical capacities of their soldiers.[17] Medical scientists turned to measures of physical size as part of their attempts to understand individual and population health; height and weight came to be used widely as a screening tool for child health.[18] Many of the other essays in this collection suggest the broad range of uses to which such measurements and assessments of the fat (or thin) body might be put.

Another institution that collected systematic information about the human body was the prison. A key step in the evolution of prison records was a decision in 1791 by the sheriffs of London and Middlesex, England to maintain tabular information recording the age, place of birth, occupation, and physical description (including height) of criminals.[19] Other personal and family characteristics were added in subsequent decades. Most nineteenth-century prison registers recorded stature along with descriptions of complexion, eye and hair colour, and distinguishing marks. The first known recording of weight on a systematic basis occurred in 1842, in Pentonville Prison.[20] Easy-to-use and affordable measurement scales became available later in the century, increasing the number of prisons that could similarly measure the weight of their inmates.[21] Prison authorities used information about the physical characteristics of convicts to aid in recapturing them if they escaped, as a means to identify repeat offenders, and to understand criminality and guide criminal justice reform. Robert Shoemaker and Richard Ward observe that officials even collected information with no apparent administrative or practical purpose. They point to "the existence of a diffuse, but significant information-gathering culture among local officials" and "a desire on the part of these officials to understand their custodial subjects and their crimes as well as control them."[22] As well, the process of stripping inmates to measure and describe them was designed to be humiliating. Such gateway rituals were used as a means of putting the recently institutionalized into place.[23] Rigakos and Bishop in this volume also discuss the way some contemporaries used these measurements to define "criminal types" who posed threats to national and racial stability.

Historians have used the information collected at these institutions for a wide range of research purposes. Height and weight records for men and women in a south London jail allowed Sara Horrell, David Meredith, and Deborah Oxley to infer the existence of a gendered distribution of resources within households that, over the life cycle, greatly weakened the bodies of women, especially those who married.[24] For the same period, Ewout Depauw documents different personal characteristics for recidivists and one-time offenders in Belgian prisons; distinct patterns for men and women point to a highly gendered process of incarceration.[25] Scott Carson uses similar data from American state prisons to expose racial differences in physical well-being and a deterioration of BMI during the nineteenth century.[26] Prison records from Tasmania, in contrast, suggest that adult stature and, by inference, childhood health, *improved* during the middle decades of the nineteenth century.[27]

A number of scholars have examined the inmate registers of Canadian prisons. A sample of people held in the Mercer Reformatory examined by Carolyn Strange, for example, supports her analysis of the institution's administration.[28] John Weaver examines the Hamilton Police Court using representative samples of cases drawn over sixty years.[29] And an influential work about prison reform by Peter Oliver draws much of its insight from samples of convicts held during the nineteenth century in Ontario county jails, the Ontario Central Prison, and the Mercer Reformatory.[30] Donald Fyson and François Fenchel, however, demonstrate possible pitfalls in the records for unwary researchers by examining prisoners held in the common jails of Quebec City (1813–71) and of Montreal (1836–99).[31] The same Quebec City jail has been used to show that French Canadians born between the 1780s and 1820s were considerably shorter than men born in the English colonies to the south, although taller than their counterparts born in France.[32]

In this chapter, we examine the height and weight of prisoners born in the nineteenth century and held in Canadian carceral institutions. We review the qualitative descriptions of prison bodies made by staff at the Victoria and New Westminster gaols from 1864 to 1914 and then summarize quantitatively the average physical stature and body weight of prisoners at these and other institutions. For body weight, we rely on the body mass index (BMI), a metric developed by Adolph Quetelet to describe a "normal" increase (or difference) in body mass as height increases (or differs).[33] No single measure can adequately capture all the ways in which bone structure and accompanying muscle of taller people add to their weight.[34] And yet, BMI has become a standard way of adjusting normal or average weight for the effect of variations in height. We examine average BMI while appreciating its limitations. We also recognize that prisoners, like soldiers, comprise a particular social group that may not be representative of the wider population. Nevertheless, as long as there is some consistency over time in the circumstances that led some people but not others to be incarcerated, the prison evidence might have broader implications.[35]

Canadian Prison Registers and the Problem of Recidivism

In this chapter, we have used a recent digitization of Canadian jail and prison records to examine the height and weight of men incarcerated in five British Columbia gaols,[36] two Saskatchewan prisons,[37] the Central Ontario Prison,[38] and three federal penitentiaries (Kingston,[39] Saint-Vincent-de-Paul,[40] and Dorchester[41]). We focus on men because there were too few female prisoners to support a useful statistical summary. We examine prisoners in each province separately, because of differences between institutions in jurisdiction, policing, and judicial practice and in the social and economic circumstances that encouraged offending.

The Kingston Penitentiary opened in 1835 to house the most serious offenders in Upper Canada; county jails continued to hold people convicted of being drunk and disorderly, larceny, minor assault, and other petty offences, in addition to debtors and the mentally ill.[42] After 1867, Kingston became a federal penitentiary that, like Dorchester and Saint-Vincent-de-Paul, held offenders whose sentences exceeded two years. The Ontario Central Prison opened in 1874 for those whose sentences were greater than one month and less than two years.[43] The Victoria and New Westminster gaols, which account for the great majority of records in British Columbia, began as comprehensive colonial/provincial prisons holding a wide range of offenders, including those charged with relatively petty offences.[44] A majority of prisoners in the two Saskatchewan prisons received sentences between two weeks and two years (similar to Ontario's Central Prison). By the 1880s, federal prisons in Western Canada existed to house inmates with longer sentences, although some long-sentence prisoners continued to appear in the British Columbia and Saskatchewan prison registers.

Some people were incarcerated more than once. Indeed, nineteenth-century officials in Ontario claimed that one-third of all prisoners in the province were recidivists.[45] This is of interest because the kind of person who was jailed on multiple Saturday nights for minor offences is likely to have differed from someone imprisoned once – possibly with a longer sentence for some serious offence.[46] A particular issue is that recidivists tend to be shorter than inmates who appear to have only been convicted once.[47] A failure to identify the recidivists, especially if their presence was uneven, risks some bias in assessing change over time or differences between institutions in examining the measurements of their weights.

Canadian prison officials typically tried to keep track of repeat offenders, although they were not always successful, and this information is available only inconsistently within our registers. As researchers, we can identify recidivists simply by reviewing the names and personal characteristics of offenders, although the effort is time-consuming and thus costly. Identifying repeat offenders in British Columbia jails, for example, required us to painstakingly review more than 33,000 records, one by one.[48] For prisons in other provinces, we have adopted a different strategy; we identify repeat offenders using information science techniques of "deduplication," or internal record linkage.[49]

First, we identify records that have *exactly* the same gender, ethnicity, country of birth, and birth year (plus or minus three years). Then, within each restricted block of records, we identify pairs of records that are highly similar using first name, last name, and birth year.[50] This method balances precision in the spelling of first names against the spelling of last names, and name similarity against birth year variation to classify each record as being similar or dissimilar to every other record in the block. We are left with smaller groups of records, each of which has precisely the same gender, ethnicity, and country of birth, and *similar* birth year and names. We set a low threshold for similarity because names (and other personal details) were often reported imprecisely. Some tolerance for name variation is needed to identify the recidivists

Table 5.1. Example of the preliminary classification of prison records as "similar"

Year of Admission	Name	Birth Year	Height(in cms)	Birthplace
1924	Marc Beaubier	1904	58.5	Montreal
1924	Marc Beaubier	1904	58.5	Montreal
1925	Marc Beaulieu	1902	66.5	St Gerard de Majella
1925	Marc Beaulieu	1902	66.5	St Gerard de Majella
1925	Marc Beaulieu	1902	66.5	St Gerard de Majella

Source: Authors

although, inevitably, we incorrectly accepted some mismatched pairs. An example from one of the prisons is reproduced in Table 5.1.[51]

In this example, the preliminary classification for similarity has brought together five records describing people of the same gender and ethnicity, who were born in Quebec at roughly the same time, with names that are identical except for two characters. And yet, it seems likely we have inadvertently mixed up the records of two people. Birthplace within Quebec differs as does the year of birth. The height variation is substantial. The surnames differ by only two characters although in this case the small change is enough to create a recognizably different name. Most telling of all, the pattern of variations in all fields point to the same division into subgroups. Additionally, a specific record of scars and tattoos (not reproduced here) confirms that there really were two people.

Clearly, a more nuanced approach using additional fields of information is needed. It is impractical to individually review all records, so the goal is to isolate a subset of the records that are most in need of case-by-case examination. A simple filter or algorithm uses intra-country detail about birth location, the report of physical height, and a different measure of name similarity to identify records whose similarity is slightly suspect or is rejected by the filter. The ability to focus on a smaller number of records allows the historian to view each record in its context within the register and take account of other details, some of them hard to quantify, including reported religion, physical characteristics (height, weight, scars, and tattoos), type of offence, any comments by the record-keeper, name commonality, and the potential for transcription errors. We also take advantage of any internal references within the register that explicitly link one record to another. We accept only groupings for which no contrary considerations are visible.

Undoubtedly there was more recidivism than is detected by our method, for multiple reasons. Some entries are difficult to transcribe faithfully because of the register's physical deterioration. Some offenders had

Table 5.2. Summary of prison records and identification of repeat offenders

	Years covered	Number of records	Estimated number of people	Share (%) of records reviewed individually
Dorchester Penitentiary	1916–1936	3,034	2,628	20%
Saint-Vincent-de-Paul Penitentiary	1897–1934	5,254	4,835	23%
Kingston & Ontario Central	1843–1919	37,582	31,895	7%
Regina & Prince Albert (Sask.)	1891–1932	39,364	30,598	9%
Five British Columbia jails	1864–1919	33,297	28,192	100%

Sources:

British Columbia Archives, *Victoria Gaol records* GR-0308 Description Lists 1864–1914, *New Westminster Gaol records* GR-0309 Description Books 1875–1917, *Nanaimo Gaol records* GR-0310.4 Description Book 1911–1914, *Saanich Prison Farm records* GR-0306.10 Description Book 1914–1917, *Quesnel* GR-0042 Description Book 1915–1919.
Provincial Archives of Saskatchewan, *Regina Jail Register* 1891–1921, *Prince Albert Jail Register* 1898–1930.
Ontario Archives, *Central Prison registers*, RG 20–55–1, Books One and Two, 1874–1912.
Library and Archives Canada, *Kingston Penitentiary*, Prisoner's Records Books 1843–1890, Cell Description Registry 1890–1895, Inmate Description Ledger 1916–1919.
Library and Archives Canada, *St Vincent de Paul Penitentiary Convict Register*, RG73 vol 382 Box 193, 1897–1934 (file 33–55).
Public Archives of New Brunswick, *Dorchester Penitentiary Records*, F854-F855, 1916–1936

forgotten their true age and birthplace, changed religion for unrelated reasons, acquired new tattoos, or attempted to conceal their identity. Measurements of height are inevitably imprecise because most people shrink physically during the day (and as they age), and weight may be even more variable over time. More generally, identifying repeat appearances is less effective if the characteristics of the prison population are relatively homogenous, and reported with limited detail or inconsistently.

Our method works well with the Saint-Vincent-de-Paul records, which have highly specific information about birthplace and other characteristics. The method functions less well with the Ontario registers because birthplace detail is limited, and a large number of the offenders had relatively common names. Many of the British Columbia and Saskatchewan prisoners offended in minor ways; prison staff may have taken less care with the record of petty criminals, who themselves may have reported their information less precisely (perhaps because they were less educated).[52] In Table 5.2, we report the number of records in each prison group, the number of people recognized as distinct within each prison group, and the share of records examined individually by the historian.

Figure 5.1. Difference between share of prisoners described as being unusually thin or unusually stout (five-year moving average, New Westminster and Victoria Gaol)

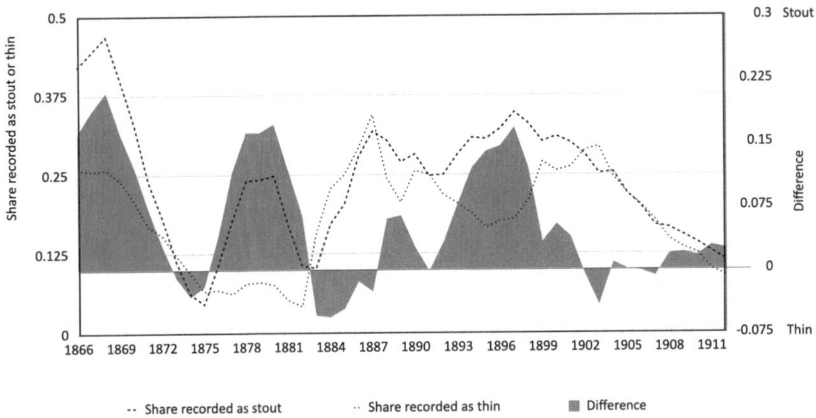

Sources: see Table 5.2

The Bodies of the Incarcerated

Nineteenth-century prison staff commonly created a record of their inmates' physical characteristics, including hair and eye colour, complexion, height, weight, and distinctive marks (tattoos, scars etc.). One additional field, "Proportions or Build," was for many years maintained by the New Westminster and Victoria provincial prisons in British Columbia. Typical responses were "Proportionate," "Stout," "Slight," "Medium," "Tall," and so on. We begin our examination of the prison registers with a review of the "Proportions or Build" information in the Victoria (1864–1914) and New Westminster (1874–1914) prison registers.

Roughly half of the comments in this field do not report some version of normal or ordinary ("medium," "proportionate," "good," etc). One-quarter of the records contain no information at all about "proportions or build." The remaining 25 per cent, however, have detail that is more interesting because the individual is described as either "stout" (or alternatives such as "heavy," "stocky," "chunky," etc.) or "thin" (with variations such as "wiry," "slight," "slender," "slim," etc.). Clearly, this information is impressionistic and imprecise, although it is still useful. We know nothing about the body shape considered by prison officials to be ordinary or common; however, we can observe the frequency with which prisoners appeared, to prison staff, as unusually thin or stout.

The share of all prison records in which the individual is described as being either thin or stout is reported in Figure 5.1 as a five-year moving

Figure 5.2. Mean adult height by birth year in Canadian prisons, for North American-born men who are not identifiably Quebec-born Catholic or of Indigenous, African, or Chinese descent

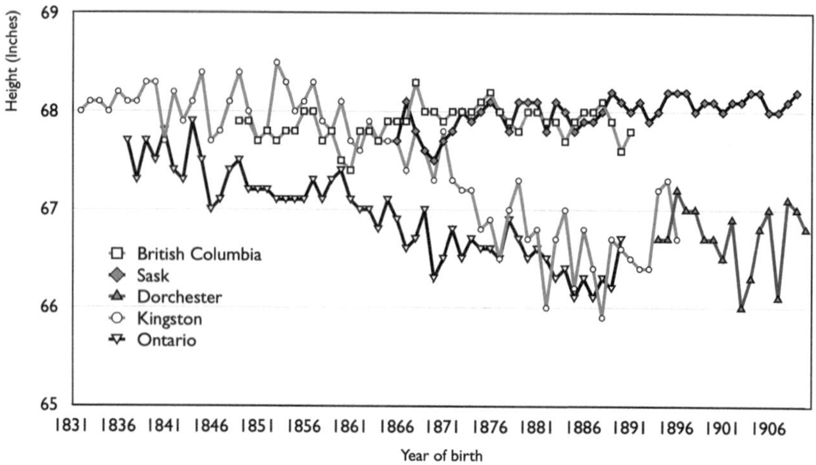

Sources: see Table 5.2

average. Over the entire period, more prisoners were described as being stout than thin, although this differential derives almost entirely from three short periods: 1866–71, 1876–82, and 1893–8. The significance of this timing is unclear, although we note that these intervals of excess stoutness correspond with short periods in which the growth of the Canadian economy is thought to have slowed.[53]

No definitive conclusions are possible without more information about the prison officials' sense of normal or usual proportions, and how that sense of normality might have changed over time. In a quest for greater precision, and information about prisoners in a wider range of institutions, we turn to the measures of height and weight reported for all prisoners (weight first becoming available in the 1870s). For this purpose, we restrict consideration to men who were between twenty-one years of age and fifty years.[54] Average height by year of birth is reported in Figure 5.2 for years that have enough observations to obtain a meaningful average (minimum 50, preferably 100 records). We use birth year rather than year of incarceration because adult height is largely determined by childhood experience. We identify prisoners of Chinese, African, or Indigenous descent, and those who had immigrated from elsewhere (mainly Europe) separately.[55] We identify French Canadians as prisoners born in Quebec who claim to have followed the Roman

Table 5.3. Number of adult male records for stature analysis, by prison and ethnicity.

Prisons	French-Canadian	Immigrant n.e.s.	African-descent	Chinese, Japanese	Indigenous	All other
British Columbia	73	9,127	221	2,461	3,554	4,917
Saskatchewan	772	11,804	395	234	1,452	11,248
Ontario	13	5,723	698	13	140	11,705
Kingston	545	1,933	280	3	77	3,753
Saint-Vincent-de-Paul	2,471	440	46	6	15	750
Dorchester	35	89	82	1	11	1,025

Sources: see Table 5.2
Note: The number of records for BMI analysis is slightly smaller.

Catholic faith.[56] A few non-French Catholics are undoubtedly captured by this definition, but unfortunately there is no easy way to identify them. We also miss any French Canadians born outside Quebec and French Canadians who no longer followed the Roman Catholic faith.

The number of available records for these groups is reported in Figure 5.2. Simple (ordinary least squares) regressions with height as the dependent variable and the ethnic indicators and year as independent variables provide an annual average height for the North American-born with no identifiable ethnicity and average (unchanging) differentials for French Canadians, Chinese, Indigenous, African-descended, and immigrants. We prevent recidivists from exerting an undue influence on the average by weighting individuals by the inverse of their frequency of appearance. The evidence in Table 5.3 describes the average stature in each prison, by birth year, of North American-born adult men who do not appear to be of Chinese, African, or Indigenous ancestry, and are not French Canadians. This "all other" group might be regarded as a "white settler" population.

The average stature of these prisoners changed little during the second half of the nineteenth century, with one important exception. Stature in Ontario's Central Prison and Kingston Penitentiary declined markedly from prisoners born in the 1850s to those born in the 1880s. Some differences between prisons are apparent. The Kingston inmates tended to be taller than those in the Central Prison, reflecting a tendency seen elsewhere for men receiving short sentences for petty offences to be shorter, on average.[57] Men in British Columbia and Saskatchewan prisons were systematically taller than those in eastern Canadian prisons – a regional contrast already familiar from historical military records.[58]

Table 5.4. Average stature differentials (inches) of men aged 21–49 years in Canadian prisons.

	Five BC prisons 1848–1890	Regina & Prince Albert 1866–1909	Ontario Central 1836–1890	Kingston Penitentiary 1831–1896	Dorchester Penitentiary 1894–1910
n	20,352	25,896	18,300	6,588	1,243
Indigenous difference	**−1.8**	**+0.4**	**+0.7**	**+0.5**	+1.3
East Asian difference	**−2.8**	**−2.8**	**−3.2**	**−2.6**	**−2.3**
African descent	**−0.5**	+0.1	−0.0	−0.1	+0.4
Quebec-born Catholic	**−0.7**	**−1.6**	+0.3	**−1.3**	**−0.7**
Immigrant not elsewhere specified	**−0.8**	**−1.0**	**−0.6**	**−1.0**	−0.1

Sources: see Table 5.2

Note: We report the average difference in stature between the identified groups and other North American-born men in an ordinary least squares regression that takes height as the dependent variable and the ethnic-birthplace indicators and birth year as independent variables, over the range of birth years indicated for each prison. Differentials that differ from zero to an extent that is statistically significantly (5% level) are in bold; the remainder are not sufficiently different from zero to permit rejection of the idea that there is no systematic difference. Most insignificant co-efficients reflect a small number of records in the relevant category (Table 5.3).

Our examination identifies an average difference, if any existed, between the benchmark white-settler population and each of the identifiable ethnicities. Large numbers of Indigenous men were incarcerated. They were taller than "all others" in the Saskatchewan and Ontario prisons but not in British Columbia. The relative shortness of the British Columbia Indigenous prisoners is striking. Immigrants, Quebec-born Catholics, and men of Chinese descent were all shorter than the benchmark group (Table 5.4). The Chinese prisoners were particularly short compared with the other groups. Further, African-descended men were half an inch shorter while French Canadians were even shorter. In the Saint-Vincent-de-Paul Penitentiary (not shown in this table), French Canadians were about an inch shorter on average than the "all other" group.[59]

More pertinent to the discussion in this collection, we also examine weight adjusted for height, or "body mass index" (BMI). As with height, an ordinary least squares regression provides average BMI for each year of prison admission and fixed ethnic differentials. We examine BMI by year of incarceration rather than year of birth because an

Figure 5.3. Mean BMI by year in Canadian prisons, for North American-born men who are not identifiably Quebec-born Catholic or of Indigenous, African or Chinese descent

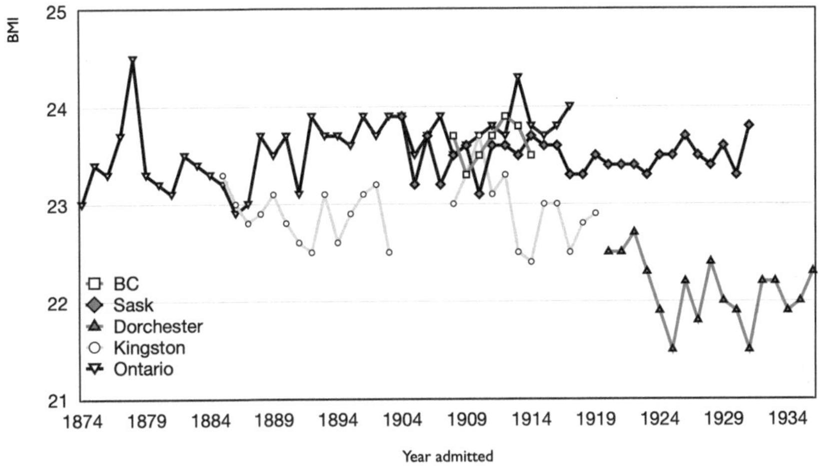

Sources: see Table 5.2

individual's weight typically reflects nutrition and energy expenditure in the recent past rather than childhood circumstance, despite the great concern about the "proper" or "healthy" weight of infants evidenced in Kennedy's chapter in this volume.

As is clear from Figure 5.3, there was no systematic tendency for the average BMI of the benchmark white settlers to increase or decrease over time. Men in the Ontario Central Prison showed a modest increase in the 1880–1910 period, while BMI in the federal penitentiaries at Dorchester and Kingston declined slightly. The overall picture, however, is one of little or no change between the late 1870s and the early 1930s. The three provincial prison systems (Ontario, British Columbia, and Saskatchewan) show broadly similar levels of BMI (between 23 and 24). Those for the three federal penitentiaries was somewhat lower (between 22 and 23).[60]

As with stature, the BMI of some ethnic groups was higher or lower than the "all other" North American-born prisoners (Table 5.5). The BMI of Chinese prisoners, in spite of being relatively short, was markedly lower than average, suggesting that they tended to be "underweight" as well as under the average height. In contrast, French Canadians, African Canadians, and Indigenous prisoners tended to have higher

Table 5.5. Average BMI differentials of men aged 21–49 years in Canadian prisons.

	Five BC prisons 1908–1914	Regina & Prince Albert 1904–1931	Ontario Central 1874–1912	Kingston Pen 1885–1898 & 1908–1919	Dorchester Penitentiary 1920–1936
n	2,179	25,855	18,854	3,394	1,701
Indigenous difference	+0.7	+0.1	+0.6	+0.2	-0.3
East Asian difference	−1.9	−2.1	−1.9	−3.5	−0.2
African-descent difference	−0.8	+0.1	+1.2	+1.1	+0.8
Quebec-born Catholic	−0.4	+0.2	+0.3	+0.6	+0.4
Immigrant not elsewhere specified	+0.3	+0.3	+0.0	+0.3	+0.6

Sources: see Table 5.2
Note: The average BMI differentials are determined with an ordinary least squares regression on BMI with ethnic-birthplace indicators and year as independent variables. Differentials differing from zero with statistical significance are in bold.

than average BMIs, although many of these differences were small and/or statistically insignificant.[61] The relatively high BMI for the Indigenous outside British Columbia prisons is noteworthy, because they were also relatively tall; their body mass was large enough to survive a particularly large adjustment for height.

Significance of the Patterns

Although this study suggests potential methodologies for understanding the measurements and physical realities of the body in the late nineteenth and early twentieth centuries, any attempt to extract broader historical meaning from the summary patterns of height and weight must recognize a number of limitations. We have said nothing about women. There were female prisoners, of course, although not in sufficient numbers to permit us to make robust generalizations. Perhaps more important, identifying average height and weight for men is useful for summary purposes even as, inevitably, it conceals important diversities. We expose some of this diversity by examining particular groups, but our analysis relies on prison authorities attributing ethnicity rather than the prisoners themselves. The use of fixed ethnic differentials means that we do not see any changes over time *within* the Indigenous, Chinese, or African-descended prison populations. The pattern of year-to-year changes provides a useful description of changes among the white settlers, i.e., North American-born prisoners of largely European ancestry, but it cannot really tell us about the evolution of other groups.

The significance of patterns identified in this chapter would be greater if we knew that prisoners were representative of the broader population. Unfortunately, this is not yet clear. We only know the particular group described by our evidence – men aged 20 to 49 years who were (i) tempted into behaviour identified as criminal, (ii) unlucky enough to be caught, (iii) successfully prosecuted, and (iv) incarcerated in a penal institution whose records have survived. Participation in this select group may have varied over time as society, the economy, policing, and penal institutions themselves evolved.[62] In the absence of other evidence, we cannot know how closely the prisoners represent the Canadian population.

The composition of the prison population itself was not static, even among men aged 20 to 49 years. Fortunately, the rich information recorded within the registers will allow us, eventually, to investigate the patterns associated more precisely with defined birthplace, occupation, the offence or crime, sentence length, and other markers for relevant experience and characteristics. Whether or not compositional change in any of these dimensions would alter, qualitatively, the patterns visible in this paper remains to be investigated. Keeping in mind these caveats, we speculate briefly about the possible significance of our brief, summary description of prison bodies.

The average stature of adults is often interpreted as an indicator of changing health and living standards during childhood.[63] This literature builds on the idea that children realize their individual genetic potential for physical growth only if they have good nutrition and are protected from debilitating infections and the energy expenditure of heavy labour. Departures from these ideal conditions, which were more common in the past, especially among the poor, can lead to a degree of child stunting that reduces adult stature. For this reason, a systematic difference (or change) in height between two large groups may reflect differences (or changes) in childhood living conditions. Because individual genetic inheritance accounts for much of the variation in physical characteristics within a population, we are not interested in the height of one or two people; rather, we seek a group average that may reveal the presence of some stunting within the group.

The absence of increases in stature, in any of the prisons, suggests that the kind of person who ended up in prison did not share in the gains from economic growth in this period.[64] Indeed, the declining stature of prisoners in the Central Ontario Prison and Kingston Penitentiary, both located in Canada's industrial heartland, points toward a decline in their standard of living. This is consistent with growing contemporary concern for public health at the end of the century[65] and evidence elsewhere that early industrialization, especially for the poor,[66] damaged human health.

The short stature of imprisoned immigrants suggests that living standards were lower in Europe, at least among men who were prepared to emigrate to Canada. Of course, this is not surprising. Like immigrants from Europe, the African-descended were shorter than the North American-born whites and their BMI was comparable or higher than that for whites – possibly indicating a degree of deprivation during childhood but not adulthood. Deteriorating economic conditions in nineteenth-century China suggest a similar interpretation for the short stature of the Chinese (most of whom were immigrants).[67] The Chinese were particularly short, and also light for their height, in all prisons. This pattern points toward a degree of malnutrition more extreme than in the other groups.

Indigenous prisoners appear to have been relatively tall everywhere except in British Columbia. The tallest Indigenous prisoners were held in the two Saskatchewan prisons. Those whose prison record reveals evidence of mixed ancestry were shorter, on average, than those with no evidence of mixed ancestry.[68] The nutritional distress experienced by particular Indigenous groups in later decades is not visible in the average size of prison bodies.[69] The Plains People living to the south are thought to have been the tallest Indigenous Peoples in the United States.[70] Their stature and that of the men incarcerated in Saskatchewan is consistent with a presumption of relatively good health before the loss of the buffalo and before the full effects of land loss and industrialization were felt.[71]

The relative shortness of the Indigenous men in British Columbia prisons is more puzzling. Our ability to contextualize this finding in a broader literature is limited, as most discussions of Indigenous health in British Columbia focus either earlier or later.[72] There has been relatively limited discussion of the mid- and late-nineteenth-century birth cohorts, which contribute most of the prison records in this study.[73]

Finally, Quebec-born Catholics were shorter than average in all prisons.[74] A similar pattern is seen in other historical sources.[75] The lower socioeconomic status of francophones and, with it, weaker childhood health, undoubtedly contributed to the differential.[76] An unexpected complication is cross-country variation, illustrated

Table 5.6. Average stature (inches) of French-Canadian prisoners (men 20–49 years, born 1883–1909.

	stature	n	s.e.
Quebec-born Catholics in Saint-Vincent-de-Paul Penitentiary	65.4	2035	0.06
Quebec-born Catholics in Saskatchewan prisons	66.5	582	0.11
Self-described French Canadians in Saskatchewan prisons, born in Quebec	66.4	237	0.15
Self-described French Canadians in Saskatchewan prisons, not born in Quebec	67.9	241	0.15
Self-described French Canadians in Saskatchewan prisons, not born in Quebec, with no evidence of Indigenous ancestry	67.2	70	0.26

Sources: see Table 5.2

in Table 5.6. The average stature of Quebec-born Catholics in the Saskatchewan prisons was more than an inch higher than those held in Montreal's Saint-Vincent-de-Paul Penitentiary. Admittedly, "Quebec-born Catholic" is an imperfect way to recognize French Canadians, insofar as it ignores those who did not practise Catholicism and includes those who ceased to identify as French Canadian as well as non-French Catholics from Quebec. An alternate identification is available. Some men in the Saskatchewan prisons were described explicitly as "French Canadian" or some related recognition of French ancestry.[77] This allows us to examine a group defined by its public identity rather than by Catholicism.

The two groups overlap substantially and had roughly the same stature (Table 5.6). Regardless of definition, it seems clear that French Canadians who relocated to Western Canada were taller than those who remained in Quebec. This points to the possibility of a selective migration of the tallest. The alternate way to identify French Canadians reveals one additional observation – men identified as French Canadians born *outside* Quebec were even taller than the Quebec-born who moved to Saskatchewan. These patterns are consistent with a healthier childhood experience in Western Canada *and* a greater premium on physical size, making it more likely that taller Quebec-born Catholics would relocate westward.[78]

French-Canadian BMI also differed by location; average BMI for Quebec-born Catholics in Saskatchewan was 23.8 compared with 22.7 in the Saint-Vincent-de-Paul Penitentiary.[79] It would appear that Quebec-born Catholics who migrated to Western Canada were either the kind of person naturally inclined to be heavier for their height, or the western environment afforded them access to superior nutrition. Or both.

Conclusion

Our preliminary review of the height and weight of men in Canada's prisons from 1874 to 1935 identifies a number of patterns that invite further investigation. We do not yet know the extent to which patterns among the prisoners may reflect the experience of Canadians more generally. Of course, this is characteristic of almost all historical sources.[80] One way to assess the limitations of particular evidence is to triangulate across different sources. In our case, the patterns of body size among prisoners in different regions, at different times, and in different kinds of penal institutions, were broadly similar. Moreover, the evidence of regional and temporal variation among prisoners is consistent with that of men who enlisted in the First and Second World Wars, even though men became prisoners and soldiers for very different reasons.[81] These observations are not definitive. However, they do encourage further investigation into the representativeness of the prisoners.

The prison evidence reveals sizeable differences by ethnicity. French Canadians were particularly short although the differential was smaller for those who relocated to Western Canada and even less for those born in the West. Indigenous Canadians in prisons west of the Rocky Mountains were shorter than those to the East. Of course, there is no reason to expect the different First Nations, each with its own culture and resources, to be similar.

The most dramatic evidence from the prison registers might be what we do *not* see: change among the white settlers. There was remarkably little change over time in the average height and weight of North American-born whites (excepting stature decline in the two Ontario institutions). This is unexpected, largely because we know the human body has the capacity to change and in fact it had changed greatly during the twentieth century. The visceral concern over the overweight and the expressed need for dieting that emerged in the culture of the late nineteenth and early twentieth century seemed to indicate a ballooning of body size. That bodies were not obviously gaining in mass perhaps suggests deeper social concerns and meanings rather than a simple reaction to a measurable weight gain.[82]

In Figure 5.4 and Figure 5.5, we report the average height and BMI of men aged 20 to 29 years in each of our historical sources and in recent health surveys. The juxtaposition of these figures alongside Figure 5.2

Figure 5.4. Average height (inches) of men aged 20–29 years.

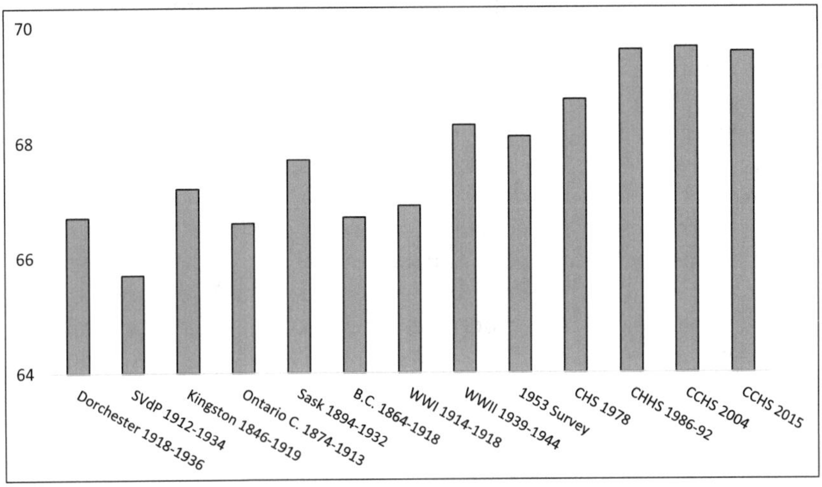

Sources: see Table 5.2

Figure 5.5. Average BMI of men aged 20–29 years

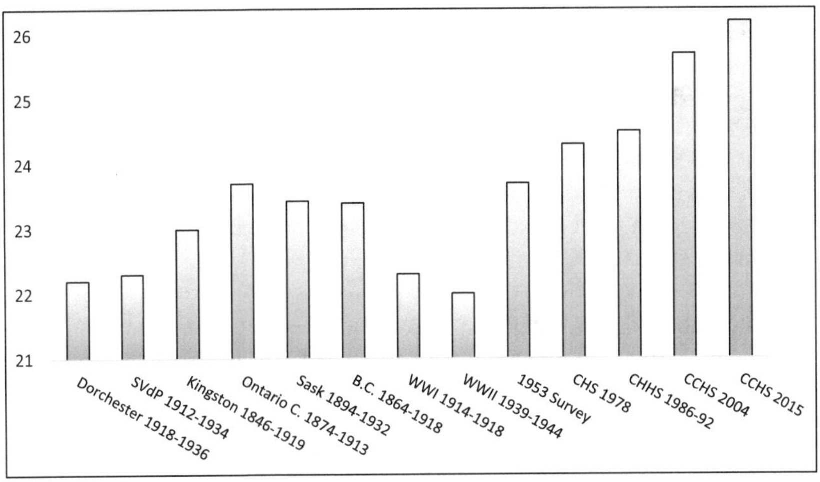

Sources: see Table 5.2

and Figure 5.3 highlights two important observations: (i) Prisoners during the long nineteenth century were shorter and lighter than Canadians today; (ii) The steady increase of both stature and BMI since 1953 has no counterpart in earlier decades.

The growth of adult stature during the twentieth century is already well documented.[83] Less evidence has been available for weight. The BMI of men in American prisons declined modestly from the middle decades of the nineteenth century to the early decades of the twentieth century.[84] The great twentieth-century rise of obesity within the United States did not get underway until, at the earliest, the 1920s.[85] Our evidence suggests that the Canadian experience may have been similar. None of the prisons, not even those with records as late as the 1930s, show any sign of rising BMI, much less the steady increase seen in recent health surveys. The most dramatic difference between the bodies of prisoners born in the long nineteenth century and those of today is the complete absence of anything like the "obesity epidemic" of recent decades.

NOTES

1 We acknowledge financial support from the Social Sciences and Humanities Research Council of Canada Awards #435–2017–1002, and #895-2019-1014, assistance with Statistics Canada data from Pat Newcombe and with the historical prison records from Georgia Dale. Vincent Geloso read the paper and provided helpful comments. The Saskatchewan data were developed jointly with Dr Ben Hoy at the University of Saskatchewan.
2 As quoted in the *Christian Science Monitor*, 18 May 1977, no. 22.
3 Margaret Atwood, *Lady Oracle* (New York, Simon and Schuster, 2012).
4 Deborah McPhail, *Contours of the Nation: Making Obesity and Imagining Canada, 1945–1970* (Toronto: University of Toronto Press, 2017); Wendy Mitchinson, *Fighting Fat. Canada, 1920–1980* (Toronto: University of Toronto Press, 2018).
5 The 1953 survey collected weight, height and skinfolds from a representative sample of the population using a sampling procedure developed by the Dominion Bureau of Statistics using 1951 census data. See Lionel Bradley Pett, "A Canadian Table of Average Weights for Height, Age, and Sex," *American Journal of Public Health* 45 (1955): 862–8; L.B. Pett and G.F. Ogilvie, "The Canadian Weight-Height Survey," *Human Biology* 28 (1956): 177–88; L.B. Pett and G.F. Ogilvie, "The Report on Canadian Average Weight, Height and Skinfolds," *Canadian Bulletin on Nutrition* 5 (1957): 1–81.

6 Ora Kendall, Tammy Lipskie and Shauna MacEachern, "Canadian Health Surveys 1950–1977," *Chronic Diseases in Canada* 18 (1997): 70–90; R.D. Hoppa & T.N. Garlie, "Secular Changes in the Growth of Toronto Children During the Last Century," *Annals of Human Biology* 25 (1998): 553–61; G.M. Torrance, M.D. Hooper, and B.A. Reeder, "Trends in Overweight and Obesity Among Adults in Canada (1970–1992): Evidence from National Surveys Using Measured Height and Weight," *International Journal of Obesity* 26 (2002): 797–804; Peter T. Katzmarzyk, "The Canadian Obesity Epidemic: An Historical Perspective," *Obesity Research* 10 (2002): 666–74.
7 Mitchinson, *Fighting Fat*, 66.
8 Alan Brown and G. Albert Davis, "The Prevalence of Malnutrition in the Public School Children of Toronto," *Canadian Medical Association Journal* 11 (1921): 124–6; Leonard C. Marsh, *Health and Unemployment: Some Studies of Their Relationships* (Toronto: Oxford University Press, 1936); L.B. Pett, "Malnutrition in Canada," *Canadian Medical Association Journal* 50 (1944): 9–14.
9 Mitchinson, *Fighting Fat*, ch. 2.
10 John Cranfield and Kris Inwood, "The Great Transformation: A Long-Run Perspective on Physical Well-Being in Canada," *Economics and Human Biology* 5 (2007): 204–28.
11 The decline is especially surprising given that at enlistment First World War soldiers were not well-nourished, judging by their sizeable weight gain during service. See John Cranfield, Kris Inwood, and J. Andrew Ross, "Before the Obesity Epidemic: The Body Mass Index of Canadians in World War One and World War Two," *Canadian Bulletin of Medical History* 32 (2015): 319–35 and Nic Clarke, John Cranfield, and Kris Inwood, "Fighting Fit? Diet, Disease, and Disability in the Canadian Expeditionary Force, 1914–18," *War and Society* 33 (2014): 80–97.
12 James Allen Young, "Height, Weight, and Health: Anthropometric Study of Human Growth in Nineteenth-Century American Medicine," *Bulletin of the History of Medicine* 53 (1979): 214–43; James M. Tanner, *A History of the Study of Human Growth* (Cambridge: Cambridge University Press, 1981).
13 Patricia Cline Cohen, *A Calculating People: The Spread of Numeracy in Early America* (Chicago: University of Chicago Press, 1982); Alfred W. Crosby, *The Measure of Reality: Quantification and Western Society, 1250–1600* (Cambridge: Cambridge University Press, 1997); Edward Higgs, *The Information State in England: The Central Collection of Information on Citizens since 1500* (Basingstoke: Palgrave Macmillan, 2004).
14 Saul Stahl, "The Evolution of the Normal Distribution," *Mathematics Magazine* 79 (2006): 96–113, 108.
15 Roderick Floud and Kenneth W. Wachter, "Poverty and Physical Stature: Evidence on the Standard of Living of London Boys 1770–1870," *Social*

Science History 6 (1982): 422–52; Thomas E. Jordan, *The Degeneracy Crisis and Victorian Youth* (Albany: SUNY Press: 1993).

16 Young, "Height, Weight, and Health": 222–3.

17 Benjamin A. Gould, *Investigations in the Military and Anthropological Statistics of American Soldiers* (Cambridge: Riverside Press, United States Sanitary Commission, 1869); Bernard Harris, *The Health of the Schoolchild* (Buckingham: Open University Press, 1995): 15–16.

18 Jeffrey P. Brosco, "Weight Charts and Well Child Care: When the Pediatrician Became the Expert in Child Health." In *Formative Years: Children's Health in the United States, 1880–2000*, ed. Stern Alexandra Minna and Markel Howard, 91–120 (Ann Arbor: University of Michigan Press, 2002).

19 Robert Shoemaker and Richard Ward, "Understanding the Criminal: Record-Keeping, Statistics and the Early History of Criminology in England," *British Journal of Criminology* 57 (2017): 1442–61.

20 Shoemaker and Ward, "Understanding the Criminal," 1444.

21 Kris Inwood and Evan Roberts, "Longitudinal Studies of Human Growth and Health: A Review of Recent Historical Research," *Journal of Economic Surveys* 24 (2010): 801–40, 817.

22 Shoemaker and Ward, "Understanding the Criminal," 1450.

23 Hamish Maxwell-Stewart and James Bradley, "'Behold the Man," Power, Observation and the Tattooed Convict," *Australian Studies*, 12, no. 1 (1997): 71–97, 75.

24 Sara Horrell, David Meredith, and Deborah Oxley, "Measuring Misery: Body Mass, Ageing and Gender Inequality in Victorian London," *Explorations in Economic History* 46 (2009): 93–119.

25 Ewout Depauw, "There and Back Again: The Selectivity of Recidivism in Belgian Prisons," *Social Science History 44* (2020): 445–62.

26 Scott Carson, "The Body Mass Index of Blacks and Whites in the United States during the Nineteenth Century," *Journal of Interdisciplinary History* 42 (2012): 371–91.

27 Kris Inwood, Hamish Maxwell-Stewart, Deborah Oxley, and Jim Stankovich "Growing Incomes, Growing People in Nineteenth-Century Tasmania," *Australian Economic History Review* 55 (2015): 187–211.

28 Carolyn Strange, *The Velvet Glove: Maternalistic Reform at the Andrew Mercer Ontario Reformatory for Females 1874–1927*, unpublished MA thesis, University of Ottawa, 1983.

29 John Weaver, *Crimes, Constables and Courts: Order and Transgression in a Canadian City, 1816–1970* (Montreal & Kingston: McGill-Queen's University Press, 1995).

30 Peter Oliver, *"Terror to Evil-doers": Prisons and Punishment in Nineteenth-Century Ontario* (Toronto: University of Toronto Press and Osgoode Society, 1998).

31 Donald Fyson and François Fenchel, "Prison Registers, Their Possibilities and Their Pitfalls: The Case of Local Prisons In Nineteenth-Century Quebec," *The History of the Family* 20 (2015): 163–88.

32 A. Arsenault Morin, V. Geloso, and V. Kufenko, "The Heights of French-Canadian Convicts, 1780s to 1820s," *Economics & Human Biology* 36 (2017): 126–36. These contrasts reinforce other evidence about the standard of living in different North Atlantic societies at the end of the eighteenth century; see Vincent Geloso, "Distinct within North America: Living Standards in French Canada, 1688–1775," *Cliometrica* 13 (2019): 277–321; and Vincent Geloso and Peter Lindert, "Relative Costs of Living, For Richer and Poorer, 1688–1914," *Cliometrica* 14 (2020): 417–42.

33 Young, "Height, Weight, and Health."

34 Stanley M. Garn, William R; Leonard and Victor M. Hawthorne, *American Journal of Clinical Nutrition* 44 (1986): 996–7; Frank Q. Nuttall, "Body Mass Index: Obesity, BMI, and Health: A Critical Review," *Nutrition Today* 50 (2015), 117–28; Roy J. Shepherd, "How Should We Assess Body Fatness?" *The Health and Fitness Journal of Canada, 10* (2017): 23–44. One important advantage for BMI is its simplicity.

35 For a brief discussion of the ubiquity and importance of selection biases, see Kris Inwood and Hamish Maxwell-Stewart, "Selection Bias and Social Science History," *Social Science History* 44 (2020): 411–16.

36 British Columbia Archives, *Victoria Gaol records* GR-0308 Description Lists 1864–1914, *New Westminster Gaol records* GR-0309 Description Books 1875–1917, *Nanaimo Gaol records* GR-0310.4 Description Book 1911–1914, *Saanich Prison Farm Records* GR-0306.10 Description Book 1914–1917, *Quesnel* GR-0042 Description Book 1915–1919.

37 Provincial Archives of Saskatchewan, *Regina Jail Register* 1891–1921, *Prince Albert Jail Register* 1898–1930.

38 Ontario Archives, *Central Prison registers*, RG 20–55–1, Books One and Two, 1874–1912.

39 Library and Archives Canada, *Kingston Penitentiary*, Prisoner's Records Books 1843–1890, Cell Description Registry 1890–1895, Inmate Description Ledger 1916–1919.

40 Library and Archives Canada, *St Vincent de Paul Penitentiary Convict Register*, RG73 vol 382 Box 193, 1897–1934 (file 33–55).

41 Public Archives of New Brunswick, *Dorchester Penitentiary Records*, F854-F855, 1916–1936.

42 Peter Oliver, *"Terror to Evil-doers": Prisons and Punishment in Nineteenth-Century Ontario* (Toronto: University of Toronto Press and Osgoode Society, 1998): 48, 93; John Weaver, "Crime, Public Order and Repression: The Gore District in Upheaval 1832–1851," *Ontario History* 78 (1986): 175–207.

43 Oliver, *"Terror to Evil-doers,"* 388–463.

44 Kris Inwood and Evan Roberts, "'Indians are the majority of the prisoners'? Historical variations in incarceration rates for Indigenous Women and Men in British Columbia," *The Howard Journal of Criminal Justice* 59 (2020): 350–69.

45 Oliver, *"Terror to Evil-doers,"* 379.

46 Boritch provides clear evidence of this differentiation; see Helen Boritch, "The Criminal Class Revisited: Recidivism and Punishment in Ontario, 1871–1920," *Social Science History* 29 (2005): 137–70.

47 Kris Inwood, Hamish Maxwell-Stewart, and J. Stankovich, "The Prison and the Colonial Family," *History of the Family* 20, no. 2 (2015), 231–48.

48 Inwood and Roberts, "'Indians are the Majority of the Prisoners'."

49 Peter Christen, *Data Matching: Concepts and Techniques for Record Linkage, Entity Resolution, and Duplicate Detection* (Springer-Verlag Berlin Heidelberg, 2012). A Canadian example with historical census records is reported by Luiza Antonie, Kris Inwood, Dan Lizotte and J. Andrew Ross, "Tracking People over Time in 19th Century Canada," *Machine Learning* 96 (2014): 129–46.

50 Blocking by gender, ethnicity, and country of birth reduces the number of record pairs that must be compared and, with it, processing time. We search for duplicates across prisons in the same province but not between provinces. The interprovincial transfer of prisoners was limited.

51 We have modified names and do not identify the prison to respect the privacy of the individuals.

52 See Fyson and Fenchel, "Prison registers" for a useful example of the care with which heights were measured in the Quebec City prison.

53 M.C. Urquhart, "New Estimates of Gross National Product, Canada, 1870–1926: Some Implications for Canadian Development," in *Long-Term Factors in American Economic Growth*, ed. Stanley Engerman and Robert Gallman (Chicago: University of Chicago Press, 1986), 9–88.

54 People at these ages typically have ceased growing and have not yet begun to shrink discernibly due to the backbone compacting.

55 African, Chinese, and Indigenous men are identified by explicit reference in one or more of the columns for physical description, religion, occupation, and name. Some registers reported "race," "nationality," or "ethnology."

56 A few non-French Catholics undoubtedly are captured by this definition. Unfortunately, there is no easy way to identify them. We also miss any French Canadians born outside Quebec and French Canadians who no longer followed the Roman Catholic faith.

57 Inwood, et al, "Growing Incomes, Growing People," Table 6; Depauw, "There and Back Again."

58 Cranfield and Inwood, "The Great Transformation"; John Cranfield and Kris Inwood, "A Tale of Two Armies: Comparative Growth in the Mirror of World War One," *Australian Economic History Review* 55 (2015): 212–33.

59 The Saint Vincent de Paul Penitentiary regression with birth years 1883–1911 takes French Canadians as the benchmark group. The "all other" category (North American-born who are not Indigenous, Chinese, or African-descended) is estimated to be 0.98 inches taller (t-statistic 8.45). The Indigenous were taller and east Asians shorter than French Canadians with magnitudes and significance levels similar to other prisons. African Canadians and other (mainly European) foreign-born prisoners were significantly taller than French Canadians.

60 A BMI today of between 18.5 and 24.9 is considered normal or healthy. There is, however, currently a great deal of debate about whether this figure accurately denotes anything about the health of an individual. The Centre for Disease Control and Prevention, https://www.cdc.gov/healthyweight/assessing/bmi/adult_bmi/index.html.

61 Higher BMI for men of African descent mirrors evidence from American prisons. See Scott Carson, "Body Mass, Wealth, and Inequality in the 19th Century: Joining the Debate Surrounding Equality and Health," *Economics and Human Biology* 11 (2013): 90–4; Scott Carson, "Biology, Complexion, and Socioeconomic Status: Accounting for 19th Century US BMIs by Race," *Australian Economic History Review* 55 (2015): 238–55; Scott Carson, "Body Weight and United States Economic Development 1840–1940," CESIFO working paper 7573 (2019).

62 Gregory Price, "Obesity and Crime: Is There a Relationship?," *Economics Letters* 103 (2009): 149–52; Howard Bodenhorn and Gregory N. Price, "Crime and Body Weight in the Nineteenth-Century: Was There a Relationship between Brawn, Employment Opportunities and Crime." *Économies et Sociétés, Série AF, Historie Economique Quantitative* 41 (January 2010), 1–20.

63 Richard H. Steckel, "Biological Measures of the Standard of Living," *Journal of Economic Perspectives* 22 (2008): 129–52 and "Heights and Human Welfare: Recent Developments and New Directions," *Explorations in Economic History* 46 (2009): 1–23.

64 M.C. Urquhart, "New Estimates of Gross National Product, Canada, 1870–1926: Some Implications for Canadian Development," In *Long-Term Factors in American Economic Growth*, ed. Stanley Engerman and Robert Gallman (Chicago: University of Chicago Press, 1986): 9–88.

65 David Gagan and Rosemary Gagan, "Working-Class Standards of Living in Late-Victorian Urban Ontario: A Review of the Miscellaneous Evidence on the Quality of Material Life," *Journal of the Canadian Historical Association* 1 (1980): 171–93; Michael J. Piva, *The Conditions of the Working-Class in Toronto, 1900–1921* (Ottawa: University of Ottawa Press, 1979).

66 Michael Haines, "Growing Incomes, Shrinking People: Can Economic Development Be Hazardous to Your Health," *Social Science History* 28 (2004): 249–70. The American evidence is contested. See H. Bodenhorn, T. Guinanne, and T. Mroz, "Sample-selection Biases and the Industrialization Puzzle," *Journal of Economic History* (2017): 171–207; John Komlos and Brian A'Hearn (2019) "Clarifications of a Puzzle: The Decline in Nutritional Status at the Onset of Modern Economic Growth in the United States," *Journal of Economic History* 79 (2019): 1129–53; Ariel Zimran, "Sample-selection Bias and Height Trends in the Nineteenth-Century United States," *Journal of Economic History* 79 (2019): 99–138.

67 Stephen Morgan, "Stature and Economic Development in South China, 1810–1880," *Explorations in Economic History* 46 (2009): 53–69; and Joerg Baten et al., "Evolution of living standards and human capital in China in the 18–20th centuries: Evidence from Real Wages, Age-Heaping," *Explorations in Economic History* 47 (2010): 347–59. A similar pattern is observed among Chinese emigrants to other countries; see Scott Carson, "Statures of 19th century Chinese males in America," *Annals of Human Biology* 34 (2007): 173–82. Peter Ward reports that stature by birth year among Chinese immigrants to Canada rose toward the end of the century; see his "Stature, Migration and Human Welfare in South China, 1850–1930," *Economics and Human Biology* 11 (2013): 488–501.

68 This is true for each birth decade. Average height for Indigenous people with some evidence of mixed ancestry was 67.8 inches for those born in the 1870s, 68.0 for the 1880s, 68.7 in the 1890s, and 67.9 for those born 1900–9. For those with no evidence of mixed ancestry, the averages by birth cohort 68.7, 68.5, 68.8, and 68.6 inches. Small samples implies that some of the decadal contrasts were not statistically significant.

69 James Daschuk, *Clearing the Plains: Disease, Politics of Starvation and the Loss of Aboriginal Life* (Regina: University of Regina Press, 2013); Maureen Lux, *Medicine That Walks: Disease, Medicine and Canadian Plains Native People, 1880–1940* (Toronto: University of Toronto Press, 2001).

70 Richard H. Steckel and J.M. Prince, "Tallest in the World: Native Americans of the Great Plains in the Nineteenth Century," *American Economic Review* 91 (2001): 287–94; Richard H. Steckel, "Inequality amidst Nutritional Abundance: Native Americans on the Great Plains," *Journal of Economic History* 70 (2010): 265–86.

71 Donna Feir, Rob Gillezeau and Maggie Jones, "The Slaughter of the Bison and Reversal of Fortunes on the Great Plains," *Federal Reserve Bank of Minnesota Working Paper* January, 2019.

72 Robert Boyd, *The Coming of the Spirit of Pestilence: Introduced Infectious Diseases and Population Decline among Northwest Coast Indians, 1774–1874*

(Seattle and Vancouver: University of Washington Press and UBC Press, 1999); Mary-Ellen Kelm, *Colonizing Bodies: Aboriginal Health and Healing in British Columbia 1900–1950* (Vancouver: UBC Press, 1998).

73 An exception is Kris Inwood and Ian Keay, "Indigenous Prisoners in British Columbia's Jails, 1864–1916: Evidence of Bioeconomic Well-Being and Sample Selection," unpublished paper presented to the Canadian Economics Association at its 2021 annual meeting.

74 The only exception, Ontario's Central Prison, arises because Quebec-born Catholics account for less than 0.1 per cent of men in the Ontario Central Prison.

75 For soldiers, see John Cranfield and Kris Inwood, "Genes, Class or Culture? French-English Height Differences in Canada," 231–53 in *Lives in Transition: Longitudinal Research from Historical Sources* (Montreal & Kingston: McGill-Queen's University Press 2015), Figure 11.1 and Table 11.3. For prisoners in the Quebec City Jail, see Arsenault Morin, Geloso and Kufenko, "The Heights of French-Canadian Convicts." For representative surveys in a later period, see Pett and Ogilvie, *The Report on Canadian Average Weight, Height and Skinfolds*, 29, and Cranfield and Inwood, "Genes, Class or Culture."

76 Lower francophone earnings in the 1901 census is documented by Alan Green, Mary MacKinnon and Chris Minns, "Conspicuous by their Absence: French Canadians and the Settlement of the Canadian West," *Journal of Economic History* 65 (2005): 822–49.

77 Reference is most often made in the "Nationality" and "Ethnology" columns within the register.

78 Green, MacKinnon, and Minns ("Conspicuous by their absence") argue that the particular characteristics of French Canadians – who, on average, have lower literacy, are unilingual, have larger families, and smaller savings – made entry into the western labour market less attractive than migration to the American northeast. The relatively short stature of many Quebec francophones may have reinforced this effect.

79 The standard errors were 0.07 and 0.1.

80 Inwood and Maxwell-Stewart, "Selection Bias and Social Science History."

81 A similar point is made about Australian prisoners; see K. Inwood, R. Kippen, H. Maxwell-Stewart, and R. Steckel, "The Short and the Tall: Comparing Stature and Socio-Economic Status for Male Prison and Military Populations," *Social Science History* 44 (2020): 463–83.

82 Phyllis B. Eveleth and J.M. Tanner, *Worldwide Variation in Human Growth* (Cambridge: Cambridge University Press, 1976).

83 R.D. Hoppa and T.N. Garlie, "Secular Changes in the Growth of Toronto Children During the Last Century," *Annals of Human Biology* 25 (1998): 553–61; Cranfield and Inwood, "The Great Transformation."

84 Scott Carson, "Nineteenth Century Race, Body Mass, and Industrialization: Evidence from American Prisons," *Journal of Interdisciplinary History*, 42 (2012): 371–91; "Body Mass Index Through Time: Explanations, Evidence, and Future Directions" in *The Oxford Handbook of Economics and Human Biology*, ed. John Komlos and Inas R. Kelly (Oxford: Oxford University Press, 2016).

85 J. Komlos and M. Brabec, "The Trend of Mean BMI Values of US Adults, Birth Cohorts 1882–1986 Indicates that the Obesity Epidemic Began Earlier than Hitherto Thought," *American Journal of Human Biology*, 22 (2010): 631–8; J. Komlos and M. Brabec, "The Trend of BMI Values of US Adult by Deciles, Birth Cohorts 1882–1986 Stratified by Gender and Ethnicity," *Economics and Human Biology*, 9 (2011), 234–50.

SECTION III

Cultural Representations and Constructions

Cultural productions of all sorts became much more widely available in the nineteenth century. Art prints, photographs, literature, fashion, and all sorts of material ornaments were increasingly consumed by the general public. In this context, the body was not just, or even mainly, subject to medical discourse in the nineteenth century – equally important to the weigh-scale was the pen, the paintbrush, and eventually the camera. Through these representations, ideas about aesthetic standards and social values developed. These cultural expressions provided a means to understand the significance of fat and thin bodies, tied to questions of gender, race, and class. How the body should be represented or understood was by no means a settled matter, with the fat body being neither absolutely good nor bad in most portrayals. The perceptions of the consumers of this culture were as likely to be shaped by what they encountered in these popular representations as they were shaped by doctors and health manuals, offering a much more complex and nuanced understanding of weight and body size.

Chapter 6 by Freya Gowrley focuses on the visual representations of corpulence in the late eighteenth and early nineteenth centuries, arguing that visual depictions of such bodies were essential for constructing a popular understanding of the meaning of the fat body. The figure of Daniel Lambert, who became a sort of celebrity at the beginning of the nineteenth century, complicates current views that the fat body has been universally viewed with disgust or derision. Lambert turned his body into a source of both fame and financial security, and his image subsequently became commodified through the reproduction of art prints and all sorts of material objects. In this narrative, and other visual and material culture that used similar motifs, fat is both represented by these cultural productions and acts as a cultural phenomenon in its own right.

The chapter by Tatiana Konrad examines Joseph Conrad's 1899 novella *Heart of Darkness*, and particularly his representations of the bodies of both European colonizers and the colonized people of Africa. Unlike many previous representations that portrayed Africans as overweight due to their lack of self-control and civilization, or critiques of imperialism that portrayed colonizers rendered fat by their avarice and ambition, this study finds a complicated and conflicted relationship embodied by colonialism.

Nsima Udo's investigation into the visual representations of the mbopo fattening ritual in Nigeria provides an alternative viewpoint to the colonial relationship and representations of fat and the body. European anthropologists, photographers, and documentarians recorded their observations of these fattening rituals for young women of marriageable age. But the Ibibio/Efik people themselves brought quite a different interpretation of this ritual, one removed from a denigration of the fat body and firmly grounded in other forms of cultural expression, which challenged the Eurocentric meanings assigned to fat and the body, alongside gender and race in the colonial viewpoint.

Taken together, the myriad cultural representations of the corpulent body, or its antithesis, suggest the complexity of views about fat and the body in the long nineteenth century.

6 Visual and Material Cultures of the Fat Body, 1780–1840: Representation, Commodification, and Display

FREYA GOWRLEY

In the 1780s, a vast swathe of satirical prints were produced featuring the exaggerated likeness of Albinia Hobart, Countess of Buckinghamshire (1737/8–1816), the heiress, celebrity, and political hostess. In these images, artists such as the satirist and printmaker James Gillray consistently portrayed Hobart's body through a language of immenseness and globular rotundity (Figure 6.1). These prints focused on Hobart because of her dual noticeability; she was not only physically highly present due to her overweight body, but ideologically so, thanks to these images intruding into the public sphere of the theatre, politics, and fashionable life. Hobart's attendance at public events, her gambling addiction, and her canvassing on behalf of her relative Sir Cecil Wray in the famously vexed Westminster election of 1784, an event that many of the images relate to, all brought her reputation into disrepute.[1] We can, accordingly, read the fatness that characterizes these prints as a key narrative device within them, an essential part of the work of visual communication that these images participated in, serving to clearly denote her many personal failings. Hobart's body, with her expansive chest and stomach, rounded facial features, and chubby arms and legs, worked together with the disreputable behaviours in which she is shown to engage to convey to an audience always in on the joke, that her fat figure signalled her moral corruption. This group of prints, accordingly, demonstrates that, long before current entrenched positive and negative associations of fat bodies became so firmly established, extremes of body size were associated with the strength (or lack thereof) of character of those who inhabited those bodies.

These notably unsympathetic portrayals of fatness, however, are just one of many of its manifestations appearing in the visual culture of this period, which included both negative and, crucially, positive representations of fat men and women living at this time. The following

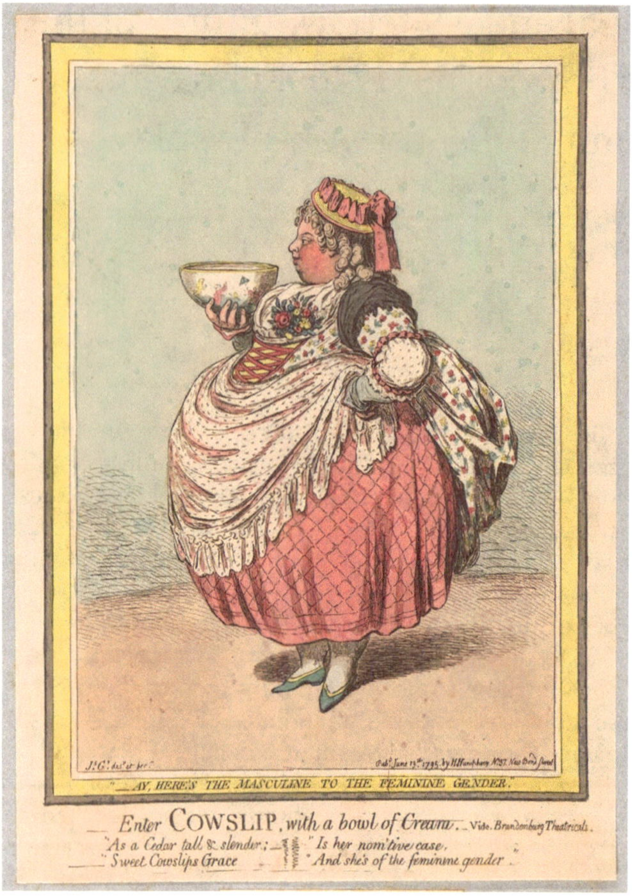
"— AY, HERE'S THE MASCULINE TO THE FEMININE GENDER."
— Enter COWSLIP, with a bowl of Cream. — Vide. Brandenburg Theatricals.
"As a Cedar tall & slender; —
— "Sweet Cowslips Grace
"Is her nom'tive case,
"And she's of the feminine gender"

Figure 6.1. James Gillray, *Enter Cowslip, with a bowl of Cream*, 1795. Etching with hand-colouring. Lewis Walpole Library, Yale University.

chapter accordingly seeks to further examine and complicate the long and complex representational history of fatness by unpacking a particular episode within that history. Focusing on images of, and objects relating to, Daniel Lambert, once known as Britain's largest man, it seeks to demonstrate the vital role played by visual and material culture in the understanding and conceptualization of the fat body throughout its history, identifying it as a cultural and historical construction with a powerful and enduring inheritance. The chapter explores how an examination of images of fatness during this period provides a more nuanced understanding of the ways in which obesity has been thought of throughout its history.[2] Paying new attention to Lambert's rich visual and material culture disrupts narratives about fatness in eighteenth- and early-nineteenth-century art and objects as rooted solely in its pejorative associations. Instead, this chapter highlights how, in the case of Lambert, fatness and its representations worked to construct identity and celebrity, facilitated commercial activities for Lambert himself, and even decorated people's homes in the form of collectable images and objects.

Eighteenth- and Nineteenth-Century Contexts

In the late eighteenth and early nineteenth centuries, body size took on unprecedented cultural currency, with fatness notably manifest across several forms of visual and material culture. As such, this period can be viewed as a unique moment during which the visual and material qualities of fatness and its conceptualization became particularly prevalent. This was due to the convergence of a number of distinctive social, intellectual, economic, and cultural contexts that characterized this period of British history. Among these factors was the apotheosis of a culture of printed satirical images, which saw the corpulent bodies of the nobility subject to constant lampooning.[3] In these images, and as we see in the case of Albinia Hobart, the mores of contemporary society – whether identifying its targets as too affected, too effeminate, too soft, too lazy, or too unattractive – were ridiculed through a visual language in which fatness and its associated effects upon the body were central.

Other relevant contexts for why fatness became so culturally prevalent in this era included the increased availability of food that characterized the period, as well as the so-called consumer revolution – which resulted in unprecedented access to luxury consumables and other forms of material culture – both of which made the eighteenth and early nineteenth centuries a period of new material profusion and indulgence.[4] This societal transformation sparked an intense discourse over the nature of needs versus desires, known as the "luxury debates," which were central to the moralizing approaches to fatness that surfaced at this time.[5] Attention to such broader discourses surrounding luxury and consumption thereby places the extensive visual and material culture of fatness in relation to much wider discourses about beauty and the body, health and medicine, religion and morality, and class and status. The last discourse manifests in the visual and material record in two distinct ways. Both satirical prints and surviving clothing preserve the lived experiences and contemporary perceptions of the fat, gout-ridden bodies of royals, such as George IV, while images of the robust bodies of the British labouring class highlight how conceptions of their healthy plumpness related to ideas of constitution and national character, particularly as articulated in the images of "John Bull," an issue also explored in a slightly later period in Bonnie Miller's essay on the Spanish-American War in chapter 9 of this volume.[6]

The second half of the eighteenth century was also the period in which the "modern self" can be said to have emerged, a time characterized by attempts to delineate identity categories such as race, class, and gender, whose ideal forms became increasingly definitive as the century progressed.[7] Images and discussions of corpulence were consistently utilized in such debates, making their analysis essential for interrogating the construction of ideas such as ideal femininity, racialized identity, and even what it meant to be human during this period. Reading these sources against the intellectual and moralizing framework of the luxury debates, one can, accordingly, use images of fatness to question how they contributed to the articulation, expression, and transgression of a range of eighteenth-century identities. This crystallization of individual characteristics was also evidenced through contemporaneous changes in beauty standards and attitudes toward the body, which subsequently shifted to begin to establish thinness as the preferred body type for women, an ideal that still resonates.[8] This preferential shift to an ideal thin body was established through medicalized texts, such as William Wadd's *Cursory Remarks on Corpulence* (1816), but was also articulated through beauty manuals, conduct literature, and fashion plates. Indeed, clothing and fatness intersected in both positive and negative ways at this time. While surviving examples of dress, underpinnings, and padding alongside fashion plates and periodicals reinforce how dress emphasized and enlarged body parts, many of these practices were also critiqued through a language of fatness and disease.[9]

This was also a period in which fatness emerged as a shared language that shaped interactions between colonized peoples and their British colonizers, with both visual images and printed texts deploying metaphors of corpulence to conceptualize and reinforce discourses of otherness and dislocation from the "home." Fatness thus became a powerful metaphor for the torrid contact zones of the British Empire, blurring what had once been strictly delineated fault lines between identities. Images of colonizers' bodies deployed fatness as a metaphor for the changes enacted by the imperial landscape and its unfamiliarly hot weather, which was presented as transforming enterprising businessmen into the lazy corpulent figures of the nabob and Johnny Newcome, the louche embodiments of the British colonist grown indolent in India and the Caribbean, respectively.[10] At the same time, painted and printed images of enslaved peoples' bodies show how figures that did not conform to standards of acceptable femininity were sexualized and dehumanized through a highly racist visual culture.[11] A key example of this is the treatment of the Khoisan woman, Sarah (Saartjie) Baartman (c.1770s–1815), once known as the "Hottentot Venus," who was sold and repeatedly exhibited in Europe. Baartman was portrayed multiple times in printed images, both straight and satirical, and she was exhibited in the Egyptian Hall of Piccadilly Circus on 24 November 1810, demonstrating how her body was also consumed through spectacularized display.[12] Although not "fat" in a traditional sense, Baartman's prominent buttocks and thighs, caused by substantial pockets of fat and tissue in these areas (a condition known as steatopygia), may be understood within a pre-existing frame of reference for fatness in contemporaneous visual culture, in which Black women's bodies were defined in contradistinction to the fashionable thinness of their white contemporaries.

Baartman's public display marks her as one of a number of famous individuals who were repeatedly visualized and commodified in portraits, prints, and decorative consumable goods on account of the fatness of their bodies. Like Baartman, those bodies marked by unusual corpulence were put on public display as spectacular objects, while the clothing that evidenced their former owners' size, and furniture made or altered to accommodate fat bodies, became desirable items and objects of renown. Baartman and her rough contemporary Daniel Lambert (1770–1809), whose case will be explored in the second half of this essay, thus exemplify how fatness was represented, commodified, and displayed during this period. From its portrayal in paintings and prints, the preservation of clothing, its appearance within published accounts, and on commemorative objects such as inkwells and glasses, the fat body was repeatedly shaped, consolidated, and created by the visual and material culture of this period.

Despite this cultural proliferation, to date there has been no sustained account of corpulence in the late eighteenth and early nineteenth centuries written from any disciplinary perspective. Although changing ideas of fatness have been sketched in broad and transhistorical terms by cultural historians such as Sander L. Gilman, Georges Vigarello, and Christopher E. Forth, attention to eighteenth- and nineteenth-century fatness has been shallow and fragmentary, and unduly focused on its pathologization through medicalized discourse.[13] Likewise, although Elena Levy-Navarro's book *The Culture of Obesity in Early and Late Modernity: Body Image in Shakespeare, Jonson, Middleton & Skelton* (2008) offers a cultural model for interrogating early modern conceptions of the fat body in literature, no one has written the equivalent for thinking about fatness in art and objects.[14] Following work that firmly establishes the necessity of visual and material approaches to the body, such as Susan Bordo's *Unbearable Weight* and Bill Brown's conception of the body as a "thing among things," this chapter contends that previous accounts have fundamentally misunderstood the fat body by overlooking the crucial role played by visual and material culture in how it has been manifested, represented, and materialized.[15] It argues that visual depiction and display are central to understanding how corpulence was culturally inscribed during the long eighteenth and nineteenth centuries, while highlighting that employing surviving material objects is likewise vital for considering the everyday realities and lived experience of being overweight at this time. Taking both reality and representation into account, a richer and more nuanced account of the late-eighteenth- and early-nineteenth-century body emerges. Adding methodologies from art history and material culture to existing cultural historical approaches that have previously characterized histories of fatness thereby creates a deeper understanding of a condition that is characterized by the co-opting of visual space and the perceived undisciplined materiality of the body.

Representation, Display, and Commodification: The Case of Daniel Lambert

Nowhere is the close relationship between fatness and its visual and material cultures clearer than in the case of Daniel Lambert, whose body was repeatedly portrayed, consumed, and visually experienced both during his life and posthumously. Lambert, a Bridewell Prison keeper and animal breeder, was famous for the large size of his body, which earned him the moniker of England's heaviest man. Born in Leicester in 1770, by the time Lambert was twenty-three he apparently weighed 32 stone (448 pounds), and by 1805 he was reputed to have weighed 50 stone (700 pounds). After the prison closed in 1805, Lambert was granted an annuity of £50, which he supplemented with income generated from selling hunting dogs and fighting cocks, and by publicly exhibiting himself in London. Here, Lambert found great fame, becoming a popular attraction for the fashionable London elite. After eventually tiring of the city, Lambert returned to Leicester in 1806, where he lived as a relatively wealthy man and continued to breed animals until his death in 1809 at the Waggon & Horses Inn in Stamford.[16]

Lambert repeatedly features in the generalized histories of fatness mentioned above but is usually mentioned only briefly. Sander Gilman gives him the most attention in his book *Obesity: The Biography*, in which he spends a few pages exploring Lambert's role as the inspiration for Charles Dickens' character "Fat Joe."[17] Although often illustrated with portraits of Lambert, these accounts have consistently ignored the implications of his repeated visualization. The first time that images of Lambert have been considered as a corpus in any real sense was 2019, with the independent publication of Roger Street's *The Daniel Lambert Picture Book*, which functions as a biography of Lambert and which attempts to gather all of the extant oil paintings, watercolours, and prints in which Lambert featured.[18] Yet Lambert's associated visual and material cultures included not merely "portraitive" representation, but a wide range of images and objects, as well as the displays of his body and its proxies in London and America, which must be considered together to fully understand how Lambert became so famously and enduringly associated with fatness during this period.[19]

In accordance with his fame, Lambert was depicted by portraitists and other artists myriad times throughout his life. Lambert's public reputation was shaped – both literally and figuratively – by a repetitive visual culture in which aspects of his physical likeness were emphasized across various forms of paint and print until they formed a recognizable silhouette.[20] In many ways, this was reminiscent of other prominent figures from this period, such as the politician Charles James Fox, and the performer and model Emma Hamilton, whose bodies were both consistently rendered grotesquely overweight in such prints, which exploited the medium's propensity for exaggerating face and figure to make assertions as to the moral characters of their subjects, specifically Fox's famously rakish behaviour and Hamilton's reputation for being sexually available.[21]

The precedent for this visual rhetoric is undoubtedly the portrait of Lambert painted by Benjamin Marshall (1768–1835), created some time around 1807 (Figure 6.2). Trained by the portraitist Lemuel Francis Abbott, Marshall specialized in the genres of sporting and animal portraiture; executing a plethora of images of fighting cocks, sportsmen, and racehorses throughout his career, many of which were engraved and published in mezzotint versions. These included sixty paintings by Marshall that were engraved by John Scott for Wheble's *Sporting Magazine*, and images of the eight types of horses by Marshall, also engraved by Scott, which appeared in *The Sportsman's Repository* in 1820.[22]

This commission provides a provocative context in which to situate Lambert's visual culture, representing a perfect culmination of Marshall's generic specialism and Lambert's own connection with the robust masculinity and physical expertise embodied by the sporting world. As the writer G.H. Wilson noted in *The Eccentric Mirror* (1806),

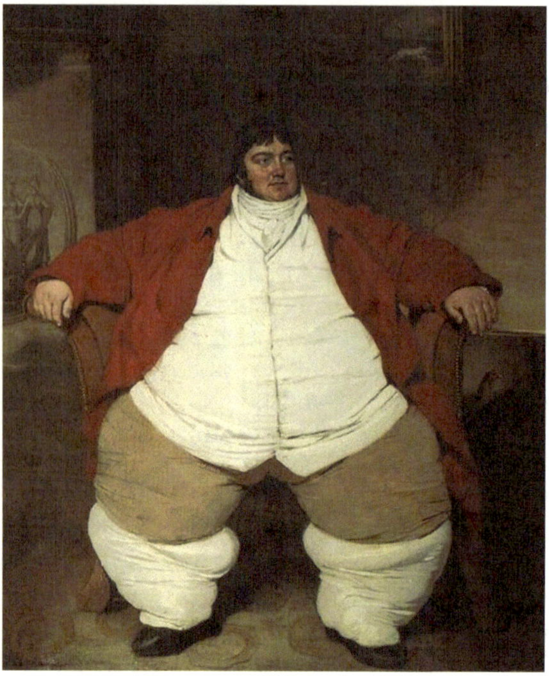

Figure 6.2. Benjamin Marshall, *Daniel Lambert*, c.1806. Oil on canvas, 76.2 x 62.9 cm. Leicester Arts and Museums Service.

Lambert was "born and bred" "among horses, dogs, cocks, and all the other appendages of sporting [...] it cannot be a matter of wonder that he should be passionately fond of all those exercises and amusements which are comprehended under the denomination of field sports, as well of racing, cocking, and fishing."[23] In the portrait, this relationship is literalized through Lambert's surroundings, with the image showing him seated in an elegant space, ornamented with paintings of a cock, horse, and dog. More metaphorically, these images signal Lambert's own position within Marshall's oeuvre, in which Lambert is not only shown as the famous sportsman he was, but as a kind of specimen worthy of visual representation. Crucially, unlike Marshall's other portraits of his hunting, and horse-riding, and animal-breeding sitters, Lambert is not shown engaging with any of these activities. Instead, he occupies a similar visual register to the cock whose image is to his right, both of which foreground the physicalities of their subjects in lieu of extraneous detailing. Here, it is Lambert's body that is the star of the show, an emphasis magnified by the stark whiteness of his waistcoat and stockings, both of which draw the viewers' eyes to the parts of his body that are perhaps most notably characterized by the condition of corpulence, that is, his stomach and calves, which appear as gargantuan forms compared with the comparatively small size of his head.

Of the painting's details that do not directly relate to Lambert's body, the neoclassicism of the space seems significant. The background of the image is somewhat difficult to discern, especially the question of the classicizing roundel to Lambert's left, which appears to be sculptural in nature, but could be part of a painting executed in *grisaille* or greyscale. However, if we are to read this part of the image as we have done the other background paintings of the cock, horse, and dog, then the inclusion is deliberate and a comment on Lambert – perhaps a device designed to contrast the lithe bodies of the diaphanously dressed women who form the subject of the roundel with Lambert's own body. Indeed, the pair appear side by side, arms outstretched, approximating something of Lambert's breadth of form between them. This was a comparison often drawn by satirists, who had long used the divergent extremes of the eighteenth- and nineteenth-century body – extreme thinness on one end of the spectrum, and extreme fatness on the other – to ridicule contemporary society. This moralizing separation of thin and fat as good and bad, respectively, has been notably consistent through the history of fatness, with such dichotomies still at the heart of much of the discourse about obesity today. Here we see a clear development of that established visual culture, executed most notably in an eighteenth-century context by artists like Gillray, adopted in this 1809 print by Charles Williams in the Wellcome Collection, which adapts that existing visual language and combines it with details from Marshall's painting in this binary of "Fat and Lean" (Figure 6.3).[24] Read together, the background inclusions within Marshall's painting might suggest that the portrait is set in Marshall's own studio, which seems particularly likely given the subjects of the images that surround him. As such, the portrait does not merely suggest that we are witnessing Lambert's physicality, but the act of representation itself, a reflexive reinforcement of the fact we are looking at a painting of Lambert, a mode of depiction that is only appropriate for a figure as represented as Lambert would become during this period.

Lambert's visual culture presence also seems to have been influenced and codified through his portrayal within a second, anonymous portrait, likely painted around the same time as Marshall's (Figure 6.4). Once again, it shows Lambert seated, although this time slightly more in profile, next to a table upon which a top hat (presumably Lambert's

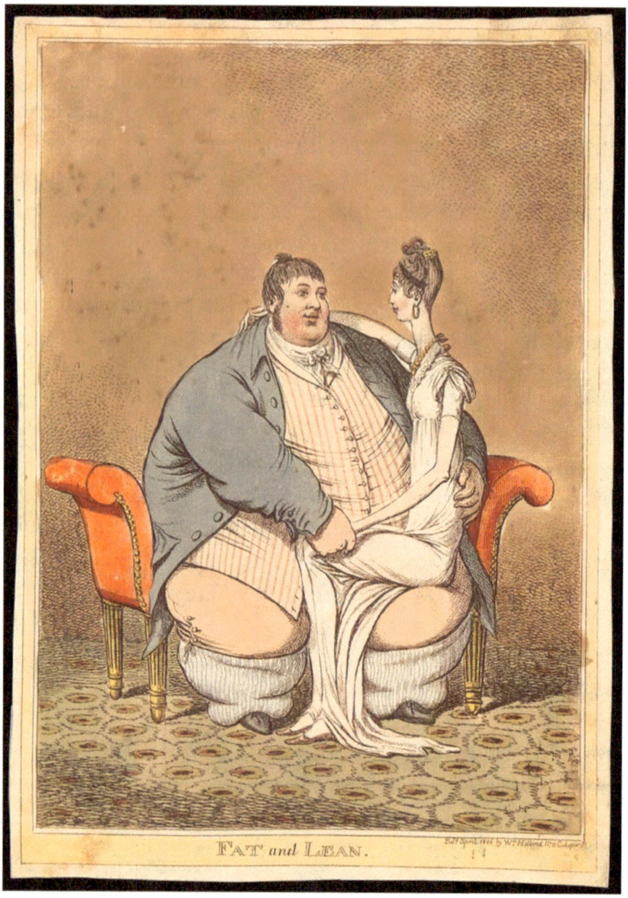

Figure 6.3. Charles Williams, *Fat and Lean*, 1806. Etching with watercolour. Wellcome Collection.

own) rests. What is remarkable about this portrait is not so much the image itself, which, like Marshall's painting, eschews distracting details in favour of a focus on Lambert's body, but the innumerable copies that exist of it, both in painted and printed form. Housed at various regional galleries around Lincolnshire, Leicestershire, Northampton, and at the Wellcome Collection, the divergent levels of quality of these copied works suggest that they were painted for financially diverse audiences, all the while reinforcing Lambert's cultural currency as a figure whom a large audience desired to see represented.[25]

Indeed, this consumer base eager for images of Lambert was reinforced by the large print culture that emerged around him. Although

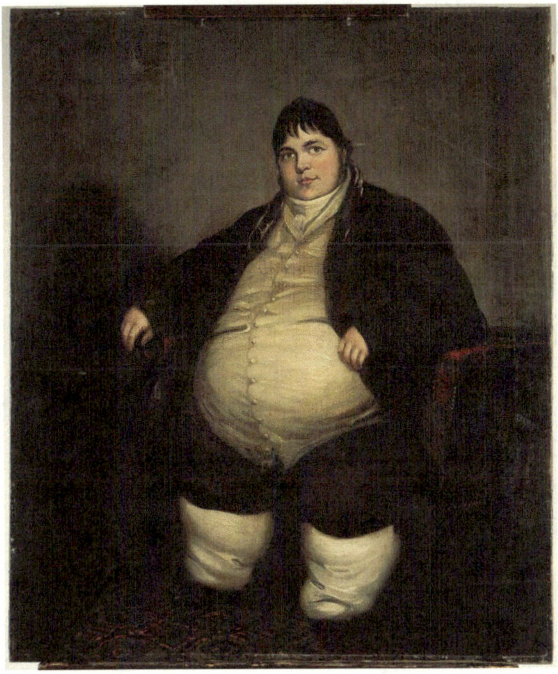

Figure 6.4. Anon. *Portrait of Daniel Lambert*, nineteenth century. Oil on canvas, 71 cm x 60 cm. Wellcome Collection.

some prints stuck closely to the archetypes provided by the two model portraits discussed above, others clearly employ an adapted mixture of the two. For example, in a relatively crude nineteenth-century etching made by an "S. Burton" (Figure 6.5), Lambert is shown face on, as in Marshall's image, but next to a table and chair, as in the other portrait type. Indeed, this composite representational form even becomes its own archetype within Lambert's iconography thanks to its repeated appearance within prints of Lambert from this period, a large number of which show him in this manner, often with the addition of a striped waistcoat. Particularly notable within these images is their use of furniture. Here, chairs and tables function as comparative visual devices designed to throw Lambert's size into the foreground. Many show Lambert in the roll-topped red chair that appears in both versions of Lambert's painted portrait, and that must have been specially made to accommodate his unusual proportions. With this extra-large chair placed next to a regular-size table, the dynamics of scale present within these images is once again heightened, with this highly

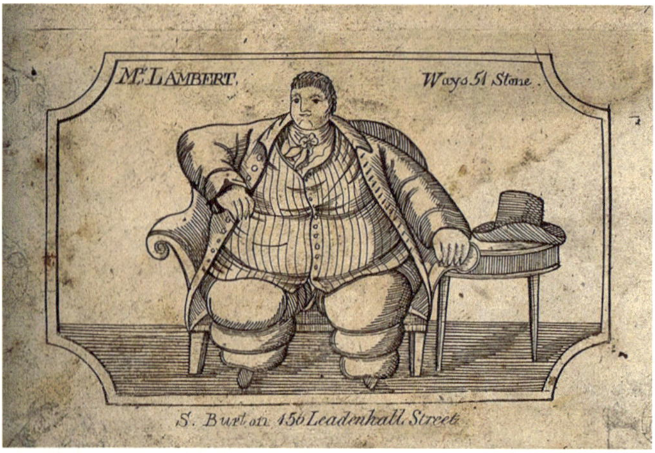

Figure 6.5. S. Burton, nineteenth century. Etching, 9 x 13.5 cm, Wellcome Collection.

ordinary, quotidian domestic material culture directly employed to reinforce Lambert's own extraordinariness. This binary is made particularly clear in one of this series of prints, in which Lambert uses a typically sized chair to prop up his arm, with the smaller example paling in comparison with his much larger seat.[26]

This interest in the accoutrements of Lambert's existence, specifically the material objects that provided him with comfort and warmth, such as his chairs and clothing, is enduring. Indeed, Lambert's clothing, including his breeches and waistcoat, are still on display in Stamford Museum in Leicestershire, while his walking stick and chair (sadly not the roll-topped example from his portraits) can still be found in the collections of the Newarke Houses Museum in Leicester. A famous photograph from the 1950s of two men holding Lambert's breeches shows how this material culture became the object of wonder and fascination, with the positioning of the much thinner men against the empty and capacious trousers echoing a nineteenth-century image of another famously fat man, Joseph Bright of Maldon, who died in 1750. Bright was a grocer who reputedly weighed 47.5 stone (665 pounds) at his heaviest.[27] In many ways, Bright's celebrity can be seen as prototypical for Lambert's own public reputation, with Bright the subject of his own body of literary and visual representation, which, like Lambert's, was both somewhat positive in tone and repetitive in nature, and which resulted in an extensive body of texts and images that together functioned to make Bright famous. An illustrated comparative account of Bright and Lambert shows the two men side by side. The right-hand corner of Bright's portrait shows an image of seven men wearing Bright's waistcoat, the result of a bet wagered following his death.[28] Throughout Lambert-related print culture, this status as a "freakish" example of the human form, whose size was marvelled at and ruminated upon was consistently emphasized. Often, this aspect of his representation took the form of his inclusion among a pantheon of late-eighteenth and early-nineteenth-century "characters" or curiosities, such as Patrick O'Brien (1760–1806). Born Patrick Cotter in Kinsale, Ireland in 1760, O'Brien grew to a height of over eight foot and became known as the Irish Giant. In 1785, he came to London where he exhibited himself for profit, a strategy that Lambert would find success with when he exhibited himself in his rooms in Piccadilly in 1806, and again in Leicester Square in 1807.[29] Of Lambert's Piccadilly rooms, Wilson noted that the apartments were more like "a place of fashionable resort" than of an exhibition, highlighting the deliberate and aestheticized gentility of his self-presentation within the capital.[30]

From April of 1806, Lambert received visitors from midday until 5 in the afternoon at 53 Piccadilly, charging them a shilling for entry, as he also would at his Leicester Square address in the following year. Far from functioning as a stereotypical "freak show" however, these exchanges were often characterized by polite and intelligent conversation, with the "qualities and endowments" of Lambert's brain often praised by his biographers.[31] Likewise, these transactions could be characterized as exhibiting genuine affection and sympathy, as the writer and editor Anne Mathews wrote of her late husband Charles's relationship with Lambert in 1860: "the half-courteous, half-sullen manner in which this 'gross fat man' received the majority of his visitors met the humour of my husband, and he liked as well as pitied him; for it was distressing sometimes to hear the coarse observations made by unfeeling people, and the silly unthinking questions asked by many of them about his appetite, &c."[32]

Alongside the "real" Lambert, a waxwork version of him was also shown in London at this time to great acclaim. The creation of this work ensured that the exhibition of Lambert's body would survive beyond its physical decay following his death in 1809. It found transatlantic fame through the display of the waxwork, first at John Mix's museum in New Haven, Connecticut, and then at P.T. Barnum's infamous Barnum's American Museum in New York.[33] Both spaces were characterized by the varied nature of their exhibits: Mix's Museum in New Haven offered to the visitor a range of curiosities, as described in an 1812 catalogue of the space, which listed wax figures "as large as life," paintings, beasts, birds, fishes, serpents, and reptiles among its exhibits, with this provocative melange highlighting how Lambert was presented here almost as a specimen of the human species.[34] Likewise, Barnum's American Museum, which was based around the natural history collection of Scudder's American Museum, acquired by Barnum in 1841, mixed scientific displays with waxworks, theatrical entertainments, zoological displays, dioramas, and a "freak show."[35]

Such exhibitionary strategies show that Lambert's visual and material cultures need to be understood as much in terms of how his body was visualized through painted and printed representations, as in terms of the histories of how that body was displayed. The connection between these two forms was literalized through the presentation of Lambert at Mix's Museum, which we know through a watercolour, graphite, and ink illustration of the waxwork done by Baroness Anne-Marguerite-Henriette Hyde de Neuville, who visited the museum in 1813. Her inscription "new-haven, mix's museum, august 30, 1813" "daniel Lambert/aged 39 Years/who died/in Stamfort (England)/on the 28th of june 1809./his Coffin measured 6 feet, 4 in. long/4 feet, 4 inches Wide/and/2 feet, 4 inch," gives a sense of what kind of information might have been on display alongside the work. It tellingly emphasizes the unusual proportions of Lambert's coffin, while the image itself demonstrates how the display conformed to the conventions of Lambert's established visual culture, powerfully recalling prints of Lambert wearing his yellow waistcoat, while seated in his roll-topped chair, small table to his left. By situating the spectacularized display of Lambert's body within the exhibitionary cultures of early-nineteenth-century London and America, such as shows of human curiosities, panoramas, and other forms of popular entertainment, as well as the large number of printed and painted portraits of Lambert, we can better understand how Lambert's body was visualized, understood, and eventually commoditized through a highly mediated and hugely consistent visual and material culture that would endure throughout the nineteenth century.

The late nineteenth century represented another key shift in Lambert's representational history, which saw a change from a visual culture of commemoration to a material one, with Lambert increasingly depicted in objects such as ceramics, metalware, and on small printed consumable objects, such as postcards depicting his portrait alongside his tombstone. In the 1880s, Staffordshire Potteries produced a figurine of Lambert, showing him as seated in a round-backed chair, his name inscribed beneath his feet. Although the figure does not specifically accord with the famous painted representations of Lambert discussed above, his buff waistcoat and trousers, and blue jacket are nevertheless reminiscent of the model portrait of Lambert. The many copies of this image included versions executed during the nineteenth century, which shows the consistency with which this representational model of Lambert was employed throughout this period, and which might therefore have provided a direct point of reference for the ceramic piece. The designer of the Staffordshire figurine sensitively rendered Lambert's face and body, with the smoothness of the ceramic form lending itself well to representing the curves of his stomach, face, and legs. The paint job further emphasizes the fatness of Lambert's body: his cheeks are delicately rouged, creating chubby rosy spheres; while brown paint is used along the edges of his clothing to denote the undulations of his form. That his surname alone ("LAMBERT") is placed so prominently at his feet shows the degree to which Lambert's body had become a synecdoche for himself and his story. This transformation of body into icon is exemplified by the faceless outline of Lambert that was used as advertising for the Leicester Festival's performance of the production "The Ghost of Daniel Lambert" in the 1980s, demonstrating how, even a century later, Lambert's seated pose and large body maintained their emblematic status.[36]

Lambert also seems to have become a reference point for the production of a series of inkwells in both salt-glaze ceramic and brass, the latter of which appears to have been mass-produced in notable quantity, given the number that survive today and have been recently sold on online auction sites such as eBay (Figure 6.6). Also made in painted cast iron, they show a Lambert-like figure seated on the floor, eating a large roasted bird with a knife and fork, the inclusion of the top hat placed at his right side recalling his earlier portrayals. Lambert's head opens to reveal the repository for the ink, his body making a suitably cavernous form for its storage. The binary of "flat versus fat," used to contrast forms of visual versus material culture seems particularly apt here; these objects take advantage of their own physicality to more tangibly represent something of Lambert's own body than can be conveyed in a simple printed or painted image.[37] While the inkwell can clearly be read against humorous models in which fatness was repeatedly satirized from the eighteenth century onwards, both these and the Staffordshire figurine were ultimately designed to be attractive domestic consumable objects, destined for display within the home. As such, these images and objects complicate contemporary understandings of the fat body as something ugly and undesirable, instead showing how the fat body could also be used as a fashionable and popular home accessory. Notably, the inkwell does not seem to accord with any extant

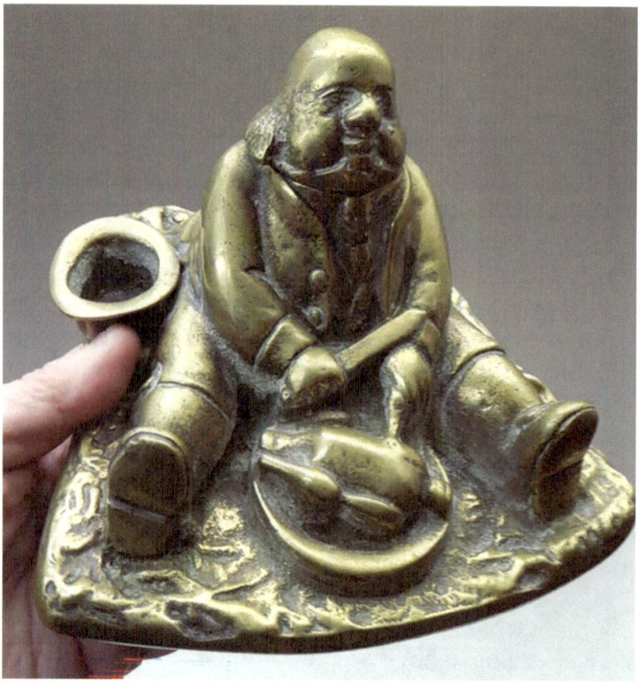

Figure 6.6. Inkwell, Victorian. Private Collection.

representational models that we associate with Lambert from the earlier nineteenth century. Nevertheless, the consistency with which this variety of inkwell is associated with him highlights the legibility of the fat body in its consumable forms as something particularly associated with ideas of celebrity. Whether showing Lambert or not, his iconic and enduring status as "'Britain's fattest man" is the crucial aspect of this transaction, in which a form of fatness that was at once generalized and particularized became bound up so powerfully with his representations in visual and material culture, that it is presumed that the inkwell could be modelled after no one else.

Issues about how fatness is, or more crucially, is not, represented culturally continue to be relevant today. In her vital feminist manifesto, *Fat is a Feminist Issue*, Susie Orbach firmly established the relationship between the image and the idea of the "perfect" female body, arguing for a damaging correlation between a glossy visual culture depicting only the thinnest women, and women's conceptions of their own bodies. As she wrote, "[I]mages aren't trivial. They work on our ideas of who we can be and these include how we need to display and present ourselves and what we can eat in order to match these images."[38] Although 2018 marked the fortieth anniversary of this important meditation on the problematic position of the media's presentation of the body, negative attitudes toward the fat body and its representations remain prevalent. This was exemplified by reactions to the UK edition of *Cosmopolitan* magazine in October of that same year, which featured the plus-size model and influencer Tess Holliday on its front cover, a choice that drew vicious criticism. Showing Holliday wearing a green swimsuit, the cover portrayed her as an unapologetically fat woman, her body representing a deliberately arresting visual intrusion into a space usually reserved for "conventionally attractive" bodies. Yet, despite its revolutionary presence on the front cover of a mainstream fashion magazine, depictions of fat celebrities, particularly positive ones, have a long and complex history, as attention to Lambert's own visual and material histories can attest.

Culminating as a complex nexus of face, space, and trace, the visual and material cultures of Lambert's body transcended individual cultural forms, geographical locations, and states of existence. They include Lambert's repeated portraitive representation, as articulated in both paint and print media, and later in brass and ceramic; as well as the exhibition of both his body and his waxen facsimile in Britain and North America; and the relics of his existence – clothing and furniture – which survived long after the corruptible body. Variously representing, spectacularizing, and commodifying Lambert, these images and objects operate as a complex visual register and material language of fatness that complicates contemporary notions of how fat bodies were not only understood but actively enjoyed. Not merely confined to the status of the freak, images of Lambert highlight his connection with the worlds of physical expertise and animal rearing, while his self-presentation while in London reveals his own agency in creating his fashionable and genteel reputation. Finally, the large number of consumable wares modelled after Lambert reinforce his status as an attractive commodity, a fact that works in opposition to models in which the fat body was viewed as inherently and irredeemably undesirable. As such, the case of Lambert exemplifies why visual and material approaches are central to the history of fatness during the long nineteenth century. Beyond communicating simple information about those who were fat during this period, they allow us to more fully comprehend the ways in which fatness culturally *worked* at this time through the processes of visualization, acquisition, and commemoration, as fully implicated within nineteenth-century cultures of print, exhibition, and commoditization.

NOTES

1 On images of Albinia Hobart, see H. Carroll, *Visualising Elite Political Women in the Reign of Queen Charlotte, 1761–1818*, unpublished PhD thesis (University of Edinburgh 2017).

2 In accordance with eighteenth-century terminologies, as well as recent attempts to reclaim stigmatizing labels, this chapter uses deliberate and specific language to refer to the overweight body during this period. This project uses the terms "fat" and "fatness" as part of the reclamation of language as characterized by A.D. Galinsky, K. Hugenberg, C. Groom and G. Bodenhausen in their article, "The Reappropriation Of Stigmatizing Labels: Implications for Social Identity," *Identity Issues in Groups Research on Managing Groups and Teams*, 5 (2003), 221–56, while also using corpulence as a term that would also have been recognizable to contemporaries. It employs the term obesity in relation to the subsequent pathologization and moralization of the fat body.

3 On eighteenth-century print culture, see D. Donald, *The Age of Caricature: Satirical Prints in the Reign of George III* (New Haven & London: Yale University Press, 2006).

4 On Britain's increased agricultural production during this period, see C. Muldrew, *Food, Energy and the Creation of Industriousness: Work and Material Culture in Agrarian England, 1550–1780* (Cambridge, 2011); and for the consumer revolution, see N. McKendrick, J. Brewer, and J. H. Plumb, *The Birth of a Consumer Society: The Commercialization of Eighteenth-century England* (Bloomington, Indiana: Indiana University Press, 1982) and J. Brewer and R. Porter, eds. *Consumption and the World of Goods* (London: Routledge, 1993).

5 For the luxury debates, see M. Berg and E. Eger, eds. *Luxury in the Eighteenth-Century: Debates, Desires and Delectable Goods* (Basingstoke: Palgrave Macmillan, 2002).

6 See the following satirical prints: James Gillray, A voluptuary under the horrors of digestion, 1792, British Museum, London; William Holland, Aristocracy and Democracy, 1794, British Museum, London.

7 On identity, see D. Wahrman, "Percy's Prologue: From Gender Play to Gender Panic in Eighteenth-Century England," *Past and Present*, 159, no. 1 (1998), 113–60.

8 On the fashion for thinness in the late eighteenth and early nineteenth centuries, see C. Day, *Consumptive Chic: A History of Beauty, Fashion and Disease* (London & New York: Bloomsbury Academic, 2017).

9 Day (2017), 82.

10 C. Northrop, "Satirical Prints and Imperial Masculinity: Johnny Newcome in the West Indies," *Nineteenth-Century Gender Studies*, 14, no. 2. http://www.ncgsjournal.com/issue142/issue142.htm.

11 On intersections between racism and fatphobia, see S. Strings, *Fearing the Black Body: The Racial Origins of Fat Phobia* (New York: New York University Press, 2019).
12 Strings (2019), 93.
13 Sander L. Gilman, *Fat: A Cultural History of Obesity* (Cambridge: Polity, 2008); Georges Vigarello, *The Metamorphoses of Fat: A History of Obesity* (New York: Colombia University Press, 2013); *Christopher E. Forth, Fat: A Cultural History of the Stuff of Life* (London: Reaktion Books, 2019).
14 E. Levy-Navarro, *The Culture of Obesity in Early and Late Modernity: Body Image in Shakespeare, Jonson, Middleton & Skelton* (London: Palgrave Macmillan, 2008).
15 Susan Bordo, *Unbearable Weight: Feminism, Western Culture and the Body* (Los Angeles & London: University of California Press, 1993); Bill Brown, "Thing Theory," *Critical Inquiry* 28, no. 1 (Things), (Autumn, 2001), 1–22.
16 For a contemporary biography of Lambert, see J. Drakard, *The Life of Daniel Lambert, With an Account of Men Noted for Their Corpulency* (Stamford, 1809).
17 S.L. Gilman, *Obesity: The Biography* (Oxford: Oxford University Press, 2013), 1–3.
18 R. Street, *The Daniel Lambert Picture Book* (Dorset: Artesius Publications, 2019).
19 For "portraitive," see E.A. Fay, *Fashioning Faces: The Portraitive Mode in British Romanticism* (Hannover & London: New Hampshire University Press, 2010).
20 Robin Nicholson, *Bonnie Prince Charlie and the Making of a Myth: A Study in Portraiture, 1720–1892* (Lewisburg, PA: Bucknell University Press, 2002); Shearer West, "Wilkes's Squint: Synecdochic Physiognomy and Political Identity in Eighteenth-Century Print Culture," *Eighteenth-Century Studies*, 33, no. 1 (Fall, 1999), 65–84.
21 See the following prints: Charles Williams, The two greatest men in England, 1806, Wellcome Collection, London, 854i; James Gillray, Dido, in despair!, National Portrait Gallery, London, NPG D13034.
22 On Marshall's career, see A. Noakes, *Ben Marshall, 1768–1835* (Leigh-on-Sea: F. Lewis, 1978).
23 G.H. Wilson, *The Eccentric Mirror* (London, 1806), 4.
24 See for example: James Gillray, *Following the Fashion*, 1794.
25 Versions of this painting are held in the Wellcome Collection (London); the Usher Gallery (Lincolnshire); Northampton Museums and Art Gallery, Compton Verney (Warwickshire); New Walk Museum & Art Gallery (Leicester); the Hunterian Museum (Glasgow); and at Discover Stamford (Leicesteshire).
26 Joseph Parry, Mr. Daniel Lambert of Leicester, 1804. Wellcome Collection, London.
27 Photograph available at Bridgeman image library.

28 Wilson (1806), 31.
29 Leary, Getz & Co. *Lives of great and celebrated characters of all ages and countries: comprising heroes, conquerors, jugglers and other curiosities of human nature* (Leary, Getz & Co: Philadelphia, 1860), 437–8.
30 Wilson (1806), 15.
31 Wilson (1806), 1.
32 A. Mathews, *The life and correspondence of Charles Mathews, the elder, Comedian* (London: Routledge, Warne and Routledge, 1860), 384.
33 J. Bondeson, *Freaks: The Pig-Faced Lady of Manchester Square & Other Medical Marvels* (Stroud: Tempus Publishing, 2006), 126.
34 See catalogue entry for "Wax Figure, Daniel Lambert, at Mix's Museum, New Haven, Connecticut, from a disassembled album," New York Historical Society, 1953.287b, https://www.nyhistory.org/exhibit/wax-figure-daniel-lambert-mixs-museum-new-haven-connecticut-disassembled-album.
35 On Barnum, see R. Wilson, *Barnum: An American Life* (New York: Simon & Schuster, 2019).
36 Poster, 1981, Victoria & Albert Museum, London, S.2361–1995.
37 V. Coltman, "Im-material Culture and History of Art(efacts)," in *Writing Material Culture History*, ed. A. Gerritsen and G. Riello (London: Bloomsbury, 2014), 17.
38 S. Orbach, *Fat Is a Feminist Issue* (London: Arrow Books, 2016), vi.

7 The Fat Body and Colonial Symbolism: Imperialism, Appetite, and Hunger in Joseph Conrad's *Heart of Darkness*

TATIANA KONRAD

In nineteenth-century Europe, the fat body was understood rather ambiguously from political, social, economic, and cultural perspectives. On the one hand, the fat body was perceived as a sign of beauty, health, and even economic prosperity. On the other hand, the well-known images and descriptions of women whose bodies were tightly corseted speak for nineteenth-century contemporaries' perception of a slim and slender female body as beautiful. Such images undermine the positive interpretations of the fat body and allow one to speculate that in certain contexts the fat body was viewed as ugly and unfashionable. The equivocacy that surrounded the fat body in the nineteenth century was further intensified by colonialism, which rather straightforwardly relied on appearance to classify individuals as good and bad, rich and poor, enslavers and the enslaved. While race and ethnicity were the primary characteristics helping colonizers visually identify certain peoples as inferior, perceptions and presentations of individual bodies also tell much about colonial and imperial policies and practices. And cultural representations only served to reinforce these social and political understandings.

This chapter focuses on Joseph Conrad's *Heart of Darkness* (1899) and examines colonial oppression through the image of the fat body. My major concern here is the interaction between colonizers and the colonized: the main characters of Kurtz and Marlow on the one hand and the locals on the other. The novella frequently contrasts colonizers and the colonized through the depictions of their bodies. The constant hunger that the locals feel is juxtaposed with the insatiable appetite of the colonizers. The healthier, nourished bodies of the white characters thus functions as a direct symbol of colonialism and its perverse politics, robbing the locals of their land, resources, wealth, and even food. This chapter considers the references to food and the process of (non) eating, as described in the novella, and contends that the fat body is an important lens through which nineteenth-century colonialism and imperialism can be understood, not only as political and economic phenomena but also as cultural ones, for they largely define appearance in the nineteenth century – not only from the perspectives of race and ethnicity but also, evidently, physically, through the idea of being (or not being) *fat*.

The Body and Colonialism

Heart of Darkness is one of the best-known narratives on colonialism and imperialism. It is the story of insatiable greed and endless consumerism, racial discrimination and economic abuse, mental illness, and oppression. All these notions are brought to the fore, in part, through very distinct descriptions of the characters' bodies, the ways these bodies are treated and nourished, and what ultimately becomes of the bodies.

Before delving into the analysis of the body, however, it is important to foreground the critical debate surrounding *Heart of Darkness*. Written over a century ago, the novella has been both recognized as one of the most important literary works of the nineteenth century as well as heavily condemned for its blatant racism. While much of this chapter's analysis draws on imperialism and the multiple metaphors that Conrad uses to communicate its horror and ultimately critique it, it is crucial to emphasize that, along with imperialism, racism permeates the novella and thus has to be recognized. Chinua Achebe's response to *Heart of Darkness* in the 1970s pointedly reveals the wrongs of the novella, calling not only for seeing racism in the work but, on a more profound level, questioning texts (and specifically Conrad's novella) that have been recognized as key literary works that must be included in university curricula. Achebe calls Conrad "a thoroughgoing racist," and claims that this has not been acknowledged earlier because "white racism against Africa is such a normal way of thinking that its manifestations go completely unremarked."[1] These very politics of oppression, but also the image of "Africa" that Conrad draws in *Heart of Darkness*, promote "dehumanization of Africa and Africans," and, as Achebe writes, "the question is whether a novel which celebrates this dehumanization, which depersonalizes a portion of the human race, can be called a great work of art."[2] Achebe condemns the imperialism and racism that made *Heart of Darkness* so popular and important, and emphasizes the significance of dealing with the racism of and in the novella.[3]

Achebe also recognizes potential obstacles that might convincingly limit his claims:

> There are two probable grounds on which what I have said so far may be contested. The first is that it is no concern of fiction to please people about whom it is written. I will go along with that. But I am not talking about pleasing people. I am talking about a book which parades in the most vulgar fashion prejudices and insults from which a section of mankind has suffered untold agonies and atrocities in the past and continues to do so in many ways and many places today. I am talking about a story in which the very humanity of Black people is called in question.
>
> Secondly, I may be challenged on the grounds of actuality. Conrad, after all, did sail down the Congo in 1890 when my own father was still a babe in arms. How could I stand up more than fifty years after his death and purport to contradict him? My answer is that as a sensible man I will not accept just any traveler's tales solely on the grounds that I have not made the journey myself. I will not trust the evidence even of a man's very eyes when I suspect them to be as jaundiced as Conrad's.[4]

Achebe concludes that "Conrad saw and condemned the evil of imperial exploitation but was strangely unaware of the racism on which it sharpened its iron tooth."[5] And it is with this important observation that I move to the analysis of the body in *Heart of Darkness*.

Conrad's novella tells the story of Charles Marlow's adventures on the African continent, which he identifies as "a place of darkness."[6] Throughout his journey, Marlow meets other colonizers, witnesses the exploitation of the local people, encounters cannibals, finds Mr Kurtz – one of the best ivory traders – and generally learns more about the continent whose image on a map seems to have fascinated him so much when he was a boy. Through these episodes, the novella outlines the horrors of colonialism in an ambiguous way, both supporting colonial exploitation and promoting racism as well as unveiling the criminal failures of this ideology and its terrifying consequences. I concur with the scholars who foreground the cultural equivocacy of the narrative, viewing *Heart of Darkness* as "a subtle and complex mixture of cultural awareness and imperialist blindness."[7] One of the ways through which to understand the novella's stance on colonialism and imperialism is through its references to the characters' bodies and their physical appearances. *Heart of Darkness*, as I will further set out, classifies bodies as fat versus slim, and via these rather plain and straightforward references identifies the characters as good and bad, privileged and abused, smart and dumb. The body serves as a signifier for the main character, Marlow, and through him for the reader, regarding the nature of people who surround him.

To put it simply, the novella seems to primarily depict the colonizers as fat and the colonized as slim. In doing so, it celebrates fatness as a unique identity category that in the times of colonization communicated a white person's superior status, revealing the complex meanings of colonialism, patriarchy, and power, and the way those intersected. Yet the exceptions that the text provides complicate this basic division and make the meaning of the "fat body versus slim body" dichotomy more intricate. The fat body in particular is portrayed rather ambiguously. Most of the white characters whom Marlow encounters in Africa are, to various degrees, overweight. Thus, for example, the reader finds out about Marlow's "white companion" who was "not a bad chap, but rather too fleshy and with the exasperating habit of fainting on the hot hillsides, miles away from the least bit of shade and water."[8] Their manager's uncle is described as follows: "He carried his fat paunch with ostentation on his short legs."[9] One person who accompanies Marlow on the steamer is portrayed in a similar fashion, as: "a little fat man, with sandy hair and red whiskers, who wore sidespring boots, and pink pyjamas tucked into his socks."[10] In general, the labelling, "[t]he fat man,"[11] appears rather frequently in the novella to characterize the appearance of white characters. Fat thus becomes an integral part of colonialism. The very project of colonialism is described in the novella as a "flabby devil,"[12] which effectively underscores the bodily appearance of those who spread and directly carry out the policy. Imperialism is thus visualized through the softness and fleshiness of the colonizers' white bodies. This is also, arguably, a reference to the enervating character of tropical lands, as they were perceived by many Europeans, who worried that time spent in the colonies would lead to indolence and feminized bodies. Even the locals who become particularly close to colonizers change their appearance accordingly, including, for instance, "an overfed young negro"[13] whose nourished appearance is indeed not representative of that of the majority of the colonized.

Through the images of fat colonizers, *fat* also becomes a metaphor for colonialism's main goals: to rob nature and the locals, consume endlessly, and profit greatly.[14] The colonizers' obsession with the region's abundant ivory is emphasized in *Heart of Darkness*. "The word 'ivory' rang in the air, was whispered, was sighed. You would think they were praying to it."[15] The aim of colonizing and exploiting the land and the peoples is thus explained with the colonizers' craving for the valuable material: "To tear treasure out of the bowels of the land was their desire, with no more moral purpose at the back of it than there is in burglars breaking into a safe."[16]

The association of fatness with colonialism foregrounds the negative characteristics of both. Fatness as an aspect of one's bodily constitution stands for the individual's incapability of controlling his/her appetite, transforming, as a result, his/her physical shape, which leads to being unable to cope with certain conditions (such as, for example, the overweight man who accompanies Marlow, mentioned earlier in this chapter). Fatness as a metaphor for colonialism stands for the colonizers' insatiable appetite, revealing that they would do anything to satisfy their hunger. Fatness becomes the face of white colonizers. In contrast to that, thinness is what characterizes the colonized.

The difference in the appearances of the colonizers and the colonized is explicitly articulated in *Heart of Darkness* through its criticism of colonialism: "The conquest of the earth, which mostly means the taking it away from those who have a different complexion or slightly flatter noses than ourselves, is not a pretty thing when you look into it too much."[17] Here, such physical peculiarities as "a different complexion" and "slightly flatter noses" are used to reinforce the visual characteristics of the locals that the colonizers do not possess. It is through the reference to their "complexion" that the novella emphasizes the differences in the way the bodies of the locals look, compared with the white colonizers (although the narrative is highlighting that some of these differences in appearance are slight). Indeed, none of the colonized individuals (except for the overweight young man mentioned above) is ever characterized as being fleshy, soft, fat, or obese. Quite the opposite. Their bodies are sharply contrasted with the well-nourished white bodies, being unhealthily slim, which reveals the abuse, deprivation of food, and overwhelming physical toil that they are forced to perform. Through bodily appearances, the novella thus condemns colonialism, illustrating that it harms both sides, oversupplying the bodies of the colonizers and undersupplying the bodies of the colonized.

In one instance, Marlow encounters a group of locals, severely exploited by the colonizers: "You could see from afar the white of their eyeballs glistening. They shouted, sang; their bodies streamed with perspiration; they had faces like grotesque masks – these chaps; but they had bone, muscle, a wild vitality, an intense energy of movement, that was as natural and true as the surf along their coast."[18] At the station shortly after his arrival, he witnesses: "A lot of people, mostly black and naked, moved about like ants."[19] It is, however, not only their physical strength and ability to perform hard work that Marlow acknowledges; he also notices how unhealthily thin these locals are:

> Six black men advanced in a file, toiling up the path. They walked erect and slow, balancing small baskets full of earth on their heads, and the clink kept time with their footsteps. Black rags were wound round their loins, and the short ends behind waggled to and fro like tails. I could see every rib, the joints of their limbs were like knots in a rope; each had an iron collar on his neck, and all were connected together with a chain whose bights swung between them, rhythmically clinking.[20]

Marlow thus witnesses the bodily transformations that the colonized go through: healthy and strong men turning into exhausted and exploited individuals.

Yet Marlow soon observes an even more horrifying sight, once he notices a group of locals literally exploited to death:

> They were dying slowly – it was very clear. They were not enemies, they were not criminals, they were nothing earthly now – nothing but black shadows of disease and starvation, lying confusedly in the greenish gloom. Brought from all the recesses of the coast in all the legality of time contracts, lost in uncongenial surroundings, fed on unfamiliar food, they sickened, became inefficient, and were then allowed to crawl away and rest. These moribund shapes were free as air – and nearly as thin. I began to distinguish the gleam of the eyes under the trees. Then, glancing down, I saw a face near my hand. The black bones reclined at full length with one shoulder against the tree, and slowly the eyelids rose and the sunken eyes looked up at me, enormous and vacant, a kind of blind, white flicker in the depths of the orbs, which died out slowly. The man seemed young – almost a boy – but you know with them it's hard to tell. I found nothing else to do but to offer him one of my good Swede's ship's biscuits I had in my pocket. The fingers closed slowly on it and held – there was no other movement and no other glance. He had tied a bit of white worsted round his neck – Why? Where did he get it? Was it a badge – an ornament – a charm – a propitiatory act? Was there any idea at all connected with it? It looked startling round his black neck, this bit of white thread from beyond the seas.[21]

While the death of the men is a terrifying view in itself, it is the way they are dying that horrifies the most. The physical appearance of the men and corpses lying together is emphasized to accentuate the way these people were treated. They were physically exploited, abused, and starved. This made their bodies shrink considerably so that Marlow even compares their unnatural and clearly unhealthy scrawniness, boniness to "air." The thinness of the dying locals reinforces the fatness of the colonizers who came to exploit and benefit from the colonized.

Symbolically, the dying man has a piece of white cloth around his neck, which stands for the suffocating, murdering effects that colonization had on the colonized populations.

It is in contrast to that unhealthy thinness of the Black man that the white body is evoked in the novella only one paragraph down: "When near the buildings I met a white man, in such an unexpected elegance of get-up that in the first moment I took him for a sort of vision. I saw a high starched collar, white cuffs, a light alpaca jacket, snowy trousers, a clean necktie, and varnished boots. No hat. Hair parted, brushed, oiled, under a green-lined parasol held in a big white hand. He was amazing, and had a penholder behind his ear."[22] While here the man is not characterized as fat, his bigness and greatness – partially what fat stands for, to characterize the power of the colonizer – are reinforced through his "big white hand" and the general appearance that emphasizes his belonging to the upper class as well as his high status. The big and healthy body dressed in rich clothing is a large contrast to the thin dying bodies of the locals dressed in rags.

Heart of Darkness clearly outlines the boundary between the colonizer and the colonized through its depiction of the characters' bodies. Yet not all colonizers are portrayed in the novella as fat, which reveals the multifaceted nature of body complexions described in the narrative, as well as emphasizing the contested meaning of fat in the nineteenth century. For example, Marlow himself is not fat, despite being a white colonizer: "He had sunken cheeks, a yellow complexion, a straight back, an ascetic aspect, and, with his arms dropped, the palms of hands outwards, resembled an idol."[23] His slimness is indeed reinforced through the description of him looking "ascetic." The captain on a steamer, a Swede, is characterized by Marlow as follows: "He was a young man, lean, fair, and morose, with lanky hair and a shuffling gait."[24] Leslie Heywood elucidates this striking emphasis on the appearance of the characters' bodies: "Most often, those with whom Marlow sympathizes are thin, and those with whom he does not are fat."[25] To be more precise, it is the division of the characters into good and bad that the novella achieves through the usage of fat/slim. Thus, Debrah Raschke notes, "those who are lean (the Swedish steamer captain, the foreman, and Marlow himself) become associated with goodness and restraint, and those who are fat (the manager's uncle and appetites, in general) become associated with badness and lack of restraint."[26] Fat is a complex metaphor for the drawbacks of colonialism; it is "the sign of some fatal flaw, or lack, or form of corruption and inefficiency, as with the metaphor 'flabby devil' to describe the imperialist project in *Heart of Darkness*."[27]

Fat also provides a powerful commentary on masculinity, for through the fat male characters, "Conrad explicitly opposes fatness and its attendant qualities to his ideal masculine universe."[28] Indeed, masculinity has always been intricately linked to the body. According to Christopher E. Forth, "[t]he masculinity of ... soft and fat males could be called into question, mainly because the gendered typology of fluids and textures could be invoked to support the supposed moral inferiority of all 'feminine' traits."[29] Sander L. Gilman observes that in the middle of the nineteenth century, one can observe the emergence of a very peculiar stereotype about fatness: "The obese ... were seen as a danger to themselves as well as to others. The general stigma associated with a potentially unhealthy body which stood out because of its size made it imperative that fat people seek treatment."[30] Fatness was thus viewed as a demasculinizing, and therefore inferior, quality.

Nevertheless, this explicit "equation between inefficiency and fat, between the imperialist project as barbaric and the fat bodies of its perpetrators"[31] that the novella vehemently brings to the fore can be read not only as a censure of certain aspects of colonialism or specific actions of the colonizers, but also as a reflection of historically transforming views on the body. The association of the fat body with "prosperity and power" – the view that was so popular at the beginning of the nineteenth century – was replaced with the perception of fat as a sign of "corruption and laziness" toward the end of the century. This, as scholars explain, was a direct reflection of industrialization and the radically transformative effects it had on people.[32] To specify: "[T]echnological innovations, economic changes, and the ideology of efficiency all conspired to reinforce the slenderized ideal. The human body – both male and female – was to be as efficient, as effective, as economical, and as beautiful as the sleek new machines, as the rationalized workplace."[33]

Slimness, however, can also be read as the state into which the colony's "darkness" brings individuals, as illustrated in the novella. Thus, Marlow talks about the lack of food in Africa in the quality and quantity that the white man is used to: "Sandbanks, marshes, forests, savages – precious little to eat fit for a civilized man, nothing but Thames water to drink."[34] The constant movement, physical activities, and the lack of food that Marlow faces in Africa turn him, in his opinion, into an individual similar to a local: "Being hungry, you know, and kept on my feet too. I was getting savage."[35] In addition, it is crucial that Mr Kurtz, for whom Marlow searches, is present in the novella only as the "disembodied voice, who surrounds himself with a wall of skulls."[36] The man is thus body-less and is surrounded by human bones – the lack of fat is evident in both instances. The transformation that Africa works on the colonizers, turning them, in the words of Marlow, into "savages," certainly reveals the novella's Eurocentrism. Moreover, even Marlow's negative attitude to fat hardly stands for his condemnation of colonialism. On the contrary, through their fat bodies, Marlow criticizes the men's inability to carry out colonialist projects in the best way possible: "Marlow's most often-voiced complaint against the imperialist project is the inefficiency and laziness of its white participants, rather than its violence and cultural annihilation."[37] Jennifer Brown makes a similar observation, claiming: "It is not that the idea of imperialism is wrong but rather the way that it is imposed."[38] Marlow thus does not disapprove of colonialism, as it might seem through his at times empathetic thoughts on the dying locals, for example, but rather he disapproves of certain methods and ways it is carried out. While he might be interpreted as *"white, but not quite,"*[39] to rephrase Homi Bhabha, for his attempts to sympathize with the locals or recognize humanity in them, he remains a colonizer and a racist throughout the novella.

In turn, the slim body of the colonized is a direct sign of oppression. Certainly, the exhausted bodies of the exploited people reflect the way the colonized were treated by colonizers. But the images of slim white women in Europe can be effectively juxtaposed with the images of colonized people to understand how the physical state of the body can emerge as a signifier of oppression. Of course, the abuse that the colonized populations experienced cannot be compared with the inconvenience of tight corsets that were so fashionable in the nineteenth century, yet colonialism and fashion were two ways through which white patriarchy could abuse certain groups of people. In *Victorian Literature and the Anorexic Body*, Anna Krugovoy Silver accentuates: "Victorian conduct literature consistently reinforces the idea of beauty as woman's special duty and domain."[40] It was impressed on a woman that being beautiful – which could, to a considerable degree, be achieved with the help of a fashionable dress – was one of her key goals. And while fashion had been changing throughout the nineteenth century, having a thin body (including with the help of a corset) was always fashionable: "Even those writers at the end of the century who wrote against tight lacing or corseting in general, in favor of a more 'natural' appearance took care to differentiate a fashionable fullness from 'downright vulgar' fatness."[41] Tight corsets, however, not only made female bodies look beautiful but they also made them unhealthy, transforming them in a dreadful manner. For example, "preventing the ingestion of food, stay laces created many starving women."[42] The slim body was thus the sign of oppression, as shown both through the instances of abuse, exploitation, and emasculation of men in the colonies, and through promoting gender inequality in Europe. The slim body emerges as a weak, feminized body, making the fat body, despite certain drawbacks, be the sign of power, stability, prosperity, and superiority.

Cannibalism and the Appetite Metaphor

Through the body, the issue of hunger and appetite are evoked in the novella both explicitly (for food) and implicitly (for the land, its resources, and wealth). The very process of consumption is discussed in *Heart of Darkness* not only through overfed and undernourished bodies and colonialism as a practice of robbing someone, but also, and perhaps even more vividly, through the issue of cannibalism. Brown underlines cannibalism as an effective tool through which "racism, degeneration, ideological ambivalence, and orality"[43] are explored and pinpointed in the novella. Yet it is through cannibalism, I argue, that *Heart of Darkness* continues to explore the consumerist nature of colonialism, drawing on the issues of hunger, appetite, and the body.

The cannibals that Marlow meets on his journey are interpreted by him in a rather positive light. First of all, Marlow notes: "Fine fellows – cannibals – in their place. They were men one could work with, and I am grateful to them."[44] Such a view (although evidently racist, for the cannibals are good only when they are "in their place") largely contrasts with Marlow's perception of the white men in the colony, who are fat, lazy, slow, and incompetent. Yet, an even more ambiguous speculation regarding the cannibals is provided later, when Marlow wonders why the cannibals did not eat the white people:

> Why in the name of all the gnawing devils of hunger they didn't go for us – they were thirty to five – and have a good tuck-in for once, amazes me now when I think of it. They were big powerful men, with not much capacity to weigh the consequences, with courage, with strength, even yet, though their skins were no longer glossy and their muscles no longer hard. And I saw that something restraining, one of those human secrets that baffle probability, had come into play there. I looked at them with a swift quickening of interest – not because it occurred to me I might be eaten by them before very long, though I own to you that just then I perceived – in a new light, as it were – how unwholesome the pilgrims looked, and I hoped, yes, I positively hoped, that my aspect was not so – what shall I say? – so unappetizing.[45]

Retelling his encounter with the cannibals, Marlow primarily focuses on the bodies of the people. The cannibals are described as "big powerful men" despite, what Marlow believes to be, their lower mental abilities and rather weary bodies. Compared with these men, the white men look "unwholesome," which for Marlow is perhaps the lack of physical strength as a result of their fat complexions. The body of the cannibal is celebrated as a beautiful body, whereas the white man's body is characterized as shameful. Marlow even puts his own appearance into question, wondering if he is as "unappetizing" (read: fat and weak) as his fellows.

The desire to be like a local seems to intensify the deeper Marlow goes into the jungle. And this desire is realized through Kurtz who, as Marlow soon finds out, has managed to become the leader of the cannibals. As Marlow goes deep into the jungle, the image of the fat body disappears completely. He discovers the place where Kurtz lives, which is surrounded by human heads. Marlow describes one of such heads as follows: "[A]nd there it was, black, dried, sunken, with closed eyelids – a head that seemed to sleep at the top of that pole, and, with the shrunken dry lips showing a narrow white line of the teeth, was smiling, too, smiling continuously at some endless and jocose dream of that eternal slumber."[46] The dryness of the head reinforces the ascetic nature of the locality, the locals, and Kurtz. As Marlow finally meets Kurtz, his attention is drawn to the body of the man: "He looked at least 7 feet long. His covering had fallen off, and his body emerged from it pitiful and appalling as from a winding-sheet. I could see the cage of his ribs all astir, the bones of his arm waving ... I saw him open his mouth wide – it gave him a weirdly voracious aspect, as though he had wanted to swallow all the air, all the earth, all the men before him."[47]

While intensifying the thinness of the bodies in the jungles, the novella powerfully comments on consumerism. Hunger becomes the central issue: the colonizers are hungry for ivory that brings them wealth and consequently *fat* on their bodies; the cannibals are literally hungry for food. Yet it is crucial that while the colonizers rob the people and the land, abusing and murdering everyone on their way, the cannibals show a striking power to control their hunger, by not attacking the white men. Marlow, himself a colonizer and thus with an appetite for what does not belong to him, is bewildered and practically offended that he is not *appetizing* enough for the cannibals. Brown notes: "In a novel so concerned with appetites, this restraint is highly valued."[48] It is valued, I argue, not only because through it the novella holds back on dehumanizing the locals but also because it helps reinforce the horrifying, monstrous nature of colonialism. Indeed, cannibalism seems to be rather trivial compared with the atrocities committed by the white colonizers.

Cannibalism becomes a metaphor for consumption. Brown, for example, notes that "the land itself is described as cannibalistic, swallowing intruders into its darkness."[49] At the same time, "colonialism itself [is] … a cannibalistic system, devouring territories and races, as well as the morals of its supporters."[50] Both Marlow and Kurtz are the representatives of cannibalistic colonialism. For them, the locals are genderless, ageless, and nationless beings.[51] Indeed, as Brown correctly observes, "Marlow attributes more human characteristics to the jungle than to the natives."[52] Kurtz in particular is the most horrifying character. Having merged with the locals, he has become their leader, exercising his colonial superiority. He, in the words of Brown, is "[t]he ideal imperialist with an appetite for success, ivory, and profit, his appetite overpowers him and becomes an appetite for Africa itself."[53] Indeed, Marlow's description of Kurtz's wide-open mouth overtly hints at this slim man's great appetite. Kurtz is "a more terrifying cannibal who, unlike the native cannibals, displays an inexhaustible desire to eat everything."[54] And it is this goal of "absolute consumption" that does not allow Kurtz (and colonizers in general) to fully "satisfy [his] desire."[55] Cannibalism is a particularly effective prism through which to look at colonialism because of the relationship between the cannibal and its victim. John P. Anderson specifies: "Cannibals treat their human victims as objects, dehumanize them, refuse to grant them value as spiritual beings."[56] Essentially, this is how colonizers treat colonized peoples and lands. In its discussion of colonization and consumerism, however, *Heart of Darkness* continuously evokes the image of the body. The image of the fat body becomes an important symbol through which the novella both celebrates colonialism and condemns certain actions of colonialists. It is crucial that cannibalism (i.e., the lifestyle of the locals) becomes the force that destroys Kurtz. He becomes, in the words of Marlow, "mad."[57] His body is physically degraded, judging by his bony appearance. And it is pivotal that, despite the evident horrors of colonialism, *Heart of Darkness* manages to veil the "shameful reality of European behaviour" and instead foregrounds the "idea of what is evil and hell" as exclusively "African."[58] The image of Kurtz's unhealthy body, curiously enough, helps reinforce the power of the fat male body. The interaction with the locals and life in the jungles exhaust and destroy Kurtz's body. Kurtz's fate suggests that the colonial environment can ruin the colonizer's healthy (fat) body and thus must be conquered, subjugated, and transformed.

Conclusion

In consuming food, we do more than merely satisfy our hunger. In *Carnal Appetites: FoodSexIdentities*, Elspeth Probyn argues that "in eating we find ourselves in various assemblages, produced and producing ourselves anew."[59] To a large degree, eating shapes our bodies. What we consume, in which portions, and how often greatly influences the appearance of our bodies. Consumption in general is what makes the body look as it does. The fat body, being often associated with wealth, stability, and prosperity for much of the nineteenth century, was the body that stood for power. It is, as I have demonstrated in this chapter, one of the most evocative symbols of colonialism in Joseph Conrad's *Heart of Darkness*, illustrating the economic, political, and cultural potency of the invaders, as contrasted to the powerlessness of the colonized. In the novella, the fat body is both celebrated and judged. Curiously, some scholars claim that today's associations of fatness with such qualities as being "lazy, gluttonous, lacking willpower, primitive" stems from the nineteenth-century interpretation of the term as "a key sign of the barbarism and primitivism of an inferior people."[60] Moreover, because of this, the fat body is frequently associated with "the African and … the homosexual."[61] *Heart of Darkness*, however, uses the fat body to discuss certain flaws of white male colonizers, and never the locals. In doing so, the novella generates stigma about fatness and contributes to the ongoing public ostracism of corpulent bodies and obesity as such. But its focus on the fat *white* body helps explicate the mechanisms and ramifications of colonialism and imperialism. The fat body thus becomes the prism through which to understand the horrifying policies through which colonialism was exercised, bringing wealth, i.e., *fat*, to colonizers, and depriving the colonized of what belonged to them and even more. Being fat, according to the novella, is what defined the *well-fed* culture of colonialism.

NOTES

1 Chinua Achebe, "An Image of Africa: Racism in Conrad's 'Heart of Darkness,'" *The Massachusetts Review* 57, no. 1 (2016): 21. Accessed on 7 July 2022. https://www.jstor.org/stable/43821495.
2 Achebe, "An Image of Africa," 21.
3 Achebe, "An Image of Africa," 22.
4 Achebe, "An Image of Africa," 23.
5 Achebe, "An Image of Africa," 26.
6 Joseph Conrad, *Heart of Darkness*, 1899 (London: Arcturus, 2017), 16.
7 Jennifer Brown, *Cannibalism in Literature and Film* (London: Palgrave Macmillan, 2013), 33.
8 Conrad, *Heart of Darkness*, 29.
9 Conrad, *Heart of Darkness*, 41.

10 Conrad, *Heart of Darkness*, 51.
11 Conrad, *Heart of Darkness*, 43.
12 Conrad, *Heart of Darkness*, 30.
13 Conrad, *Heart of Darkness*, 31.
14 For more on the relationship between colonialism and the body, please consult the chapters in this collection written by Amy Shaw, Nsima Udo, and Bonnie Miller.
15 Conrad, *Heart of Darkness*, 32.
16 Conrad, *Heart of Darkness*, 40–1.
17 Conrad, *Heart of Darkness*, 15.
18 Conrad, *Heart of Darkness*, 22.
19 Conrad, *Heart of Darkness*, 24.
20 Conrad, *Heart of Darkness*, 24.
21 Conrad, *Heart of Darkness*, 26.
22 Conrad, *Heart of Darkness*, 26–7.
23 Conrad, *Heart of Darkness*, 11.
24 Conrad, *Heart of Darkness*, 23.
25 Leslie Heywood, *Dedication to Hunger: The Anorexic Aesthetic in Modern Culture* (Berkeley: University of California Press, 1996), 122.
26 Debrah Raschke, *Modernism, Metaphysics, and Sexuality* (Selinsgrove: Susquehanna University Press, 2006), 78.
27 Heywood, *Dedication to Hunger*, 114.
28 Heywood, *Dedication to Hunger*, 114.
29 Christopher E. Forth, *Fat: A Cultural History of the Stuff of Life* (London: Reaktion Books, 2019), 34.
30 Sander L. Gilman, *Fat: A Cultural History of Obesity* (Cambridge: Polity, 2008), 4.
31 Heywood, *Dedication to Hunger*, 121.
32 Heywood, *Dedication to Hunger*, 123.
33 Roberta Pollack Seid qtd. in Heywood, *Dedication to Hunger*, 123.
34 Conrad, *Heart of Darkness*,14.
35 Conrad, *Heart of Darkness*, 32.
36 Raschke, *Modernism, Metaphysics, and Sexuality*, 78.
37 Heywood, *Dedication to Hunger*, 123.
38 Brown, *Cannibalism in Literature and Film*, 32.
39 Homi Bhabha, "Of Mimicry and Man: The Ambivalence of Colonial Discourse," *October* 28 (1984): 126, 130, italics in original. Accessed on 20 January 2020. https://www.jstor.org/stable/778467.
40 Anna Krugovoy Silver, *Victorian Literature and the Anorexic Body* (Cambridge: Cambridge University Press, 2004) 29.
41 Silver, *Victorian Literature and the Anorexic Body*, 34.

42 Laurence Talairach-Vielmas, *Moulding the Female Body in Victorian Fairy Tales and Sensation Novels* (Aldershot: Ashgate, 2007), 37.
43 Brown, *Cannibalism in Literature and Film*, 34.
44 Conrad, *Heart of Darkness*, 45.
45 Conrad, *Heart of Darkness*, 52.
46 Conrad, *Heart of Darkness*, 70.
47 Conrad, *Heart of Darkness*, 72.
48 Brown, *Cannibalism in Literature and Film*, 36.
49 Brown, *Cannibalism in Literature and Film*, 34.
50 Brown, *Cannibalism in Literature and Film*, 34.
51 Brown, *Cannibalism in Literature and Film*, 36.
52 Brown, *Cannibalism in Literature and Film*, 37.
53 Brown, *Cannibalism in Literature and Film*, 41.
54 Brown, *Cannibalism in Literature and Film*, 41.
55 Peter Hulme, "Introduction: The Cannibal Scene," in *Cannibalism and the Colonial World*, ed. Francis Barker, Peter Hulme, and Margaret Iversen (Cambridge: Cambridge University Press, 1998), 36.
56 John P. Anderson, *Conrad's* Heart of Darkness*: Rebirth of Tragedy* (Boca Raton: Universal Publishers, 2005), 44.
57 Conrad, *Heart of Darkness*, 80.
58 Brown, *Cannibalism in Literature and Film*, 38.
59 Elspeth Probyn, *Carnal Appetites: FoodSexIdentities* (London: Routledge, 2000), 4.
60 Amy Erdman Farrell, *Fat Shame: Stigma and the Fat Body in American Culture* (New York: New York University Press, 2011), 173.
61 Farrell, *Fat Shame: Stigma and the Fat Body in American Culture*, 173.

8 Visualizing the Body: The *Mbopo* Ritual and the Politics of Fatness in Southern Nigeria in the Late Nineteenth and Early Twentieth Centuries

NSIMA UDO

Among the Ibibio/Efik of southern Nigeria, fatness represented physical, spiritual, psychological, and material wellness. While there were different rituals about fattening and seclusion for men and women, this study centres on the mbopo ritual, a cultural institution and a rite of passage for young women, who were secluded, circumcised, fattened, and pampered for anywhere between three months and three years, as part of traditional preparation for marriage in the late nineteenth and early part of the twentieth century.[1]

This study analyses fatness as an inclusive, multilayered, political tool and ritual phenomenon that signified feminine spirituality, morality, etiquette, character, and vocation.[2] This is represented by the different kinds of corporeal and extra-corporeal activities (and their spiritual significations) that went on in the mbopo seclusion space. Further, I consider mbopo ritual as an educational space, where the expected bride was temporarily removed from familiar persons and activities and secluded for the purpose of spiritual immersion and cultural education. Mbopo ritual points to the ways in which society tries to control the sexuality of young women. For the Ibibio/Efik, the mbopo fattening ritual was also seen as an attempt to preserve the particularity and uniqueness of each local community, in the face of scarcity and the challenge of survival.[3]

This study defines the mbopo institution as a transitional space, a site of bodily and personal transformation, and a ritual of an "inclusive" fattening. Through a close study of documents and a visual analysis of photographs from the historical texts of early anthropologists, more recent works in ethnography and art history, and selected photographs and documentary films, this chapter tracks a "visual narrative" that points to the politicization of fat and the "inscriptions of the past"[4] in the changing history of the mbopo ritual. I take very seriously the ways in which visual sources have a privileged space of recreating a sense of the ritual and its symbolic meanings, in relation to some eccentric narratives of fat and its cultural representations by colonial anthropologists.

Pre-colonial Nigeria was riddled with diverse forms of inter-tribal relations, cultural affinities, and political and religious tensions among people with a wide range of heterogeneity. The almost 250 ethnic groups, who spoke about 500 languages, travelled, traded, and warred among themselves to establish independent chiefdoms and kingdoms across the four corners of the country. The intrusion of the West by European explorers, traders, missionaries, and political overlords culminated in the British colonialism of the nineteenth century. Through trade contacts, Christian evangelizations, missionary/colonial education projects, and colonial officiations and officialdoms, the English language came to be widely introduced into Nigeria.[5] By the beginning of the twentieth century, the English language had become a homogenizing apparatus that unified the once heterogenous enclave into an amalgamated political bloc.

While the western world was experiencing a form of *corporeal transition* in the long nineteenth century – "a change in body ideals,"[6] in which corpulence was seen as ugly and pathological,[7] corpulence came to be seen as desirable in Africa, north, south, and west: as a symbol of aesthetics, bodily wellness, and a measure of spiritual agility.[8] In Cameroun, Mauritania, Ivory Coast, Niger, several regions in Nigeria, and a host of other African communities, "body ideals are still very important" aspects of aestheticizing of the body, and rituals of fattening are deliberate markers driven by the mechanisms of culture. For instance, Rebecca Popenoe's study among the Nigerien Arabs in Niger in the 1990s found that the village Arabs forcefully fed their children with lots of milk and millet from a very tender age so as to develop voluptuous bodies that would be ideal for early puberty.[9]

While the motivation for deliberate rituals of fattening among Africans differs, this chapter asserts that among the Ibibio/Efik people, the "pathologizing discourse"[10] of fatness and the "lipophobic" obsession of contemporary society did not exist.[11] Rather, the Ibibio/Efik conceptualized fatness as a symbol of spiritual, emotional, sociocultural, and corporeal aesthetics and well-being. This traditional ritual of "fatness" came to be challenged during the colonial period in Nigeria by missionaries and government officials and later by the Nigerian government itself in the post-independence era. It became a contested site of internal cultural politics, not least because of the female circumcision associated with the ritual.

In the traditional Ibibio/Efik culture of southern Nigeria, as in other African societies, girls who were attested by traditional matriarchs to be chaste before marriage were viewed with pride. They were celebrated through a ritual of fattening in the mbopo institution. Those who these matrons claimed were not chaste were barred from participating in the mbopo fattening ritual and stigmatized with pejorative names and folksongs.[12] Among the Ibibio/Efik men, marrying a fattened mbopo bride engendered social and political status and instituted patriarchal autonomy.[13] This was predicated on the belief that a fattened bride represented sacredness, status, and aesthetics, thereby engendering ancestral and spiritual connection, social acceptability, fertility, and wealth.[14]

Spiritual Initiation

In the late nineteenth and early twentieth centuries, mbopo still had a deep sense of secrecy and spiritual mystery and a degree of vibrancy. The ritual was described in great detail by pioneering ethnographer Dorothy A. Talbot in her study, *Woman's Mysteries of a Primitive People: The Ibibio of Southern Nigeria* in 1914. While there are of course theoretical limitations in ethnographic studies produced on Africa in this early period, Talbot was able, in a way not possible for male counterparts like her husband, Nigerian colonial officer Percy Talbot, to gain access to the stories and sites of this women's secret ritual. I lean on her ethnography although I am assessing it from a critical perspective, particularly in my rereading of the photographs included in this work.

Certain forms of corporeal requirements were needed before initiates could pass through the fattening seclusion and its intended spiritual immersion. Before initiation, a girl had to attain certain forms of corporeal maturation. "The coming of the new and full breast," referred to as *mbobi*[15] was a sign of puberty and was one of the major considerations for a girl's participation in the pre-nuptial seclusion rite. Thereafter, intense ritual practices preceded the actual admission of the initiate into the seclusion space. For coastal communities, "sacred streams or rivers," believed to be inhabited by "naiads," (water goddesses) were revered.[16] Thus, the seclusion rite began with the initiate being led down to the edge of the stream where prayers and sacrifices were offered to the "naiads" for their protection and the success of the ritual process.[17] For some communities in the hinterlands, spiritual consecration for the initiates were conducted at the centre of the village, where old trees were special sites set aside and revered as shrines inhabited by divinities, ancestors, and other spiritual guardians. These streams and trees were carefully managed to evoke the aura of an enduring presence of these deities.[18] The streams and tree shrines were believed to possess cleansing, invigorating, and fertilizing powers for the initiates. Here, sacrifices and prayers were made to their ancestors and other divinities, asking for help and guidance for the initiate.

For the Ibibio/Efik, fatness represented fertility and symbolized an expected increase in productivity in farming. The mbopo fattening ritual was usually observed before a new planting season began, to draw blessings of fertility and productivity for new crops that could benefit the initiate, the expected new family she represented, and the community at large.[19] The success of the seclusion and fattening rite was tied to the idea that the ritual was overseen and sanctioned by deities and ancestors, who were perceived as spiritual custodians and a source of succour for individual families and the community.[20]

Unlike Egyptian women, who "performed arts of fattening" to satisfy their "male's desire for the fleshiest and the fattest of women,"[21] the mbopo fattening ritual had strong spiritual connotations expressed through animal sacrifices and libations up to the early part of the twentieth century.[22] Dorothy Talbot observed that "from a cord round the neck of each of the initiates dangled a live chicken, freely fluttering against the bare brown breasts of its bearer."[23] These kinds of ritual aesthetics were items of animal sacrifice used as a spiritual channel to consecrate the initiates to their deities and ancestors.[24] Another colonial anthropologist, Mervyn Jeffreys, described the mbopo outing ceremony, which marked the conclusion of the fattening rite and seclusion period and the presentation of the initiate in a public ceremony, as overwhelmingly grounded in Ibibio/Efik spirituality. He describes how the arena for *urua mbopo* (the market square for the outing ceremony) included shrines and altars to different ancestral deities, and was arrayed with different concoctions used as mediums for spiritual invocation. Mbopo initiates were dressed with ritual materials hanging around their necks and their ankles were decorated with a newly hatched white chicken "still fluttering, their wings having been partly severed through the neck with a knife."[25] These were animal sacrifices used as spiritual insignias to consecrate the initiates before and after fattening seclusion, and to appease the ancestors, seeking their support during the ceremony.

Two "fattening house women" (Figures 8.1 and 8.2) are among forty-four images that Dorothy Talbot used in her text *Woman's Mysteries of a Primitive People*, to illustrate the so-called esoteric practices of the Ibibio women.[26] The photographs use both frontal and side portrait techniques, which were part of the language of ethnographic and anthropological photography of the time.[27] The two photos are different scenes

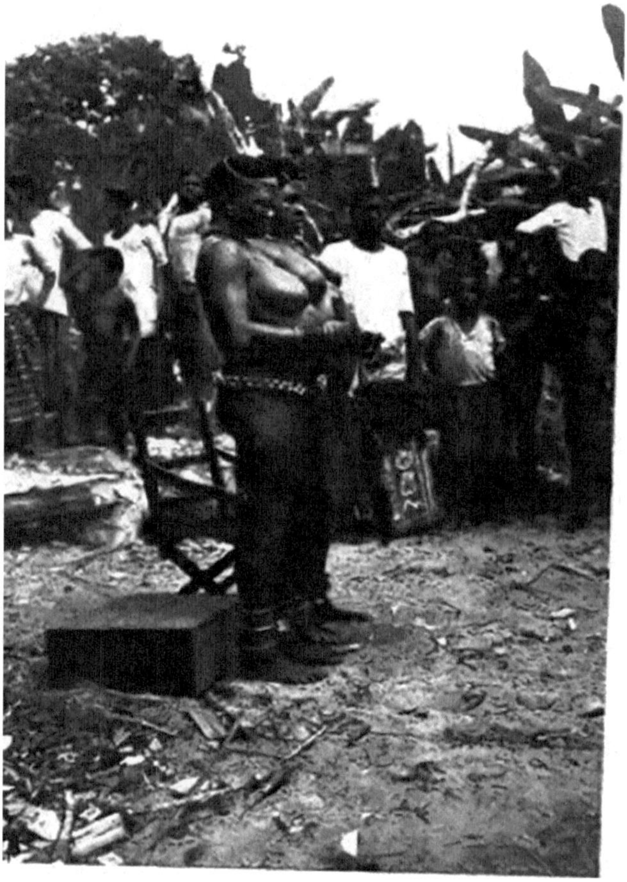

Figure 8.1. "Fattening House Women": circa 1914, photographs from D.A. Talbot, *Woman's Mysteries,* frontispiece.

taken on the same occasion. The initiates in the centre frame (Figure 8.1) appear half naked and viewed from the side, embodying signs of their recent seclusion. Their oily skins and plump bodies resonate with the "fattening house" appellation. These photographs present the viewer with a mix of dressed and undressed people, a sign of cultural hybridization.[28] The initiates face the camera with an apathetic look and have very few decorated ornaments. No specific analysis accompanies the photos in Talbot's text except for the captions. Talbot's photographs are used to illustrate, and to reinforce a reading of, how "fattening house women" looked in the early decades of the twentieth century.

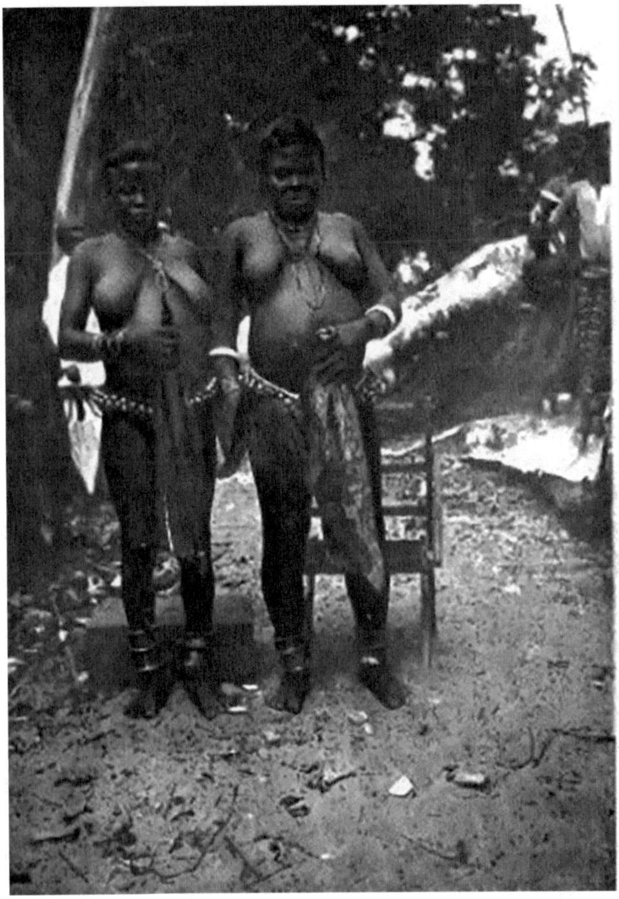

Figure 8.2. "Fattening House Women" circa 1914, photographs from D.A. Talbot, *Woman's Mysteries*, frontispiece.

The frontal view of this photograph (Figure 8.2) engages our attention. It reveals the rounded stomachs and rotund breasts of the initiates that foreground their experience of having been fattened up in their seclusion space. The armchair and the box in the background symbolize the moment of honour when the fattened initiates would take a sitting position at the centre of the market square. In the patriarchal and endogamous Ibibio/Efik society of the nineteenth century, this sitting position represented prestige and honour for the initiates.[29] The box could be an improvised seat provided for the younger initiates, to depict the seniority of the elder initiate who might sit on the armchair in a more exalted position. The fattened girl on the right side in the photograph is bigger and taller, and she appears to be the elder of the two initiates. Their facial resemblance suggests that they may be sisters or relatives, perhaps from the same polygamous family. During the early twentieth century, it was customary to find two or more sisters or relatives being secluded at the same time, perhaps for the purpose of managing resources and organizing time.[30]

The photographs reveal certain commonalities that were inherent in Ibibio/Efik cultural practices. They help us to visualize and historicize the sociocultural dynamic that materialized within the mbopo fattening practices in the Ibibio/Efik nation. The metallic leg bands, waist beads, and hand-held cloths that serve as flywhisks, were status symbols.[31] They were also used for bodily beautification at the time.[32] The sparse ornamentation of the "fattening house women" in these photographs, compared with other photographs of mbopo initiates of the 1890s, indicates their relatively modest economic situation.[33] At the same time, it points to the high value and worth that was attached to the mbopo seclusion rite up until the first few decades of the twentieth century as a female rite that should be upheld regardless of one's economic circumstances.[34]

Inside the Seclusion Chamber

After intense spiritual immersion, the initiates were admitted into the seclusion room. Talbot did not gain access into this intimate space. The popular perception of mbopo seclusion among societies outside the Ibibio/Efik cultural circle is that it was particularly a "fattening" ritual that concentrated on the corporeal alone, as mirrored in the "fattening house women" captions. But fattening-up, which was broadly symbolic, was just one of the activities the initiate went through in her seclusion. While the fattening process symbolized corporeal beautification and spirituality in Ibibioland and other parts of Africa, weight consciousness grew in the West with divergent interpretations. On the one hand was a "pathologizing [of] corpulence as ugliness, gluttony … vices of the intemperate."[35] Fat was at "the least unattractive and inconvenient but in all likelihood a positive danger as well," and resulted in "declining social prestige."[36] On the other hand, some westerners of this period perceived corpulence as "an inherited trait," a sign of good composition and a marker for inward rectitude and virtue."[37] In 1914, Talbot asserted that the Ibibio/Efik thought of the mbopo fattening ritual as necessary for the overall well-being of the initiate.[38]

Such positive views among the Ibibio/Efik persisted well into the twentieth century, even as attitudes toward the fat body became increasingly negative in much of the rest of the English-speaking world. John and Betty Messenger's ethnographic study of the 1950s, for example, shows that among the Ibibio/Efik communities, corpulence was perceived as a mark of good health, longevity, and successful childbearing.[39] Fattening was deemed necessary because it was thought to create broader hips and a larger birth canal so babies could be delivered more easily.[40] In a society where the threat of mortality at birth was high, where laborious farming activities were the bedrock of the subsistence economy, and where women were active in farming, fattening was conceived as a way to protect the would-be bride. It was also a kind of a premarital "bridal holiday" for the expected bride, and a preserving mechanism for the particularity and uniqueness of each local community.[41]

The common assumption in some anthropological literature and the print media is that the mbopo initiates were force-fed to become rotund. While consumption played an important role in the fattening-up process, other practices were believed to have sped up fattening. The Egyptians used warm baths, injecting clysters of bran, sesame oil, and animal fat to cultivate corpulence.[42] The mbopo initiates were made to lie on a wooden bed made with rounded bamboo or raffia branches without any bed covering.[43] It was believed that the direct contact of the flesh and skin on the hard bamboo bed aided in massaging the flesh of the initiate, thereby breaking up the tissues and opening up the flesh for freshness and fatness. Talbot asserts that miniature bamboo beds and fish racks were hung up as signposts to signify an ongoing seclusion rite in 1914. This practice of the "food and the flesh" being channels through which corpulence could be achieved endured into the early decades of the twentieth century.[44] Furthermore, initiates were massaged daily with local oils and herbs, and with a local chalk-like substance called *ndom*. This was targeted at accentuating fatness in certain parts of the body. Fatness around the hips, the pelvis, the backside, and the chest were the main targets, with an overall corpulence a sign of a successful seclusion.[45]

Massaging the body of the initiate was perceived by the Ibibio/Efik as a process of softening, breaking up, and remodelling the initiate corporeally. When combined with other corporeal practices within the seclusion space, it translated into an "emotional, intellectual, and spiritual reshaping and refining until she (the initiate) emerges as the ideal."[46] They also point to the carefully orchestrated attention the

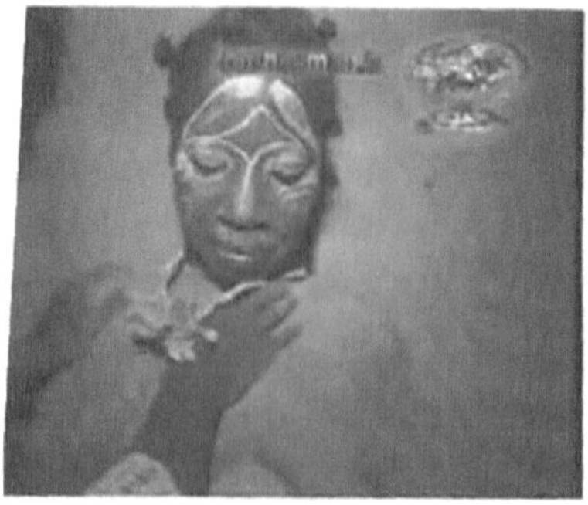
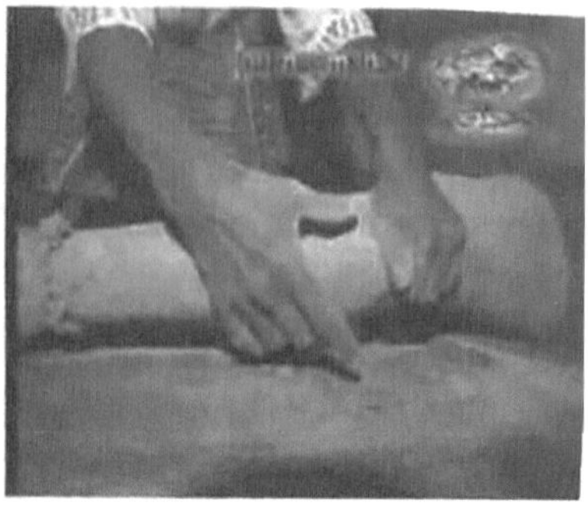

Figures 8.3 and 8.4. Young mbopo initiate being massaged with white chalk and herbs. Source: Imeh, *Daughters of Seclusion* (2012).

initiates received at the hands of traditional matriarchs through massaging. The massager's hand was to follow a certain trajectory across the body: from the leg area through to the hips and up to the chest and back. The synchronizing movement of the massager's hands reveals the energy, attentiveness, and importance of massaging as a complementary ritual to assist the flesh in gaining weight. It was also meant to help tone the flesh and to enhance a sound psychological self-image during seclusion. Local chalks and other herbal concoctions were used in this process as a form of "softening, breaking-up and rebuilding" the initiates so that they would emerge as beautiful women (Figures 8.3 and 8.4).[47]

The weight increase of mbopo initiates during seclusion was treated as evidence of the beauty of character, ethical formation, and the creative ideas that the initiate had acquired. Fatness therefore embodied the high moral standards, social etiquette, and work prowess that the initiate was expected to garner during the rite. Great care and effort were taken to ensure that the initiate was made fat through sumptuous feeding and massaging.[48] As well, other complementary rituals were advanced to articulate fatness as an all-inclusive and multilayered extra-corporeal and ethical outcome of a fattened bride. These included lessons on beauty treatments, and in ethics and social education. Thus, in addition to fattening, the initiates were taught the art of self-beautification by experienced matrons: self-beautification that would enhance their self-image, and at the same time would make them attractive to their husbands and wider community.

Skin care and decorative hairdos were important aspects of the ritual of fattening and beautification. Skin care was seen to be a very important aspect of the ritual, considering the harsh weather and environmental conditions of the tropical rainforest region that women were exposed to while farming.[49] Ornamental coiffures were also part of the practice and performance of feminine beautification, of identities and status representation, and symbols of spiritual power and connectivity.[50] Nsentip Udeme asserts that, for the Ibibio/Efik people, hairdos invoked meaning in terms of Indigenous identities and showcased creativity and skills. Hairstyles such as *mkpuk eba* (new breasts), *eba nkaifere* (full breasts), *Idet ubot* (hand weaving without artificial extensions), *effiom Inyang* (crocodile), *wobo* (gather into one bunch), or *ibuot ekong* (the head of a warrior) were expressions of love, sexuality, status, identity, and the aura of extravagance that surrounded the mbopo institution up to the early decades of the twentieth century.[51]

Scarification, tattooing and skin decoration with chalks, dyes, and special herbs, as well as clitoridectomies were also prominent bodily practices that carried strong ritual and spiritual connotations. Up until the 1930s, clitoridectomies were performed in the first part of the seclusion period in some communities. Scarification came immediately after circumcision. This was done to allow the skin incisions to heal along with the cut on the clitoris, which were treated with herbal concoctions.[52] Circumcision was believed to improve fertility and aid childbearing.[53] In relation to the fattening process, circumcision was also conceived as a mechanism for social value: a symbolic bodily inscription for the celebrated virgin girl – and as "the sign of a blameless maidenhood."[54]

Facial scarification was not elaborate, but it was strategically placed: in dotted or pinched scars on both cheeks or at the side of the eye. These were referred to as *ntoi uyai* (beautiful dots).[55] *Ntoi uyai* came along with elaborate skin decoration with designs made with *ndom* and *odung* (local dyes and chalks), signifying birth status through particular motifs. Skin decorations and inscriptions, which were believed to contribute to enhancing the overall beauty and softness of the skin, endured across the century. They were not permanent tattoos, but temporary skin inscriptions with local dyes. They were consistently but intermittently inscribed, and later washed off during occasions of celebrating the bride. This happened during the mbopo seclusion, pregnancy and post-natal treatments, and during other women's rituals.[56]

Social Induction and Intellectual Robustness

The fattening seclusion was a comprehensive learning space as well as a corporeal experience. The mbopo initiate was expected to learn special values and skills while in the "fattening room." These skills and values epitomized her social and intellectual robustness, which was in turn thought to enhance her effectiveness as wife and mother, energize her socializing skills, and empower her economically to connect with the rest of the community efficiently.[57] The political economy of the Ibibio/Efik society of the early twentieth century demanded an elaborate form of learning that went on in what I interpret as an educational bedchamber. These practices probably started well before the late nineteenth century and continuously endured into the second quarter of the twentieth century. These were among the "woman's mysteries" that Dorothy Talbot and Mervyn Jeffreys encountered in the 1910s and 1920s, as described earlier. The anthropologist John Messenger also documented these rituals, particularly those relating to sexuality, in the 1950s. The fattened body he argued, aestheticized "sexual politics." As wives to be, the initiates were taught about sex: sexual mannerisms and tonal "romantic" gestures to excite and please their husbands. "Sexual education and techniques" were transmitted to the initiates in the seclusion chamber based in part on the belief that women were the repository of sexual knowledge. They were expected to know about sex so they could pass this knowledge on to their husbands.[58]

Within the seclusion bedchamber, initiates were also told how to manage the outcome of pregnancy. Though there were professional midwives called *abia uman,* the seclusion rite offered the initiate some basic knowledge on how to manage pregnancy and childbirth. Messenger, Brink, Imeh, and Akpapan all highlight the fact that the mbopo ritual and the fattening process prepared initiates for fertility, conception, delivery, and the successful suckling of their babies.[59] While the Ibibio/Efik believed that an ample female figure was necessary for fertility and eventually breastfeeding their offspring, the mbopo initiate was also taught that certain herbs and practices could reduce labour pains or induce milk secretion for lactation.[60] Fatness was seen as a gynaecological apparatus for easy conception, delivery, and suckling for the newborn.

The Ibibio/Efik attached great importance to fertility and still do. Another form of seclusion, a fattening ritual known as *nwo-nwo*, was prescribed as a spiritual healing process to ward off evil spirits that hindered conception and to appease the deities to respond favourably to the needs of the barren.[61] Fattening was also perceived as a "physiological panacea" to cure a married woman diagnosed with infertility.[62] The mbopo rite then offered the expected bride a site for sex education and fertility induction before marriage. Because nutrition played a central role in the fattening-up process of the mbopo initiate, she had the privilege of feasting daily on sumptuous and delicious meals like *ekpang nkukwo, afia afere ebot* etc. which are rich in starch, vegetables, seafood, and animal protein. Furthermore, since the Ibibio/Efik attach great importance to what they eat and how it is cooked, the initiates were given culinary lessons by an experienced elderly woman on the technicalities of preparing these local meals.[63] For the Ibibio/Efik, food, nutrition, and sex were interlinked, and culinary interest continues to be deeply entrenched within the fabric of their sociocultural economy.

The period of seclusion also allowed the initiates to learn and develop artistry. The "fattening rooms" were centres for arts.[64] This vocational training and the type of crafts they learned were culturally specific, depending on the communities to which they belonged. For example, some groups specialized in basket weaving, or clay wall and floor painting. Others were skilled in making raffia mats, cloths, and roofing rafts.[65] The Efiks specialized in comb making, embroidery, and making symbolic cloth called *mbufari*. Robert Thompson asserts that *mbufari* cloth originated from initiates' innovations during seclusion and dated from before the nineteenth century. Such embroidery art highlights Ibibio/Efik cultural and artistic skills that utilized colours and patterns, and a decorative *nsibidi* ideogram and motifs (Figure 8.5) to depict feminine artisanship, fertility, grandeur, autonomy, and power within the Ibibio/Efik social economy.[66]

Other forms of cultural education and literacy also went on within the seclusion chamber. Initiates received lessons in folklore, folksongs, and stories that carried strands of history, fetishized ethical taboos, moral lessons, and cultural literacy. *Nsibidi,* a highly secretive hieroglyphic form of writing specific to southeast Nigeria, which was particularly popular with powerful male groups like *ekpe, ngbe,* and *ekpo* men's societies, also resonated with mbopo ritual.[67] Several recent scholars assert that mbopo initiates received some measure of literacy in *nsibidi,* a form of hieroglyphic writing and reading, from experienced elderly women: a robust form of Indigenous intellectuality.[68]

The image in Figure 8.5 is used by Imoh Imeh to analyse the artistic literacy and "practices that reveal female agency in learning and reproducing important designs" within mbopo fattening ritual spaces. The image, photographed by Dorothy Talbot's husband Percy in 1912, is repositioned by Imeh to show the aesthetic prowess of mbopo initiates

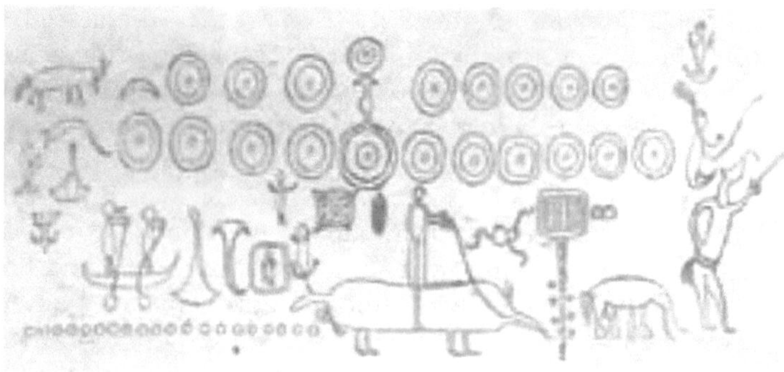

Figure 8.5. *Nsibidi* wall drawing by mbopo initiate, c.1912. Source: Imeh, *Daughters of Seclusion* (2012).

through "youthful rumination and imagination."[69] The mural shows the seclusion space as an engaged and thoughtful space where mbopo initiates undertook reproductive thinking. They were engaged in creative art, body decoration and drawing, and learning and writing the *nsibidi* ideograms.[70]

Mbopo initiates could document their journey in seclusion through murals and writing. The various images in the mural appear as complex symbols, articulating different forms of activities that took place in the society to which the initiate belonged. The men riding on a boat on the left side of the drawing, the different kinds of animals, and the beast of burden in a central position could denote a complex economy based on fishing, farming, hunting, and pastoralism in the initiates' community. The images might also point to the different kinds of culinary "gumbo" that garnished the initiates' meals, with reference to a society that hunted game in the Ibibio/Efik tropical rain forest.[71] The three human images can be said to represent the different kinds of men's masquerade cults, like *ekpo*, *ekpe*, and *ekong*, who were responsible for maintaining social order in the society. These masquerades aestheticized mbopo outing ceremonies, as part of their performing cultural tropes.

The triangular-shaped images and the guitar-type symbol (central-right in the picture) might be references to musical instruments in Ibibio/Efik land. We can discern the *nkruk ubok*, the hand gong, and the *ikon etto*, the xylophone, both of which were important in producing sonorous music for initiates during their outing ceremony.[72] Akpapan and Akpapan have shown how music was used as a form of learning, entertainment, and transmission of moral values to the initiates during seclusion.[73] The mural fuses pictorial images to record the diverse experiences of the initiate during seclusion, and to articulate some of the sociocultural features of the society to which she belonged at that time. While initiates were cosseted and inducted into the art of corporeal beautification and fattening, the fattened body and its sociological outcomes clearly mediated a wide and complex range of spiritual, psychological, aesthetic, affective, and intellectual forms.

Changes, Cultural Continuity, and Challenges

Over the years, the culture of the Ibibio/Efik of southern Nigeria has experienced some dynamic changes and acculturation. Its ideas, customs, philosophy of life, worldview, and social behaviour have been modified, moving away from what were considered as traditional practices and beliefs at the beginning of the nineteenth century – the result of encounters with external forces like colonialism, as well as its own internal dynamics over time, as younger generations were constantly being exposed to western education and the influences of Christianity. The conception of fat and its embodiment in the mbopo ritual has dramatically shifted. In the long nineteenth century, fatness still represented spirituality, status, wellness, and aesthetics. It became an instrument for survival, sustenance, and belonging, with associated political resonance among Ibibio/Efik people. In the later part of the century, the establishment of European rule and the extension of Christianity "demoralized" fat and the mbopo ritual. By the beginning of the twentieth century and after, tension had built up, and fatness began to be pathologized as undesirable and risky.

Nonetheless, certain aspects of this culture remained vibrant, thus producing a modified version that is still being perceived as culturally normative. William Bascom and Melville Herskovits in their edited volume, *Continuity and Change in African Cultures,* analysed the effect of external forces on African cultures, submitting that "there is no African culture which has not been affected in some ways by European contact, and there is none which has entirely given way before it."[74] While African cultures maintain strong residual elements that define their unique identities and connect them with their ancestry, they have been challenged in new and unsettling ways. This complex dynamic is evident from the consolidation of Christianity, with well-established mission stations across Ibibio/Efik land in the 1910s, which saw Indigenous practices and values, including spiritual and cultural beliefs, challenged.[75]

The mbopo fattening ritual was not spared this turmoil. In 1926, Jeffreys reported that the traditional customs of mbopo seclusion and other women's rituals were breaking up under intense missionary pressure. Through missionary education and religious proselytizing, the missions were creating a new clan of young Indigenous literate Christian men and women, who joined them to contest, challenge, and resist the validity and the practice of the fattening rituals.[76] African Christians, following the missionaries, came to represent Indigenous rituals and cultural practices of spirits and ancestors as a "barbarous and hurtful custom." These practices were denounced as markers of paganism and idolatry.[77] The mbopo women's rite was perceived as a ritual invested with animistic and non-theistic beliefs, which allegedly undermined the dignity of women, and was said to be resisted by them.[78] The result was that the mbopo fattening rite was progressively modified. From the first quarter of the twentieth century, European contact, and particularly the proliferating Christianizing project of the western missionaries, led to cultural hybridization within the Ibibio/Efik sociocultural economy.

Apart from the sacrifices and the spiritual connotations of mbopo, other traditional aspects of the rite were also challenged by the missionaries and their converts. For example, mbopo was grounded in certain established ritual forms. Seclusion was specifically designed around *usen ibed*, sacred days and periods for performance of these rites. These also stipulated when the initiate should be unveiled at her outing ceremony. Talbot plausibly insists that significance was attached to the ritual when the initiate enters or emerges from seclusion.[79] This continued up to the 1920s and 1930s. Jeffreys holds that for those Ibibio groups in Ikot Ekpene region, *anantia* season (a stipulated ceremonial period that began around the month of July after the ritual ceremony of *Nyama*, a women's matriarchy cult), was set aside for the initiates to enter into seclusion.[80] Since these days and periods were dedicated to certain deities and localized naiads, Christian converts who were interested in modifying the seclusion rite began to challenge the authenticity of such days and periods.

Among their contentions was their perception that the mbopo seclusion was a harmful process. The epidemiological characterization of fat that had existed in other parts of the English-speaking world, which hitherto had not been part of the Ibibio/Efik social consciousness, began to be championed by the Christian churches. In addition, European missionaries and their African converts claimed that the half-naked parade of initiates associated with mbopo outing ceremonies was a show of uncivilized sensuality and barbarism. Indigenous people countered that fat was an embodiment of social belonging, and that the nakedness of unmarried virgins was a sign of "blameless maidenhood." The missionaries' unrelenting campaign against the fattening ritual and traditional spirituality as "esoteric" uncivilized sacrifices and practices had undermined and irrevocably altered the practice of mbopo by the mid-twentieth century.[81]

The missionary campaigns against mbopo came to be expressed in intergenerational tension within Ibibio/Efik communities. Jeffreys records that between 1926 and 1932, he received several reports by local chiefs who complained that some of their countrymen were not willing to seclude and fatten their children on *anantia*, but proposed instead to celebrate their daughters' seclusion rites over Christmas. They claimed that "it was the Church who altered the season."[82] The Christianization of Indigenous people was therefore slowly modifying Indigenous beliefs and producing a continually changing version of mbopo that tried to accommodate Christian concepts while maintaining some form of Indigenous authenticity. This was not possible without sociocultural tension.

The colonial government and its European agencies supported some of these practices as long as they did not challenge colonial administrative proceedings. This sometimes brought the colonial government into tension with the Church. The Colonial Court was always careful how it mediated over matters that were connected with cultural practices. Jeffereys reports on how, in 1930 and 1931, he was asked by the Nigerian colonial government to write reports on the mbopo seclusion and fattening rite, in response to the petitions forwarded to the central government by the missionaries. His response was that the missionaries' condemnation was a result of them misunderstanding Ibibio/Efik concepts of virginity, fattening, and marriage. The government supported the continuation of the practice, which it perceived as an effective social tool for indirect rule, whereby local chiefs were empowered by the colonial government to keep the people obedient. Upholding aspects of African traditions, and avoiding tensions, was an effort to work with chiefs to consolidate colonial rule and authority.[83] But this effort was not capable of saving the fattening ritual from weakening cultural appreciation and devaluing its spiritual connotations.

As religious acculturation heightened during the late colonial period, the spiritual vibrancy and social rigour of the mbopo seclusion and fattening ritual had begun to wane. In his 1950s study of religious acculturation among the Annang, John Messenger shows the extent of social change in Ibibio/Efik cultural life, particularly in the area of religion. He estimated that in 1951, over half of the population of the Annang, and perhaps the entire Ibibio/Efik, had converted to Christianity. He reveals that some Ibibio/Efik groups preferred to maintain their cultural practices along with their new Christian creed,[84] which hybridized culture and diluted the sociocultural and spiritual energies that Indigenous practices, like the fattening ritual, evoked. These social dynamics remodified indigeneity and allowed the mbopo institution to drift into a practice focused on corporeal aesthetics and the politics of wealth.

Conclusion

The mbopo seclusion and fattening ritual of the Ibibio/Efik people gave attention to corpulence for the purpose of beauty, health, spirituality, social status, and fertility. While in seclusion, other forms of physical wellness and prettification were also emphasized. Initiates received treatments and training on skin and hair enhancing skills, and other forms of ornamental decoration. Nubile virgin girls, who had attained a certain level of maturity, were intentionally secluded, cosseted, and schooled on important components of the Ibibio/Efik sociocultural dynamics. Through a detailed study of documents, and textual and visual materials, I show that colonial ethnographies can be an enormously rich resource for an Africanist reading of the past. While I do not share Dorothy Talbot's framework of this women's ritual, her descriptions and visuals, when read in a different and deeply empathetic way and context, and in relation to other writing, provide a rich resource in understanding African cultures and history. Here, from these colonial ethnographies, I try to tease out a sense of the complexities and the symbolisms of the mbopo fattening ritual: its spirituality, socialization, gender attitudes, ethics, aesthetics, and vocation, in a new Africanist orientation.

Among the Ibibio/Efik, fatness was conceived as a multilayered symbolic representation of a symbiotic relationship between fleshiness, corporeal aesthetics, and different components of the Ibibio/Efik political economy. The ritual of fattening included the performance of corpulence, corporeal beautification, and sociocultural induction in sexual and health education including Indigenous gynaecological practices of managing pregnancy, child conception, labour, and parturition. Initiates received lessons on how to use certain herbs to enhance easy delivery of their babies, and how to induce milk to suckle their young ones. The fattening rite became one avenue through which social order, decency, and the preservation of society, was instituted. It became a celebrative mechanism before marriage for virtuous women.

Significant changes in emphasis regarding these different aspects of the mbopo ritual and their popular reception began to occur in the early decades of the twentieth century. The early ethnographies, from the 1910 and 1920s, suggest that the secrecy and spiritual emphasis were very strong in the nineteenth century and when colonial agents and missionaries were documenting and challenging Indigenous cultural practices. From the 1930s through to the 1950s, anthropological studies point to its weakening spiritual relevance, occasioned by the consolidation of Christianity and the emergence of a new clan of young literate Christian men and women in Ibibio/Efik land.

At the time when the mbopo ritual still maintained its vibrancy, the Ibibio/Efik social philosophy perceived fatness as an embodiment of corporeal and social well-being: that which encompasses spiritual, physical, material, as well as affective and emotional wellness. The successful conclusion of the mbopo ritual, the fattening of the initiate, signified the favourability and approval from the water goddesses, ancestors, and other deities that were revered. Consequently, fertility, sustainability, and productivity were expected divine blessings for the initiate, her prospective new family, and the community at large. Fatness was seen as a cure for infertility, and as a resource for the preservation of their community. At the same time, men derived social standing for marrying mbopo initiates who had been educated and fattened.

The modifications that have attended the practice of mbopo have been a result of historical events, particularly European colonization and Christianization. The intense religious acculturation among the Ibibio/Efik in the first decades of the twentieth century affected all aspects of Ibibio/Efik cultural life, but not without tension. European contact, particularly the missionaries' efforts of the late nineteenth and early twentieth centuries, redefined fatness among Ibibio/Efik toward an epidemiological viewpoint that centred primarily on the health implications of fatness. In the 1950s, the popularity of the mbopo ritual began to wane as a result of intense Christianization projects coupled with the impetus of literacy in southern Nigeria. By the 1960s, the political tension in Nigeria, and the effect of global connectivity, fundamentally disrupted cultural traditions in southern Nigeria and the mbopo became morally suspect.

NOTES

1 D.A. Talbot, *Woman's Mysteries of a Primitive People: The Ibibio of Southern Nigeria* (London: Casel and Company, 1915), 83.

2 I. Imeh, *Daughters of Seclusion: The Revelation of the Ibibio "Fattened Bride" as the Icon of Beauty and Power* (New York, Lang Publishing 2012), 8.

3 I. Imeh, *Daughters of Seclusion*, 2.
4 E. Edwards, "Photography and the Performance of History" in *Kronos* (Special Issue: Visual History), *Journal of Cape History*, no. 27 (2001), 15.
5 A. Ayandele, "External Relations with Europeans: Explorers, Missionaries and Traders" in *Groundwork of Nigerian History*, ed. O. Ikimi (Ibadan, Heinemnn Educational Books, 1980), 367–89.
6 K. Walden, "The Road to Fat City: An Interpretation of the Development of Weight Consciousness in Western Society" in *Historical Reflections / Réflexions Historiques* 12, no. 3 (1985), 332.
7 K. Walden, "The Road to Fat City," 332.
8 C. Forth, "Fat, Desire and Disgust in the Colonial Imagination" in *History Workshop Journal*, 73 (2012), 211–39.
9 R. Popenoe, "Ideal" in *Fat: The Anthropology of an Obsession*, ed. D. Kulick and A. Meneley (New York, Penguin Group, 2005), 10–11.
10 C. Santolin and Luiz C. Rigo, "The Birth of Pathologizing Discourse of Obesity" in *Movimento, Porto Alegre* 21, no. 1, 77.
11 In some parts of Africa, intentional fattening cuts across gender and class. In Mauritania, young girls as young as eight years were force-fed and fattened to be sized up for marriage. In Uganda, women were fattened by their husbands to satisfy the appeal for obese wives: and these women were exploited as "instrument of her husband's economic prosperity" through the sex trade. In Nigeria and Cameroun, fattening seclusion was part of an initiation rite into men's secret cults and a show of wealth. Some women were also fattened as a cure for some infirmities, including infertility.
12 M. Jeffreys, "The Nyama Society," *African Studies* 15, no. 1 (1956), 15–28, 16. See also J. Messenger and B. Messenger, "Sexuality in Folklore in a Nigerian Society," *Central Issues in Anthropology* 3, no. 1 (1981), 29–50.
13 Wilker Jackson, *Eyen Akpabuyo Mme ma Ido Afo*: https://www.youtube.com/watch?v=kqy6oCi18ig&start_radio=1&list=RDEMiDza5crckbvoNr69mQkbEw, accessed on 2 October 2018.
14 P. Brink, "The Fattening Room among the Annang of Nigeria," *Medical Anthropology* (1999), 12, 132.
15 D.A. Talbot, *Woman's Mysteries*, 76.
16 A. Essien, "The Sociological Implication of the Worldview of the Annang People: An Advocacy for Paradigm Shift," *Journal for Emerging Trends in Educational Research and Policy Studies* (JETERAPS) 1, no. 11, 31.
17 D.A. Talbot, *Woman's Mysteries*, 76.
18 A. Essien, "The Sociological Implication," 32.
19 D.A. Talbot, *Woman's Mysteries*, 80.
20 D.A. Talbot, *Woman's Mysteries*, 76.
21 C. Forth, "Fat, Desire and Disgust," 214.

22 P. Brink, "Fertility and Fat: The Annang Fattening Room" in *Social Aspects of Obesity*, ed. I. de Garine and N. Pollock (Amsterdam; Overseas Publishers Association, 1995), 75.
23 D.A. Talbot, *Women's Mysteries*, 83.
24 A. Essien, "The Sociological Implication," 36–7.
25 M. Jeffreys, "The Nyama Society," 21.
26 Talbot's book was framed around James Fraser's colonial anthropological viewpoint, which considered non-Western cultures, such as secret societies and religious cults, and ritual practices as being shrouded in magic and esoterism, and, as such, unsophisticated.
27 A. Bank, "Anthropology and Portrait Photography: Gustav Frisch's 'Natives of South Africa,' 1863–1872" in *Kronos: Journal of Cape History*, Special Issue: Visual History, no. 27 (2001), 43–5.
28 D.A. Talbot, *Woman's Mysteries*, 2.
29 J. Messenger and B. Messenger, "Sexuality in Folklore," 35.
30 Jill Salmons, "Foreword," in I. Imeh, *Daughters of Seclusion*, xv.
31 I. Imeh, *Daughters of Seclusion*, 218.
32 I. Imeh, *Daughters of Seclusion*, 218.
33 See "Akenta Bob in wedding dress, c.1898," one of the photographs taken by Jonathan A. Green in 1898 published in M. Anderson and L. Aronson, "Jonathan A. Green: An African Photographer Hiding in Plain Sight" in *African Arts* 44, no. 2 (2011), 38.
34 J. Messenger and B. Messenger, "Sexuality in Folklore," 32–6.
35 C. Santolin and Luiz C. Rigo, "The Birth of Pathologizing Discourse," 78.
36 K. Walden, "The Road to Fat City," 335.
37 K. Walden, "The Road to Fat City," 336.
38 D.A. Talbot, *Woman's Mysteries*, 76.
39 J. Messenger and B. Messenger, "Sexuality in Folklore," 36.
40 P. Brink, "Fertility and Fat," 77.
41 I. Imeh, *Daughters of Seclusion*, 3.
42 C. Forth, "Fat, Desire and Disgust," 214.
43 D.A. Talbot, *Woman's Mysteries*, 82. See also P. Brink, "The Fattening Room," 132.
44 D.A. Talbot, *Woman's Mysteries*, 82.
45 I. Imeh, *Daughters of Seclusion*, 3.
46 I. Imeh, *Daughters of Seclusion*, 3.
47 I. Imeh, *Daughters of Seclusion*, 131–3.
48 I. Imeh, *Daughters of Seclusion*, 131–3.
49 J. Akpapan and M. Akpapan, "Mbopo Institution and Music," 51.
50 N. Udeme, "Mbopo Institution," 4–5.
51 N. Udeme, "Mbopo Institution," 4–5.

52 M. Jeffreys, "The Nyama Society," 16.
53 M. Jeffreys, "The Nyama Society," 16.
54 M. Jeffreys, "The Nyama Society," 16. Pamela Brink asserts that clitoridectomy was practised in high secrecy: up until the 1970s, when Brink did fieldwork among the Ibibio/Efik, no person was allowed to view or photograph the operation. See P. Brink, "The Fattening Room," 131.
55 I. Imeh, *Daughters of Seclusion*, 115.
56 N. Udeme, "Mbopo Institution," 3.
57 J. Akpapan and M. Akpapan, "Mbopo Institution and Music," 51.
58 J. Messenger and B. Messenger, "Sexuality in Folklore," 34–6.
59 P. Brink, "The Fattening Room," 139.
60 P. Brink, "The Fattening Room," 139.
61 I. Imeh, *Daughters of Seclusion*, 6.
62 I. Imeh, *Daughters of Seclusion*, 6.
63 See my honours mini thesis "Imagining Home and Identity: Narratives of Members of the Ibibio/Efik Ethnic Association of Cape Town, 2014–2016" (Unpublished Honours Mini-thesis, History Department, University of the Western Cape, 2016), 50–1.
64 R. Thompson, *Flash of the Spirit: African and Afro-American Arts and Philosophy* (New York, Knopf Doubleday Publishing 1984), 230.
65 R. Thompson, *Flash of the Spirit*, 230–3.
66 R. Thompson, *Flash of the Spirit*, 230–3.
67 I. Imeh, *Daughters of Seclusion*, 75.
68 I. Imeh (2014), Thompson (1984) and Munoz (2015).
69 I. Imeh, *Daughters of Seclusion*, 56–7.
70 I. Imeh, *Daughters of Seclusion*, 75.
71 For a photograph of a "hunting scene" taken around 1915, See D.A. Talbot, *Woman's Mysteries*, 13.
72 J. Akpan and M. Akpan, "Mbopo Institution and Music," 51.
73 J. Akpan and M. Akpan, "Mbopo Institution and Music," 51.
74 W. Bascom and M. Herskovits, "The Problem of Stability and Change in African Culture," in *Continuity and Change in African Cultures*, ed. W. Bascom and M. Herskovits (Chicago: University of Chicago Press, 1959), 3.
75 A. Afigbo, "The Eastern Provinces under Colonial Rule" in *Groundwork of Nigerian History*, ed. O. Ikimi (Ibadan, Heinemann Educational Books, 2004), 423–5.
76 M. Jeffreys, "The Nyama Society," 24.
77 See Jan Nederveen Pieterse, *White on Black: Images of Africa and Black in Western Popular Culture* (Yale University Press, 1995).
78 A. Afigbo, "The Eastern Provinces," 425.
79 D.A. Talbot, *Woman's Mysteries*, 85.

80 M. Jeffreys, "The Nyama Society," 24.
81 M. Jeffreys, "The Nyama Society," 24.
82 M. Jeffreys, "The Nyama Society," 24.
83 T. Tamuno, "British Colonial Administration in Nigeria in the Twentieth Century" in *Groundwork of Nigerian History*, ed. O. Ikimi, 398–9.
84 J. Messenger, "Religious Acculturation among the Annang Ibibio" *Continuity and Change in African Cultures*, ed. W. Bascom and M. Herskovits, 291.

SECTION IV

Imperialism, Colonialism, and the Body Politic

Imperialism and colonialism fundamentally shaped the late nineteenth century. The chapters in this section reveal that imperial views of fat were closely tied to views of racial identity. They also show fat to be about the possession and consumption of resources, and thus ultimately about power. Control of access to food was political, shaping the physical size of various groups in ways that reflected power within the imperial/colonial framework. These expressions of fat as indicative of imperial power and success conflict with the stereotype, in which Indigenous people (particularly in Africa) were portrayed as fat to indicate their lack of self-control and civilization.

The nineteenth century drew to a close with two wars of territorial acquisition: the Spanish-American/ Philippine-American War and the South African War. These wars, fought at nearly the same time, between 1899 and 1902, had notable similarities in their motivations, the discourse about them, and the means by which they were fought. Both the conflict in the Philippines and in South Africa extended longer than intended and involved civilians being interned in concentration camps, and widespread death from hunger and disease, drawing attention to the control of resources, including food, that sustained both the body and imperialism. Together they provide interesting insight into the shifting nature of the colonial project and the language with which it was promoted, which included a significant emphasis on the bodies of those colonizing and those being colonized.

The conflicts took place at a time of rapprochement between Britain and the United States, and the countries sometimes presented their imperial goals as part of a joint Anglo-American project. These were shaped by the popularity of social Darwinism, according to which this group's position atop a hierarchy of races justified both countries' expansion across the globe. The imperial success that in earlier centuries had been read as due to divine favour was now increasingly seen as the result of some largely biological fitness. While this put the excesses of imperialism in a flattering light, as inevitable and necessary, it also caused anxiety. Such superiority, imprinted on its enforcers' bodies, could be lost, either through regressing to a more primitive state or through succumbing to the fruits of success and becoming decadent. As such, constant attention to bodies was integral to nineteenth-century imperialism, and the fatness or thinness of those bodies was of immense symbolic and sometimes literal importance.

In chapter 9, Bonnie Miller examines political cartoons that use the figure of Uncle Sam to express judgments about the United States' imperial ambitions and behaviour. Miller shows that the discourse of fatness was widespread enough that it provided immediately understood visual cues. The traditionally lanky Uncle Sam was getting fat on new colonies, and that imagery was dense and evocative enough to express a battery of political and racial hopes and anxieties.

Amy Shaw's chapter also shows that by the late nineteenth century fat functioned as a trope, this time in a written, rather than visual way. Her examination of letters home from Canadian soldiers during the War in South Africa indicates that the language of fat carried a variety of symbolic meanings – about health, safety, and success – that were more important than their literal veracity.

The symbolism of both fat and imperialism was malleable but they shared a recognition that political ideas can be written on the physical body.

9 Colonial Engorgement in the Pictorial Arts: "Fat" Uncle Sam in the Imperialist Debates, 1898–1902

BONNIE M. MILLER

As the Spanish-American War came to a close, graphic artist Charles Nelan of the *New York Herald* penned a cartoon taking a cheap shot at former president Grover Cleveland, an outspoken critic of imperial expansion. Depicting Cleveland as exceedingly corpulent next to Uncle Sam, Nelan captioned his drawing: "The big man is telling the little fellow that he is opposed to 'expansion,' except in his own case" (Figure 9.1). The basis of the cartoon's humour lies in the cultural backdrop of the imperialist debates: most viewers would have been familiar with the word play of "expansion" in both a corporeal sense and a territorial one. Numerous cartoons published before Nelan's imprinted American overseas expansion on the body of Uncle Sam through the visual trope of weight gain, providing the context for comprehending this "fat" joke. Beyond making fun of Cleveland's heft, Nelan was tapping into broader discussions about the implications of American imperialistic designs in the aftermath of Spanish defeat in this war.

Just eight months earlier, on 11 April 1898, President William McKinley had asked Congress for the authority to use force to end the Cuban colonial crisis. His war message outlined the "exercise of cruel, barbarous, and uncivilized practices of warfare" that have "offended the humane sympathies of our people" and caused Cuba's "people [to perish] by tens of thousands from hunger and destitution."[1] Congress granted McKinley's request, propelling the nation into a brief war that transformed American foreign policy and thrust the United States onto the world stage. In the Treaty of Paris ending the war, McKinley demanded that Spain cede Cuba, the Philippines, Puerto Rico, and Guam to the United States in exchange for a $20 million payment. The war also created the political conditions for Congress to pass a bill officially annexing Hawai'i during the summer of 1898. As evidenced by McKinley's war message, pervasive privation of food for the Cuban

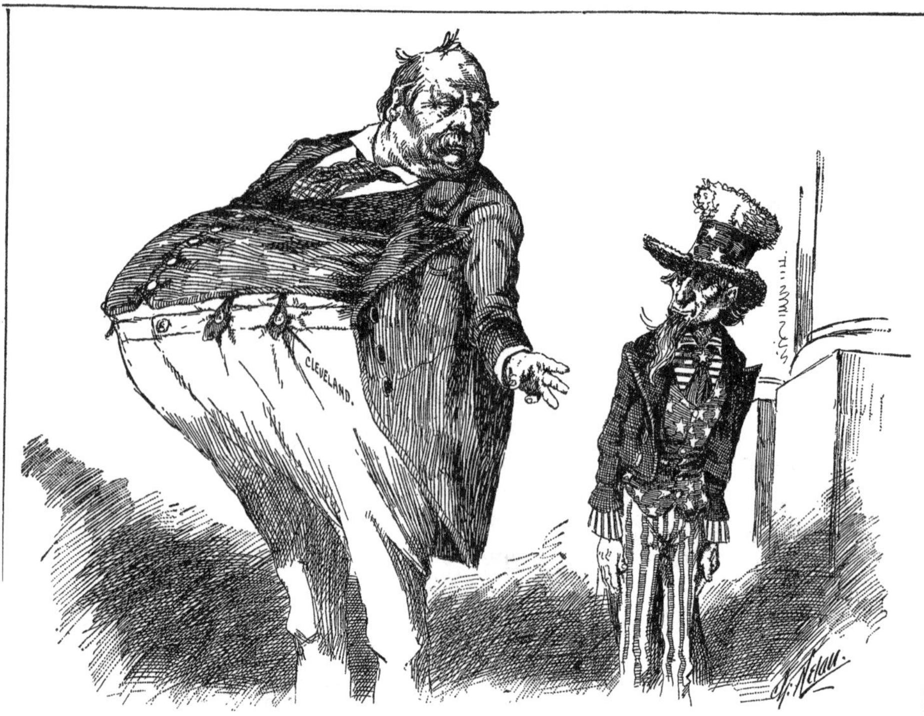

THE BIG MAN IS TELLING THE LITTLE FELLOW THAT HE IS OPPOSED TO "EXPANSION," EXCEPT IN HIS OWN CASE.

Figure 9.1. In this political cartoon published in the *New York Herald*, cartoonist Charles Nelan pokes fun at former president Grover Cleveland's anti-colonialist stance by calling attention to his expanding waistline. Uncle Sam comments, "The Big Man is Telling the Little Fellow that He is Opposed to 'Expansion,' Except in his Own Case." Charles Nelan, *New York Herald*, 19 December 1898, 3.

population was central to the war's rationale, and accordingly, the physical act of eating became a contested metaphor in the iconographic battle over imperialism in American print and visual culture.

This essay examines pictorial representations of Uncle Sam in the context of the imperialist debates of the Spanish-American and Philippine-American Wars in the popular press. Political cartoonists were practitioners of a social art, creating and recirculating images with politically contested meanings. To produce effective cartoons using only sparse text, cartoonists relied on familiar images, allusions, references, and symbols that would be readily apparent to viewers, with little to no explanation.[2] Cartoonists on both sides of the imperial debate embodied the stakes of empire in the figure of Uncle Sam, the visual incarnation of the American national body, fattening his formerly tall and lanky frame into a globular shape that encompassed his new acquisitions (Cuba, Puerto Rico, Guam, Hawai'i, and the Philippines).

In this embodiment, cartoonists deliberately juxtaposed Uncle Sam with his British national counterpart, John Bull. Artist John Arbuthnot had first introduced the character of John Bull in a 1712 political satire titled *Law is a Bottomless Pit; or, the History of John Bull.* In the earliest prints, John Bull was most often portrayed as a bull or other animal. Slowly he evolved into a human figure, often cast in the social station of English common folk. By the 1790s, the John Bull character appeared broadly in print, representing an array of English classes and interests. Satirists associated John Bull's personality with the traits of frankness, steadfastness, and decency. Physically, images of John Bull varied considerably, but after 1780, he was generally portrayed as a well-fed British commoner, often eating beef or drinking ale, as the English dinner table was used as a symbol for the domestic polity.[3] From the 1860s onward, graphic artist Sir John Tenniel transformed the figure of John Bull on the pages of *Punch;* unlike earlier versions from artists such as Isaac Cruikshank, James Gillray, or John Leech, Tenniel's John Bull appeared fatter and more self-satisfied. His expanding girth correlated to England's growing wealth, though John Bull only rarely appeared in cartoons with an imperial context.[4] Most cartoonists preferred using the John Bull figure when discussing domestic fiscal issues, like taxation.

By the late 1890s, the short, stocky John Bull character was a familiar figure in the graphic arts of the American popular press as England's national symbol. His American foil – Uncle Sam – emerged during the War of 1812, a hybrid of two earlier graphic characters: Yankee Doodle (the American patriot) and Brother Jonathan (the witty, rural American farmer). John Tenniel and John Leech of the British magazine *Punch* helped to crystallize Uncle Sam's physical form and attributes during the mid-nineteenth century, but it was cartoonist Thomas Nast of *Harper's Weekly* who turned Uncle Sam into a recognizable character before a broad American audience during the second half of the nineteenth century. Uncle Sam's figure took shape in visual contrast to John Bull: tall and lanky, not short and stocky, with his signature top hat, white beard, striped pants, and vest.

When President McKinley decided to acquire the former Spanish colonies in 1898, he was breaking with the nation's longstanding foreign policy of isolationism. He was seeking not only to have more influence in the Western hemisphere (extending policies like the Monroe

Doctrine), but also to occupy and govern colonies beyond America's continental borders. The United States and Britain had found common ground in their shared imperialistic projects throughout the world. Proponents of imperialism often rooted the affinity between American and English empires in their shared racial heritage – a racial formation they called Anglo-Saxonism – as the basis of their congruent political, economic, and cultural interests. This climate of Anglo-American rapprochement provided the impetus for cartoonists to depict John Bull and Uncle Sam more as friends than foes, and this camaraderie no doubt influenced Uncle Sam's physical transformation: he now looked more like John Bull than he ever had before, particularly in the growing size of his body.

While pro-expansionists celebrated Uncle Sam's bulk as evidence of his rise to global power, Uncle Sam's weight gain did not go uncontested, allowing anti-colonialists to register their concerns about the future of the nation upon his body.[5] Cartoonists on both sides of the debate used the visual metaphor of "fatness" to reflect on how imperial expansion would affect the health of American political culture. Such images varied in tone, from representing self-sustaining prosperity to grotesque overindulgence and gluttony. As Uncle Sam embarked upon a new diet of imperial ingestion, cartoonists regularly employed pictorial vocabularies of food to symbolize the colonies, available for Uncle Sam's gastronomic pleasure. "Fat" Uncle Sam gained currency as a symbol in these debates because of the cultural inconsistencies over the ideal body weight for men in that moment.[6] It is notable that there were no corresponding images in this period of an overweight Columbia, the female counterpart to the nation's symbol of Uncle Sam. Columbia did not generally appear heavier than she had in previous years, and rarely was she depicted in the act of eating, perhaps because that would have compromised popular ideals of feminine beauty and delicacy. Uncle Sam, however, epitomized national power and masculinity, making his body the ideal visual terrain to debate the prospects of empire. Which figure would prevail as the embodiment of the nation: the lanky or the portlier Uncle Sam?

This essay puts this pictorial theme into political and racial context by examining how cartoonists manipulated imagery of consumption and its bodily impacts in the debates surrounding American imperialist actions abroad. As in some of the essays of the previous section, it explores the visual trope of "fatness," in this case as a metaphor for the embodiment of the United States, thus reflecting not only on debates about empire/foreign policy at the turn of the twentieth century but also revealing the contested social perceptions of men's weight as, on the one hand, symbolic of power, confidence, and poise; and on the other hand, symbolic of overindulgence, engorgement, and greed.

Food as the Basis for American Intervention

Access to food shaped the power struggle in Cuba, inducing the United States into a war with Spain. Beginning in early 1896, Spanish Governor-General Valeriano Weyler's strategy to suppress Cuban colonial resistance was to institute a policy of reconcentration, forcing Cuban civilians from the countryside into camps to prevent them from supplying the rebel army with food, shelter, and supplies. It was a similar situation to what motivated the British concentration camps in the South African War only a few years later, as discussed by Amy Shaw in this volume. These Cuban concentration camps were ill equipped to provide for these civilians, resulting in rampant starvation, disease, and death. The American press reported widely on the humanitarian crisis, stirring sentiment in support of US intervention in the colonial conflict. In short, it was food, or the lack of it, that helped to create the pretext for bringing worldwide attention to how Spain was negligently administering its empire and mistreating its subjects.

Consequently, in the newspaper coverage of Cuban affairs in the year leading up to the outbreak of war, one of the most important and recurring visual representations was the image of emaciated, starving Cubans, particularly women and children. One such example appeared six months before the war began on the front page of the *New York World* portraying a gaunt fourteen-year-old boy whose mother had just died (Figure 9.2). The *World* made a special point of noting how this was "typical" and not even an "extreme" example of the devastation *World* photographers had been witnessing. The *New York Journal* launched a comparable series of articles that they called their "Human Documents" campaign, featuring similar images of emaciated women, children, and babies. Their selection of the term "documents" reflects their investigative style, as they intended these images as documentary proof of Spanish inhumanity. "The pictures of human misery which the *Journal* publishes are drawn from photographs," the *New York Journal* explained. "They are selected from a hundred or more in the possession of this paper, and are far from being the most ghastly, the most horrifying of all, for some are too frightful to print. Verbal exaggeration could not increase their horror, the coldest conservatism must be stirred to hot indignation by the thought of the human agony they reveal."[7] These representations were intended to shock American readers into action,

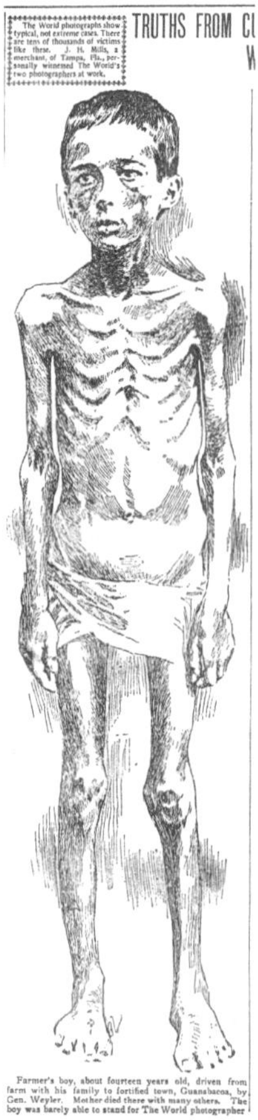
The World photographs show typical, not extreme cases. There are tens of thousands of victims like these. J. H. Mills, a merchant, of Tampa, Fla., personally witnessed The World's two photographers at work.
TRUTHS FROM C
Farmer's boy, about fourteen years old, driven from farm with his family to fortified town, Guanabacoa, by Gen. Weyler. Mother died there with many others. The boy was barely able to stand for The World photographer

Figure 9.2. Graphic illustration of a young Cuban boy suffering from extreme emaciation from Spain's reconcentration order. *New York World*, 8 November 1897, 1.

to register the severity of the starvation and the urgency of intervention by the United States.

Along with photographs, cartoon imagery showing Cuban suffering appeared not only in the big urban dailies of the *New York Journal* and *New York World*, but also in newspapers across the country. A cartoon published in the *St. Louis Republic* (and reprinted in the *Rocky Mountain News*), for example, depicted the iconic image of a weeping Lady Charity, bound to a rock as she looks away from the skeletal remains of the dead and dying Cubans of all ages surrounding her (Figure 9.3). The caption presses for action: "The Cubans are in a sense our proteges [*sic*] and it remains to be seen how long we will permit thousands of them to be condemned to starvation while Charity is held bound and helpless,

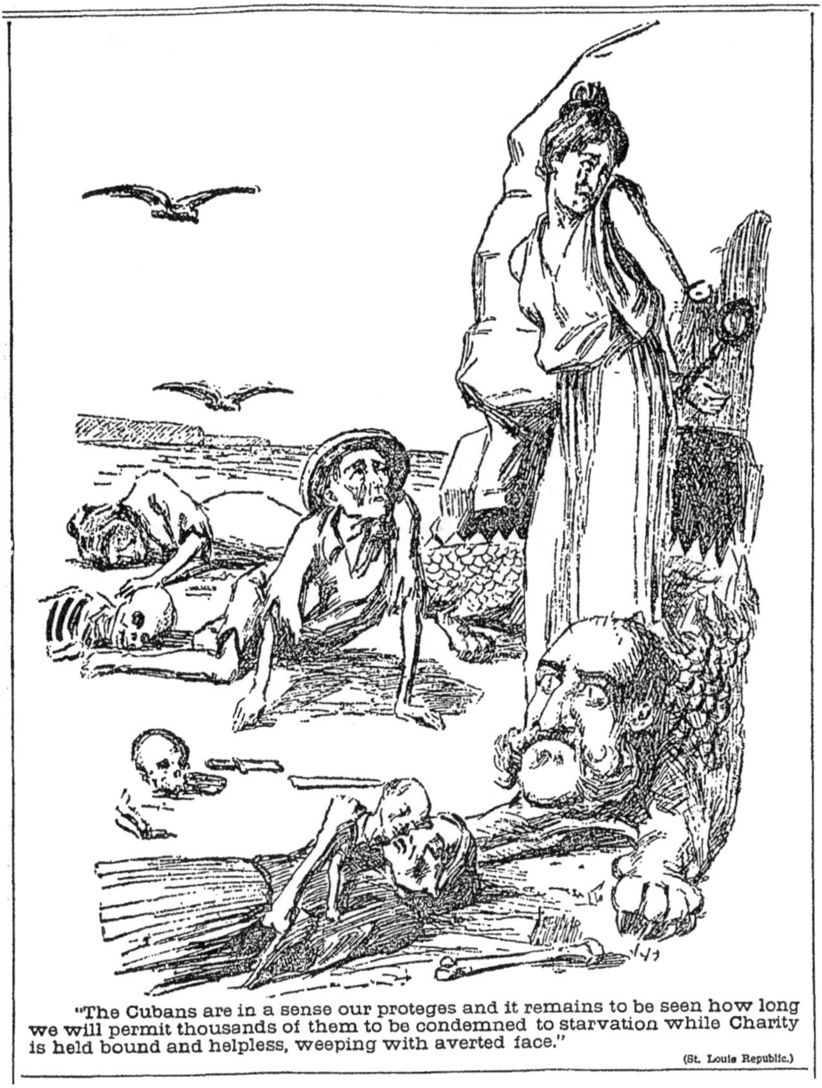

Figure 9.3. Political cartoon depicting the skeletal remains of dying Cuban civilians. It features the iconic white female victim in Grecian dress – cast as a weeping Lady Charity – chained to a rock to symbolize Spanish oppression. The architect of the reconcentration policy, Governor-General Valeriano Weyler, appears as a dragon at her feet. The cartoon prints the quote, "The Cubans are in a sense our proteges and it remains to be seen how long we will permit thousands of them to be condemned to starvation while Charity is held bound and helpless, weeping with averted face." Originally published in the *St. Louis Republic* and reprinted in the *Rocky Mountain News*, 14 June 1897, 1.

weeping with averted face."[8] US newspapers presented a scathing critique of Spanish imperial rule as one of brutal aggression, calling upon readers' sympathies to support intervention.

Senator Redfield Proctor, a Republican from the state of Vermont and ex-secretary of War under President Benjamin Harrison, made a landmark trip to Cuba in March of 1898 to survey the conditions of the camps. The speech he gave to the Senate upon his return, which was widely reprinted in the press nationwide, had broad public influence in urging military action. He described the scenes he witnessed as ones of "'desolation and distress, misery and starvation.'" He explained:

> I went to Cuba with the strong conviction that the picture had been overdrawn, that a few cases of starvation and suffering had inspired and stimulated the press correspondents, and they had given free play to a strong, natural, and highly cultivated imagination. Before starting I received through the mail a leaflet, published by *The Christian Herald*, with cuts of some of the sick and starving reconcentrados, and took it with me, thinking these were rare specimens got up to make the worst possible showing.... I saw plenty as bad and worse; many that should not be photographed and shown. I could not believe that out of a population of 1,600,000[,] 200,000 had died within these Spanish forts, practically prison walls, within a few months past from actual starvation and disease caused by insufficient and improper food.[9]

Proctor's words lent credence to the accusation that Spain was withholding food deliberately as a military strategy to quell resistance, assuring readers that what they were seeing was not merely a ploy of sensational journalism. Although other factors shaped McKinley's decision to call for a declaration of war against Spain, most notably the explosion of the *U.S.S. Maine* in Havana Harbor on 15 February 1898, the image of starving Cubans became the underlying moral rationale for US intervention – how could the United States allow a humanitarian crisis that denied people their essential needs for survival to occur so close to its own borders?

This moral imperative thus led many newspapers to frame the war as a humanitarian mission, not one fought for imperial gain. With headlines such as "Starving Cubans Welcome American Army of Invasion" or "Two Warships are to Take Supplies: Will Carry Food for Starving Cubans, and Then Return to the United States," the press established war and occupation as a humanitarian mission to feed the starving Cuban population.[10] A political cartoon published in the *New York*

Herald featured a Cuban rebel compelled not by a firearm, as one side of the cartoon beckons, but by a bakery, filled with bread rolls. "It's bread, not war, he wants."[11] A similar cartoon, published on the front page of the *Chicago Tribune*, showed a Cuban insurgent ("The Man Behind the Grub," as cartoonist HRH calls him) happily inhaling "free pie," surrounded by barrels of consumables marked as American-delivered goods such as pork, flour, canned tomatoes, marmalade, and salt. The caption reads: "Throw away the sword. States can be saved without it."[12] Such images justified Cuba's struggle for independence, not on the basis of greed, but rather for their basic survival. They implied that had Spain provided for the Cuban people and met their basic requirements, such resistance would not have been necessary. In this way, the media's framing of intervention as a fight to ensure access to food not only had the effect of demonizing Spanish colonial practices, but also of minimizing the nationalist vision and larger political and economic motivations of the Cuban rebellion – an effect that would have important consequences once US intervention turned imperialistic.

Growing Fat on Imperial Fare

Given that mass starvation helped rationalize the war, it is not surprising that political cartoonists opted to employ iconographies of eating to conceptualize the war's imperial prospects. Political cartoonists comprised a fairly small group of artists in the 1890s, and they often borrowed common tropes and ideas from each other. The pictorial motif of feasting on America's new colonial prospects gained traction among a number of leading political cartoonists of that period and across a range of popular magazines and urban dailies.[13]

Despite the humanitarian framing of the war itself, President McKinley made a critical decision to begin his military offensive against Spain not in Cuba, where hundreds of American journalists were waiting anxiously for the war to start, but in another one of Spain's colonial holdings – the Philippines. He ordered Admiral George Dewey to hit the vulnerable Spanish fleet in Manila, and the attack was swift and effective. Only three American war correspondents were stationed there and able to cover the naval battle, evidence in and of itself that the press was not expecting the war to expand beyond Cuba.[14] After the Spanish fleet was decimated in Manila, it became apparent to McKinley that the Philippines were ripe for the taking, and his administration shifted its focus away from securing Cuban independence and toward overseas acquisitions. But the imperial turn of the war came as a surprise to American news editors, who had expected that war would

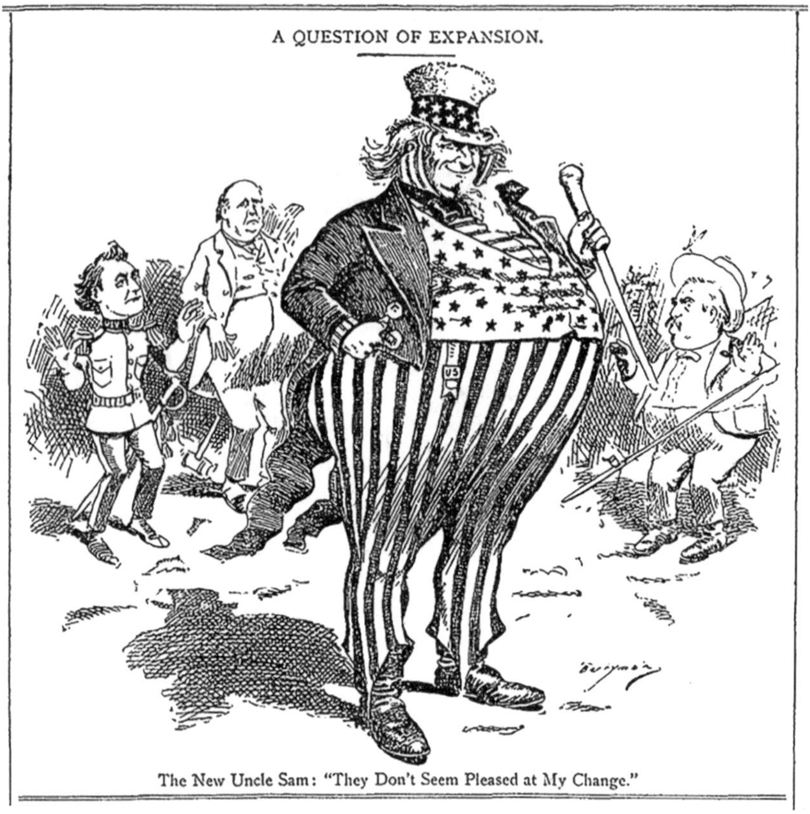

Figure 9.4. Political cartoon titled "A Question of Expansion" visually expresses Uncle Sam's foreign policy of expansion through his weight gain. Uncle Sam's gaze evokes confidence and self-assurance as he stands before members of the anti-colonialist opposition. Described by cartoonist Clifford Berryman as "The New Uncle Sam," the globular-shaped Uncle Sam comments that "They Don't Seem Pleased at My Change." Clifford Berryman, *Washington Post*, 22 July 1898, 1.

facilitate Cuban independence. As President McKinley's intention to retain the colonies became evident, anti-colonialist sentiment began to stir: would McKinley allow the Cuban nationalists to achieve the independence they had been fighting for? This unanticipated turn toward imperial acquisition inspired a debate that played out on the body of Uncle Sam in the press.

The potential for imperial gain led cartoonists to change the pictorial narrative. No longer was the war about feeding famished Cuban civilians; rather, they reframed the mission of the war to encompass empire through the physical transformation of Uncle Sam's stature and girth. Cartoonist Clifford Berryman of the *Washington Post* published a front-page cartoon in July of 1898 depicting a corpulent Uncle Sam standing tall as his anti-colonialist critics, such as William Jennings Bryan, look upon him with apprehension (Figure 9.4). Titled "A Question of Expansion," the caption indicates that anti-colonialists seemed less than pleased with Uncle Sam's weight gain. Despite their reproaches, Uncle Sam appears happy, confident, and in command, holding a weapon. He has emerged anew, ready for a new chapter of power and growth.[15]

Similarly, cartoonist Mostyn Kelly in the *Boston Herald* depicted Uncle Sam standing on a map of the Philippines, towering over John Bull, who stands over the map of England. With his full-bodied prowess, Uncle Sam looks more formidable than John Bull, who is similarly portly, but much shorter. Although this tall Uncle Sam offers John Bull a Manila cigar in a friendly gesture, John Bull looks trepidatious over Uncle Sam's sudden growth spurt. Both figures hold fishing lines to their naval fleet, and, despite England's reputation for naval supremacy, Uncle Sam's fleet appears more substantial, his new physical size signalling an amplification of American naval power. John Bull says in the caption, "Oh, My, but He is a Big Boy Now."[16] With treaty negotiations underway, a *Los Angeles Sunday Times* cover depicted Uncle Sam standing tall and fat, like a hot air balloon, as a diminutive John Bull observes him anxiously. Uncle Sam appears as if he might lift off, his cheeks bulging with air, and his hands held out to steady his large, distended body. With his buttons about to burst, he says to John Bull: "'I've grown so much lately, John, that I'm afraid I'll soon have to have a new suit.'"[17] The iconographic shift of Uncle Sam's newfound heft, whose mass was still growing, reflected the widespread perception that the war had transformed the United States into a more formidable rival of Great Britain.

But was "fat" Uncle Sam a symbol of prosperity or of gluttony? Plumpness could be interpreted as a sign of well-being or of overindulgence, as Freya Gowrley has shown in her analysis of art and material culture in chapter 6. When imagining Uncle Sam as a fat body, therefore, cartoonists were connecting their portrayals to popular ideas and anxieties about weight as it related to social status and health. Cartoonist "Boz" of the *Boston Globe* was one of many artists who expressed ambivalence on this question in a front-page cartoon in early December 1898, just days before the signing of the peace treaty ending the war (Figure 9.5). Uncle Sam stands before a mirror trying on a new suit, with President McKinley attending him as his tailor, looking most pleased at

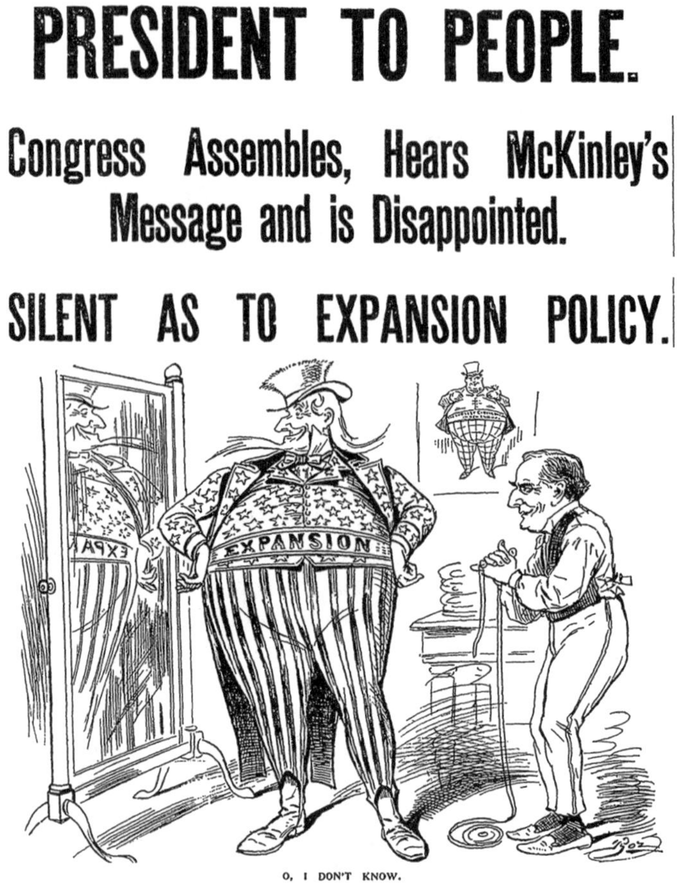

Figure 9.5. This front-page graphic spread drawn by *Boston Globe* artist "Boz" features a hefty Uncle Sam standing before a mirror getting fitted for a new suit. "Expansion" is written on his belt across his bulging midriff. His tailor, represented as President William McKinley, awaits his assessment of his new duds as he clasps his measuring tape. Uncle Sam responds, "O, I Don't Know." Boz, *Boston Globe*, 6 December 1898, 1.

the result. With his "Expansion" belt spanning his midriff, he examines himself and says, "O, I don't know."[18] Even for pro-expansionist papers, like the *Globe*, who supported McKinley's actions, the change in policy seemed sudden and uncertain. As he admires himself in the mirror, Uncle Sam seems unclear as to whether or not this change truly suited him (pun intended!).

Even when cartoonists framed Uncle Sam's weight gain in a positive light, their underlying anxieties were still evident. Illustrator Grant Hamilton in the pro-expansionist *Judge*, for example, depicted a full-page cartoon of Uncle Sam in 1901 contemplating a portrait of his younger self (Figure 9.6). He stands before the portrait short and plump, with his suspenders barely holding his pants over his rotund belly. Fat Uncle Sam not only appears bursting at the seams with his newfound size; his pockets are also lined with cash, as he stands next to a bag overflowing with money. He is fattened by wealth. When he looks at his reflection, however, the forlorn gaze returning his eye is of the "old" Uncle Sam, tall and lean. Hamilton's caption elucidates Uncle Sam's state of mind in his new body: "He is pretty well, thank you." Uncle Sam says, "Who would believe I am the same man? And yet that was a good likeness of me at the time it was painted in 1895."[19] Despite the show of wealth, a subtle ambivalence is expressed in Uncle Sam's thoughtful reflection as he gazes upon the likeness of his solemn former self: is his new look a better one? Would his newfound wealth corrupt him?

By contrast, the anti-colonialist *Life* magazine explicitly represented Uncle Sam's physical transformation as a threat to the health and longevity of the nation. *Life* delineated the history of US expansion from 1776 through 1899 as a sequence of land binges swelling Uncle Sam's girth, from the Louisiana Purchase, the Mexican cession, and the acquisition of Alaska to the colonial acquisitions of the Spanish-American War (Figure 9.7). With the map redrawn upon his trousers at each milestone, Uncle Sam embodies the evolving geographic configuration of the nation and its expanding borders. From *Life*'s perspective, at some unnamed date in the future annotated by a question mark, Uncle Sam's stomach is doomed to explode.[20] To the anti-colonialist press, the formal acquisition of a colonial empire would compromise the nation's constitutional integrity, political health, and Anglo-Saxon racial superiority. The cartoon calls into question the "digestibility" of the colonies, presenting the outcome as fatal for Uncle Sam, who is disregarding the signs of distress manifesting on his own body as he pursues a foreign policy of excess. Fears of racial contamination that might accompany long-term US occupation were at the heart of this anti-colonialist critique. *Life* was not simply pointing to fear of over-engorgement, but rather, fear that the intake of what was perceived as inferior racial stock would adulterate, and potentially obliterate, the United States' national body from within.

The variability of Uncle Sam's physical shape in these years across American print culture occurred through a confluence of factors. For these cartoons to be effective, the ambivalence manifested in Uncle Sam's weight gain had to register with viewers, which means that

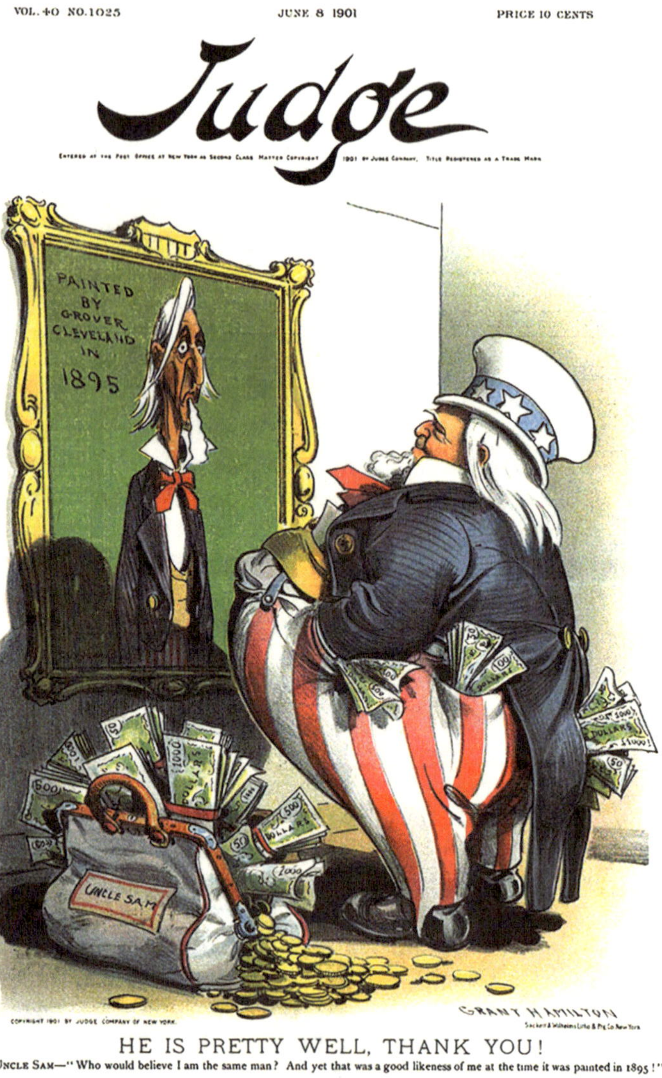

Figure 9.6. This *Judge* magazine cover featured a full-page political cartoon produced by graphic artist Grant Hamilton. A rotund Uncle Sam looks back at a portrait of his younger self labelled "Painted by Grover Cleveland in 1895," who appears tall and lanky. With his pockets and satchel overflowing with cash, the hefty Uncle Sam exemplifies financial prosperity. The caption reads, "He is Pretty Well, Thank You!" and Uncle Sam responds, "Who would believe I am the same man? And yet that was a good likeness of me at the time it was painted in 1895!" Grant Hamilton, *Judge* 40, no. 1025, 8 June 1901, 1.

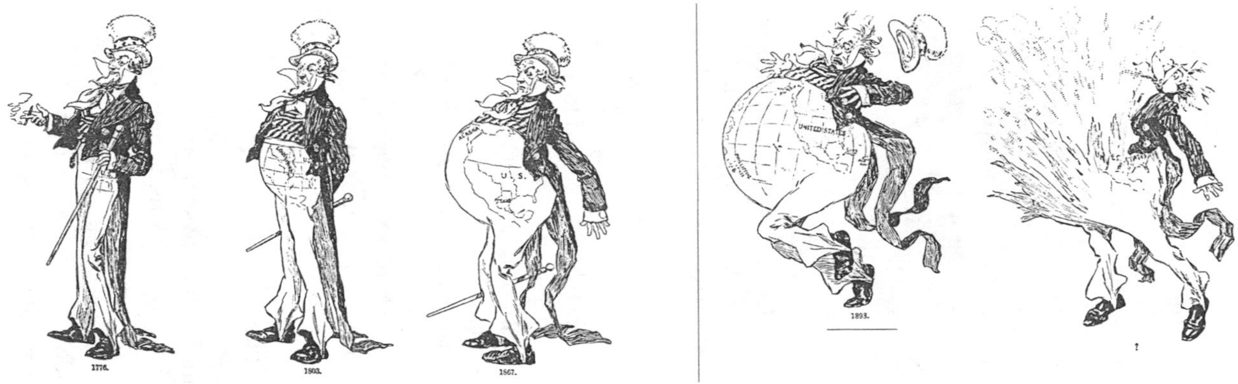

Figure 9.7. This two-page political graphic in *Life* magazine shows Uncle Sam's physical transformation due to policies of expansion. Tall and lean in 1776, he begins to grow a belly in 1803 from the Louisiana Purchase and then becomes even larger in 1867, with the acquisition of Alaska. In 1898, his stomach appears as if it were a full globe, with the new colonies mapped upon it, as Uncle Sam looks alarmed and uncomfortable. *Life* leaves the future date unspecified with a question mark when Uncle Sam implodes. *Life* 33, 26 January 1899, 72–3.

cartoonists consciously or subconsciously tapped into contemporary uneasiness over the benefits of weight gain, specifically for men. At the same time, this "fatness" theme enabled editors and illustrators to encapsulate perceptions of the sudden nature of America's shifting foreign policy and the uncertainties accompanying overseas colonialism. As Cubans bristled with a sense of betrayal at McKinley's reluctance to grant them complete independence, and Filipino nationalists countered with violent resistance, the McKinley administration (and its defenders in the popular press) felt pressed to justify their decision to retain these colonies. An editorialist in the *Richmond Times* expressed disgust that the Cubans were not eager to turn over the administration of their island to the United States: "For this body [the Cuban leadership] to puff itself up and put on airs and talk of its unwillingness to receive bounty from the United States is about upon a par with a beggar who is given a night's lodging setting up a claim to his host's establishment as soon as he has warmed his feet and got a few mouthfuls into his empty stomach."[21] The editorialist's analogy of the Cuban as a beggar is a revealing one; if the war was initially conceptualized to provide "bread" and "free pie," then the Cubans should have been satisfied by getting their "few mouthfuls" and recognized that they were not equipped for self-government. The framing here of US occupation as a show of "bounty" demonstrates a fundamental lack of understanding as to why the Cubans sought true political sovereignty and how they had sacrificed to achieve it.

Stepping out into the iconographic world as a man of great size and stature, Uncle Sam literally embodied the transformation of American military, political, and economic power on the global stage. To complete the body metaphor, cartoonists had to nourish Uncle Sam's growth with an abundant dietary regimen to sustain his hardy figure and manly vigour. Whereas cartoonists had first urged war to feed the hungry Cubans, now the Cubans would become the feed – and America's imperial appetite seemed to be growing by leaps and bounds.

Colonies as Edible Consumables

On the cartoon pages of numerous newspapers and illustrated magazines, Uncle Sam was consistently snacking and feasting, consuming a new diet of colonial edibles. In line with representations of Uncle Sam's expanding waistline came images of the former Spanish colonies and Hawai'i as Uncle Sam's new dietary regimen. McKinley's territorial acquisitions – including Cuba, Puerto Rico, Guam, the Philippines, and Hawai'i – consistently appeared in cartoons as fruit, fish, pies, sweets, nuts, meats, and stews, likening the process of colonial conquest to the physical act of ingestion.

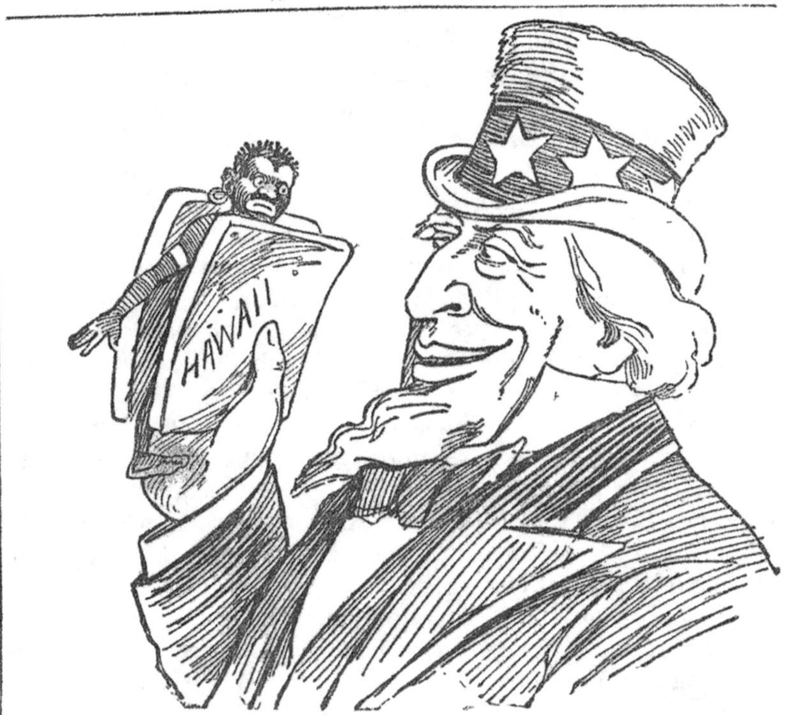

Uncle Sam—I feel like taking a Sandwich! —From the New York Advertiser.

Figure 9.8. This political cartoon depicts Uncle Sam holding a sandwich labelled "Hawaii" in which the "meat" of the sandwich is a dark-skinned, primitive native with big hoop earrings and large lips. Playing upon the nicknaming of Hawai'i as the "Sandwich Islands," Uncle Sam says, "I feel like taking a Sandwich!" Printed soon after the 1893 coup d'état, the cartoon first appeared in the *New York Advertiser* and was reprinted in the *Minneapolis Journal*, 3 February 1893, 1.

This pictorial trend had already acquired cultural currency during the debates over Hawaiian annexation preceding the Spanish-American War, setting an important precedent for imperial representations during the war. Playing upon Hawai'i's colloquial nickname of the "Sandwich Islands," some cartoonists opted to symbolize the islands as edible sandwiches. For example, in a *New York Advertiser* cartoon published soon after American citizens and Hawaiian sugar planters forced Hawai'i's Queen Liliuokalani to abdicate her throne in 1893 (Figure 9.8), Uncle Sam gleefully holds a sandwich labelled Hawai'i: "Uncle Sam – I feel like taking a Sandwich!"[22] The cartoon explicitly depicts

Hawai'i's racialized Native people as food; the meat of the sandwich in this case is as an actual Hawaiian, represented as a racialized savage, with large white lips, black skin, large hoop earrings, and kinked hair. Such images embodied the incorporation of Hawai'i as an act of cannibalistic pleasure for Uncle Sam. As Kyla Wazana Tompkins' examination of food imagery over the course of the nineteenth century has shown, those who got "eaten" on a symbolic level tended to be racially marginalized peoples,[23] so it is no coincidence that when cartoonists were representing colonies in the form of food, at the same time they were also depicting them as inferior Black subjects incapable of self-government.[24] In short, cartoonists framed colonial acquisition as America's racial prerogative to satisfy its bodily desires by consuming native peoples who were deemed subordinate.

Five years after Queen Liliuokalani was deposed, the United States formally annexed Hawai'i – an imperial "appetizer" of sorts – just as McKinley's war policy explicitly shifted toward acquiring Cuba, the Philippines, Puerto Rico, and Guam. As tropical fruits to be picked or foods served to Uncle Sam at the American table, the colonies appeared in the pictorial press as passive, available for the taking, and politically and culturally digestible. In a cartoon published in the *Boston Herald*, Uncle Sam grotesquely takes large bites out of the globe, with each bite consuming one of his new colonial additions. With Uncle Sam standing before an audience of world leaders such as China, Japan, Russia, Germany, France, and England, the cartoon marks Uncle Sam's inclusion at the table of world powers. A chorus of world leaders say to him, "Uncle Sam, give us a piece of something good." Uncle Sam responds, "Yes, boys after this next bite," as he prepares to sink his protruding teeth into the Philippines.[25] Imperial conquest, on a global scale, was represented by the act of consumption, as if colonizing empires had the right to ingest any area of the globe that delighted their palate. This simple representation of eating connoted a much deeper expression of power and privilege between the eaters and the eaten.

Cartoonist Charles Bartholomew (who went by "Bart") of the *Minneapolis Journal* regularly employed edible vocabularies to represent the colonies. In a cartoon published in August 1898 titled "A Valuable Addition to the Repast," Uncle Sam feasts at a table overflowing with tropical fruits (Figure 9.9). When depicted as foodstuffs, the colonies most often appeared in the form of fruit, raw food materials that on the one hand, gestured to the agrarian value of colonial trade, and on the other hand, signified associations of sweetness, exoticism, and pleasure. Uncle Sam sits at the "Expansion Restaurant" where "tropical fruits" are "a specialty." The abundance of Uncle Sam's fruited feast marks a stark contrast to the images of famished Cubans that had

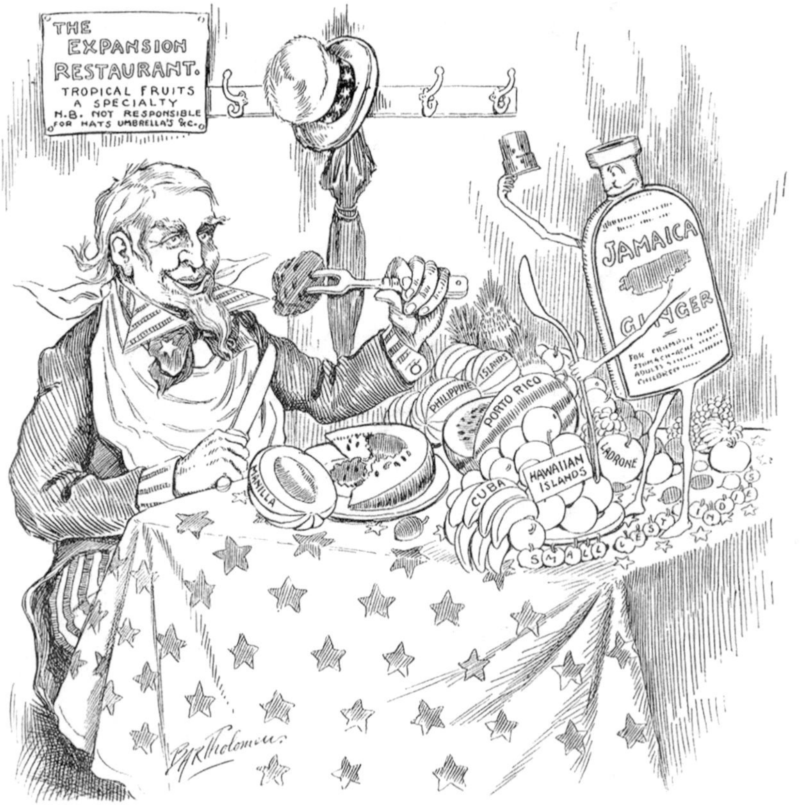

A VALUABLE ADDITION TO THE REPAST.

Jamaica-Ginger—Uncle Sam, I Thought You Would be Likely to Want Me After Absorbing All That Green Fruit.—August 24

Figure 9.9. Cartoonist Charles Bartholomew or "Bart" of the *Minneapolis Journal* in its 24 August edition pictured Uncle Sam eating a feast at "The Expansion Restaurant" comprising a bounty of tropical fruits labelled with the names of the former Spanish colonies and the Hawaiian Islands. The caption reads, "A Valuable Addition to the Repast," referring to a bottle of Jamaica-Ginger. Implying that the United States might continue its expansionist pursuit by acquiring Jamaica, the Jamaica-Ginger says to Uncle Sam, "I thought you would be likely to want me after absorbing all that green fruit." *Cartoons of the Spanish-American War, By Bart with Dates of Important Events; from the Minneapolis Journal, January 1899*, Minneapolis, Minn.: The Journal Printing Company, 1899.

mobilized the nation for war. The temptations to consume to the point of excess, Bart suggests, is so great that other potential colonies (in this case Jamaica, offering its ginger elixir), might seek out American guardianship, if for nothing else but to soothe Uncle Sam's stomach

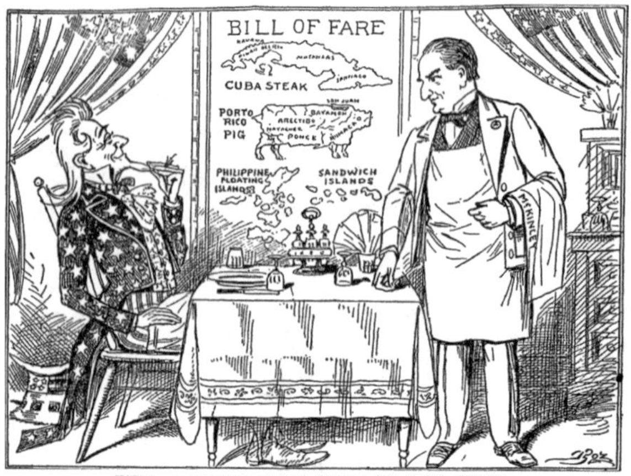

WELL, I HARDLY KNOW WHICH TO TAKE FIRST!

Figure 9.10. Cartoonist "Boz" of the *Boston Globe* depicts Uncle Sam eating at a fine dining establishment, waited on by his server, President William McKinley. The "Bill of Fare" for the meal consists of Cuba steak, Porto Rico Pig, Philippine Floating islands, or Sandwich Islands. Stroking his beard, Uncle Sam struggles to make his selection and says, "Well, I hardly know which to take first!" Boz, *Boston Globe*, 28 May 1898, 4.

after consuming large quantities of green fruit.[26] Bart's reference to the potential digestibility of the colonies is a direct response to anti-colonialist nativism that dreaded the absorption into the national "body" of subjects presumed to be racially inferior. To Bart, the best natural remedy would be for the United States to grow an even larger empire to ease consumption and nurture the national appetite. Following this theme, Bart depicts another bounteous dinner scene with Uncle Sam at a table with the Republican elephant and Democratic donkey. They feast together at "Uncle Sam's Territorial Expansion Dinner," with a variety of foods before them: Ladrone Melon, Hawaiian Poi, Spanish oxtail soup, Porto Rico coffee, Cuban bananas, Philippine fillets, and West Indian cigars. Titled, "The Expansion Policy," the elephant says to the donkey, "Better Pitch in Old Fellow and Get an Expansion on Yourself."[27]

Cartoon imagery of Uncle Sam's sumptuous feasting equated imperial gain with both gastronomic enjoyment and global prerogative. Just one month into the war, Boz in the *Boston Globe* depicted Uncle Sam faced with deciding the direction of imperial policy, which he represents as a fine dining choice (Figure 9.10). President McKinley waits on Uncle Sam at a restaurant while he considers what to order: "Cuba steak," "Porto Rico Pig," "Philippine Floating Islands," or the "Sandwich Islands." Pondering and pulling on his bearded wisps, he says: "Well, I hardly know which to take first!" Not only are the colonies depicted as entrées, but they also appear on the menu with their maps geographically reconfigured into sources of meat in the American diet (e.g., Puerto Rico appears in the shape of a pig).[28] McKinley serves the colonies up to Uncle Sam as meals to be eaten and enjoyed. Clifford Berryman in the *Washington Post* created a cartoon with a similar theme, picturing Uncle Sam at a restaurant with John Bull at an adjoining table. John Bull holds a menu offering entrées like "Conquest" and "Foreign Aggression" while Uncle Sam's menu reads "Monroe Doctrine" and "No Entangling Alliances." Uncle Sam looks bewildered, poised to make a decision that would change the course of American foreign policy. Titled "Uncle Sam's Temptation," John Bull baits Uncle Sam to adopt the new bill of fare, saying: "I say, Sam, why don't you try a change of diet and put some meat on your bones?" John Bull infers that Uncle Sam's lean figure is a sign of weakness and inaction, while a "meaty" diet of colonial acquisition would bolster his manhood and global clout. Uncle Sam must decide soon, for a waiter is about to serve him "Anti-annexation broth." Will John Bull entice him to try something new instead?[29]

Likening national politics to dining, these cartoonists were borrowing a pictorial motif that had been appearing for over a century in English prints. In these prints, a plenitude of eating and drinking had traditionally been linked to signs of prosperity while meagre portions reflected times of want or oppression.[30] Cartoonists conceptualized eating as the sustenance of national identities, and as such, English and French characters were often symbolized by the foods they ate. In English prints, the French were often denigrated with images of their petite portions and strange ingredients, like snails or frogs.[31] A Frenchman, likely an Anglophile, wrote a tract in 1889 about John Bull that exemplifies this idea: "Education, climate, and food, all help to account for the striking difference that exists between the English and French characters. The man, whose dinner consists of a pound of beef, a large slice of plum pudding, and a tankard of thick, heavy, black beer, must certainly look at things in a different light from the man who dines off oysters, chicken, fruit, the lightest of pastry, and a bottle of Pomard."[32]

Given the precedent of conceptualizing the French and English by what they ate, this same logic likely framed the thinking of graphic artists reflecting on the new foods in Uncle Sam's diet. Were the colonies digestible and healthy fare for Uncle Sam? To the anti-colonialist press, the answer was no, and they employed this analogy to critique the nation's course of territorial acquisition. The anti-colonialist *Life* magazine employed this analogy for its Thanksgiving issue of 1898. Once again, McKinley is serving a meal to Uncle Sam: "Philippine Stew," accompanied by Porto Rican wine and a Cuban side dish. Uncle Sam looks less than pleased and says, "William, I can never digest that mess without straining my constitution." With the constitutional pun, cartoonist F.G. Attwood draws a parallel between Uncle Sam's "constitution" or digestive system and the nation's political and social health.[33] His word choice invokes a central argument of the anti-imperialist movement – that a policy of colonialism would be unconstitutional and would compromise the nation's political integrity. Such cartoons suggested that certain foods, particularly those made from colonial stock, were indigestible and would compromise America's political, cultural, and racial well-being.

In one final variation to this consumption theme, numerous cartoons inverted the narrative and depicted Uncle Sam or President McKinley feeding the colonies, as an act of imperial benevolence or domination. Cartoonist Alfred C. Eastman depicted Uncle Sam feeding soup to a man with his head in the shape of a globe: "Uncle Sam Feeds the World."[34] By contrast, C.G. Bush, in the anti-colonialist *New York World,* presented McKinley feeding five Cuban children standing before him with their hands clasped, labelled the "Cuban Committee of 5" from a soup bowl labelled "Platt Amendment." With a sinister expression, McKinley instructs the children, "'Now, then, open your mouths and shut your eyes, And you'd all get something that will make you wise.'"[35] The 1901 Platt Amendment, which came attached to a US army appropriations bill, ended the era of formal US military occupation of Cuba by transferring sovereignty to the Cubans, with the stipulation that the United States reserved the right to intervene in Cuban affairs whenever it saw fit. C.G. Bush recognizes that the Platt Amendment compromised Cuban sovereignty and therefore depicts McKinley as feeding the children a mouthful of artifice intended to silence their protests and secure accommodation to American hegemony.

Conclusion

The arguments put forth in these graphic compositions harnessed cultural ideas about physical weight, gender, race, and power to justify or contest the transformation of the United States into an overseas empire. The physical body, like the national body, is not static; physical mass can fluctuate up and down just as territorial mass can be annexed or removed. As Antonio de Baecque explained, "[T]he body is not only a metaphor for the world, it is also a spectacle given for us to see."[36] Representing imperial expansion through the lens of consumption and weight gain had an explicitly visual component, making it an ideal iconographic tool for the cartoonist's pen. It had enough elasticity to allow cartoonists, even those from opposing sides of the political spectrum, to seize upon the metaphor, providing a conceptual framework to think about imperialism and its long-term effects both on the United States and on the new colonies.

Graphic artists in the 1890s were the social media influencers of their time. The compact visual statements of political cartoons appeared on the front pages of major newspapers and illustrated periodicals, serving as the first thing viewers saw when perusing a printed issue. As a result, political cartoons framed how viewers engaged with the news of the day. What is more, political caricature had the ability to distill complex arguments into simple representations and articulate political arguments in pithy, memorable ways. While viewers might not necessarily have interpreted the cartoons as their makers intended them, their messages and symbolism were reinforced through widespread repetition.[37] The ideological power of these images lies in how they represented the hierarchies of power between US imperial interests and colonial subjects (the eaters vs. the eaten) and how they reduced colonial nationalism to hunger, as a primal need, not a more complex social and political one. The privileges associated with empire were thus symbolically conveyed through metaphors of masculine appetite and gastronomic pleasures. Still, the debate over the potential political, cultural, and economic consequences of colonial acquisition was inscribed upon Uncle Sam's body, as some questioned the haste of Uncle Sam's sudden expansion, others worried about the magnitude of his enlargement, and some feared that the colonial edibles themselves did not constitute a proper and healthy diet to maintain the nation's political and racial fitness.

Once US authorities captured Filipino nationalist leader Emilio Aguinaldo in March 1901, reports about colonial resistance largely faded from the front pages, despite ongoing tensions there. With that, Uncle Sam physically transformed again, returning to his tall, lanky self in the pictorial press. The Philippines remained under US colonial control until gaining independence in 1946, Cuba received its conditional independence in 1901, Hawai'i retained territorial status until it became a state in 1959, while Puerto Rico and Guam remain American territories to this day. Uncle Sam's quick weight loss had important political implications for perceptions of the US empire; cartoonists effectively masked America's ongoing imperial commitments by hiding his "imperial weight," thus reinforcing the argument that the Spanish-American War was merely an aberration and empire was not integral to the nation's political culture.[38] Although Uncle Sam's diet and figure seemingly returned back to "normal" and anti-colonialist dissent faded, the effect of his brief dietary binge nonetheless had a lasting effect on US foreign policy, particularly in the Western hemisphere, and on the peoples, economies, and governments of Puerto Rico, Guam, Cuba, Hawai'i, and the Philippines well into the twentieth century.

NOTES

1 Fitzhugh Lee and Joseph Wheeler, *Cuba's Struggle Against Spain with the Causes for American Intervention and a Full Account of the Spanish-American War, Including Final Peace Negotiations* (New York: The American Historical Press, 1899), 208.

2 On the history and rhetorical analysis of editorial cartoons, see Martin J. Medhurst and Michael A. Desousa, "Political Cartoons as Rhetorical Form: A Taxonomy of Graphic Discourse," *Communication Monographs* 48 (September 1981): 197–236; Lucy Shelton Caswell, "Drawing Swords: War in American Editorial Cartoons." *American Journalism* 21, no. 2 (2004): 13–45; LeRoy M. Carl, "Political Cartoons: 'Ink Blots' of the Editorial Page," *Journal of Popular Culture* 4 (1970): 39–45; Robert Philippe, *Political Graphics: Art as a Weapon* (New York: Abbeville Press, 1980); Charles Press, *The Political Cartoon* (Toronto: Associated University Presses, Inc., 1981); Paul Somers, *Editorial Cartooning and Caricature: A Reference Guide* (Westport: Greenwood Press, 1998); Stephen Hess and Sandy Northrop, *Drawn and Quartered: The History of American Political Cartoons* (Montgomery: Elliot & Clark Publishing, 1996), John Geipel, *The Cartoon: A Short History of Graphic Comedy and Satire* (Newton Abbot: David & Charles, 1972); W.G. Rogers, *Mightier Than the Sword: Cartoon, Caricature, Social Comment* (New York: Harcourt, Brace & World, Inc., 1969); and Mary Campbell and Gordon Campbell, *The Pen, Not the Sword* (Nashville: Aurora Publishers Inc., 1970).

3 On the history of John Bull, see Tamara L. Hunt, *John Bull: Political Caricature and National Identity in Late Georgian England* (Burlington, VT: Ashgate Publishing, 2003); Jeannine Surel, "John Bull," in *Patriotism: The Making and Unmaking of British National Identity*, Volume III National Fictions, ed. Raphael Samuel (London: Routledge, 1989), 3–25; and Diana Donald, *The Age of Caricature: Satirical Prints in the Reign of George III* (New Haven: Yale University Press, 1996), 157–8.

4 Miles Taylor evaluated all instances of John Bull's appearance in the British press from 1712 through 1929 and found only a small subset of

representations of John Bull in prints about foreign policy or imperial concerns. "John Bull and the Iconography of Public Opinion in England c. 1712–1929," *Past & Present*, no. 134 (February 1992): 93–128.

5 I am using the term "anti-colonialists" to underscore the fact that most historical actors who opposed formal colonialism in this period were not necessarily opposed to extending American's political, economic, and diplomatic influence in other ways. They opposed US political and military occupation in a very narrowly defined sense. Most anti-colonialists would have called themselves "anti-imperialists" at the time, but it is important to acknowledge that how we understand the politics of imperialism and empire today also includes more informal modes of dominance. See larger discussion in Bonnie M. Miller, *From Liberation to Conquest: The Visual and Popular Cultures of the Spanish-American War of 1898* (Amherst: University of Massachusetts Press, 2011), 123.

6 On gender and body weight, particularly with respect to men, see Amy Erdman Farrell, *Fat Shame: Stigma and the Fat Body in American Culture* (New York: New York University Press, 2011); Joyce L. Huff, "A 'Horror of Corpulence': Interrogating Bantingism and Mid-Nineteenth-Century Fat-Phobia" in *Bodies Out of Bounds: Fatness and Transgression*, ed. Jana Evans Braziel and Kathleen LeBesco (Berkeley: University of California Press, 2001): 39–59; Lee F. Monaghan, "Big Handsome Men, Bears, and Others: Virtual Constructions of 'Fat Male Embodiment'" in *Sociology of the Body: A Reader*, ed. Claudia Malacrida and Jacqueline Low (Don Mills, ON: Oxford University Press, 2008): 57–64.

7 "Human Documents from Cuba," *New York Journal*, 14 March 1898, 6.

8 Reprinted *Rocky Mountain News*, 14 June 1897, 1.

9 "Senator Proctor on Cuba's Desolation," *Literary Digest* 16, no. 13 (26 March 1898): 361–2.

10 "Starving Cubans Welcome American Army of Invasion," *New York World*, 24 June 1898, 3; "Two Warships are to Take Supplies: Will Carry Food for Starving Cubans, and Then Return to the United States," *Boston Herald*, 3 March 1898, 1.

11 Charles Nelan, "It's Bread, Not War, He Wants," *New York Herald*, 14 May 1898, 5.

12 HRH, "The Man Behind the Grub," *Chicago Tribune*, 20 August 1898, 1.

13 A few prominent examples include Grant Hamilton (*Judge*), Victor Gillam (*Judge*), Boz (*Boston Globe*), Clifford Berryman (*Washington Post*), Charles Nelan (*New York Herald*), and Samuel E. Morss (*Indianapolis Sentinel*).

14 Miller, *From Liberation to Conquest*, 89–95.

15 Clifford Berryman, "A Question of Expansion," *Washington Post*, 22 July 1898, 1.

16 Mostyn Kelly, "John Bull –'Oh, My, but He is a Big Boy Now,'" *Boston Herald*, May 1898, 3.
17 "'I've Grown So Much Lately, John, that I'm Afraid I'll Soon Have to Have a New Suit,'" *Los Angeles Sunday Times*, 11 December 1898, 1.
18 Boz, "President to People," *Boston Globe*, 6 December 1898, 1.
19 Grant Hamilton, "He is Pretty Well, Thank you," *Judge* 40, no. 1025 (8 June 1901): 1.
20 *Life* 33 (26 January 1899): 72–3. See analyses of this cartoon in Miller, *From Liberation to Conquest*, 177; Martha Banta, *Barbaric Intercourse: Caricature and the Culture of Conduct, 1841–1936* (Chicago: University of Chicago Press, 2003), 211.
21 "The Troublesome Cubans, "*Richmond Times*, 16 March 1899, 4.
22 "Uncle Sam – I Feel Like Taking a Sandwich!" *New York Advertiser* [Reprinted in the *Minneapolis Journal*, 3 February 1893, 1].
23 Kyla Wazana Tompkins, *Racial Indigestion: Eating Bodies in the 19th Century* (New York: New York University Press, 2012), 8. See also Erica Owens and Bronwyn Beistle, "Eating the Black Body: Interracial Desire, Food Metaphor, and White Fear," in *Body/Embodiment: Symbolic Interaction and the Sociology of the Body*, ed. Phillip Vannini and Dennis D. Waskul (Burlington, VT: Ashgate, 2006): 201–12.
24 See discussion of racial imagery with additional pictorial examples in Miller, *From Liberation to Conquest*, 196–230.
25 *Boston Herald*, 21 January 1898, 4.
26 Reprinted in Abe Ignacio, Enrique de la Cruz, Jorge Emmanuel, and Helen Toribio, *The Forbidden Book: The Philippine-American War in Political Cartoons* (San Francisco: T'Boli Publishing, 2004), 61.
27 Bart, "The Expansion Policy," *Minneapolis Journal*, 11 August 1898, 1.
28 Boz, "Well, I Hardly Know Which to Take First!" *Boston Globe*, 28 May 1898, 4.
29 Clifford Berryman, "Uncle Sam's Temptation," *Washington Post*, 26 June 1898, 1.
30 See Joanne Ella Parsons, "Eating Englishness and Causing Chaos: Food and the Body of the Fat Man in R.S. Surtees' *Jorrocks's Jaunts and Jollities*, *Handley Cross*, and *Hillingdon Hall*," *Nineteenth-Century Contexts* 36, no. 4 (2014): 335–46; Annette Cozzi, *The Discourses of Food in Nineteenth-Century British Fiction* (New York: Palgrave Macmillan, 2010); Gwen Hyman, *Making a Man: Gentlemanly Appetites in the Nineteenth-Century British Novel* (Athens: Ohio University Press, 2009).
31 John Brewer, *The Common People and Politics, 1750–1790s* (Cambridge: Chadwyck-Healey, 1986), 41–3.
32 Max O'Rell [pseudonym, possibly Paul Bloüet], *John Bull and His Island*, translated from French (New York: Charles Scribner's Sons, 1889), 237.

33 F.G. Attwood, "Uncle S.: William, I Can Never Digest That Mess Without Straining My Constitution," *Life* 32, no. 833 (24 November 1898): 1; See analysis of this cartoon in Banta, *Barbaric Intercourse*, 211.

34 Alfred C. Eastman, "Uncle Sam Feeds the World," *Boston Herald*, 16 October 1898, 21.

35 C.G. Bush, "'Now, then, open your mouths and shut your eyes, And you'd all get something that will make you wise,'" *New York World*, 25 April 1901, 6.

36 Antonio de Baecque (translated by Charlotte Mandell), *The Body Politic: Corporeal Metaphor in Revolutionary France, 1770–1800* (Stanford: Stanford University Press, 1993), 10.

37 Roger A. Fischer, "Political Cartoon Symbols and the Divergence of Popular and Traditional Cultures in the United States," in *Dominant Symbols in Popular Culture*, ed. Ray B. Browne, Marshall W. Fishwick, and Kevin O. Browne (Bowling Green: Bowling Green State University Popular Press, 1990), 182, 189; Thomas Milton Kemnitz, "The Cartoon as a Historical Source," *Journal of Interdisciplinary History* 4 (Summer 1973): 85; Alton Ketchum, *Uncle Sam: The Man and the Legend* (New York: Hill and Wang, 1969), 121.

38 The work of Amy Kaplan, Louis A. Pérez, Jr., and others has gone far to revise the view of the Spanish-American War's imperial legacy from what Samuel F. Bemis in 1955 called "a great national aberration." Ernest R. May corroborated Bemis in arguing that McKinley "led his country unwillingly toward a war that he did not want for a cause in which he did not believe" and concludes that "a frightened elite retracted from resistance to acquiescence" due to the pitch of emotional fervour. See Bemis, "The Great Aberration of 1898," in *American Imperialism in 1898*, ed. Theodore P. Greene (Boston: D.C. Heath and Co., 1955), 92; May, *Imperial Democracy: The Emergence of America as a Great Power* (New York: Harcourt, Brace, & World, 1961), 147, 159. Pérez, Jr. and many others have critiqued this perspective at length, declaring that the assertion that America by chance, providence, or unforeseen circumstance "fell into empire" unjustifiably deflects responsibility for the important political, diplomatic, and economic factors underlying empire-building on excited popular passions. See Pérez, Jr., *The War of 1898: The United States and Cuba in History and Historiography* (Chapel Hill: University of North Carolina Press, 1998), 111–16; Kaplan, "Left Alone with America: The Absence of Empire in the Study of American Culture," in *Cultures of United States Imperialism*, ed. Amy Kaplan and Donald E. Pease (Durham: Duke University Press, 1993), 3–21.

10 Gaining in Flesh: Canadian Soldiers in the War in South Africa

AMY J. SHAW

Noble Jones's experience of the War in South Africa offered him rather fewer opportunities for adventure and heroism than he had hoped. The twenty-seven-year-old Canadian spent several months toward the end of his year's service in 1900 camped at Belmont, an isolated base about halfway between Johannesburg and Bloemfontein, waiting, along with hundreds of others, for the British leadership to decide what to do with them. It was an unhealthy place to be. A lack of supplies and insufficient, unsanitary drinking water meant the place was riddled with typhoid and dysentery. But Jones, writing home to his brother Joe, reassured him that he was doing all right, "I am gaining in flesh since we arrived here and getting a rest I have a great appetite and I get all I can handle."[1]

Fat has been particularly problematic when associated with the military body. It has connotations of slowness, excess, and a lack of control, where the military body is meant to be disciplined and efficient and active. As well, fat is typically individualized, viewed both as evidence of personal pleasure in food, and as leading to bodily distinctiveness which goes against the uniformity of the group expected in the military. It also challenges the expectation that a soldier, particularly one on active duty, is meant to be pared down to essentials.[2] But, as the other chapters in this collection have revealed, in the nineteenth century there was a fair bit of ambivalence and contradiction in thinking about fat, and that applied to the military body as well.

The War in South Africa, also called the Second Anglo-Boer War (1899–1902), was fought between the British Empire and the South African republics of the Transvaal and the Orange Free State as the nineteenth century turned into the twentieth. It is a particular marking point of change in ideas about imperialism, gender, and military behaviour and strategy, as well as nationalism and control, and the fat body was a locus for these ideas. Partly because of the popularity of social Darwinism at the time, these ideas were often inscribed on the bodies of those fighting or inhabiting the areas in dispute.[3] This chapter looks at the bodies of Canadian volunteers sent to fight in support of the British Empire, but also a nascent Canadian nationalism, and it particularly considers the way the volunteers presented and perceived their own bodies, and the bodies of their foes.

Imperial Anxiety

The end of the nineteenth century was, perhaps somewhat unexpectedly, an anxious time for advocates of empire. The British Empire was at its height, but worries were rife that it was also at risk. Many political, social, religious, and military leaders feared that the changes undergone over the century of tremendous growth of empire, especially greater industrialization and a growth in clerical work, meant that the physical quality of British subjects had degenerated.[4] Social Darwinism, which interpreted evolution as a fight for "survival of the fittest" among individual people, ethnic groups, and nations, provided a "scientific" and philosophical underpinning for these understandings. The British people, and the civilization they had developed, were, in their view, superior to all others; the empire on which "the sun never set" was evidence of that.[5] But commentators worried about degeneracy. Sedentary jobs, technological advancements, and the pleasures of urban life threatened to lead to a population incapable of defending British civilization and the assets its forebearers had wrested from around the world. J.L. Cranfield has described "[A] whole battery of anxieties that tied together fears of imperial decay, bodily degeneration, the growth of tertiary industry, the death of chivalry, and the uncertain future of 'Victorian' ideals"[6] that coalesced around the bodies of the empire's young men. Canada, as a settler colony, generally shared a comfortable assurance of the superiority of British civilization. Commentators also, at times, argued for the country's special role in the continued development of empire, based on the physical bodies of its nationals. Canada was less industrialized than Britain and many writers and speech-makers in the colony saw the hardier agricultural and frontier life of its inhabitants as a means of regeneration for the empire.[7] That most of the first contingent the country sent overseas was made up largely of urban clerks did little to dispel the impression Canada had of its volunteers as a contingent of imperial gentlemen cowboys.[8]

The War in South Africa, then, broke out at a time of unease. This meant, perhaps unexpectedly, that it was widely welcomed. For those concerned about physical degeneracy, it seemed a propitious means of proving mettle. A short, sharp, frontier war would shake the empire's young men out of their industrialized ease. It would give them experiences of satisfying physical action, manly comraderie, and assured victory, with themselves as proud enforcers of British dominance. This would revive manliness at home, and show the watching world that Britain was still fully deserving of its empire, and capable of defending it. For Canadians, this opportunity to prove prowess on a world stage was national as well as imperial.[9] The country was very young; the colonies of British North America had only confederated in 1867, and this was the first time it had sent a contingent of soldiers overseas. Canada was anxious that its fighting men acquit themselves well, and that they did so while also looking well. As the first Canadian soldiers the world would see, the bodies of these volunteers bore a heavy symbolic weight.

Causes of War

As with many wars, the answers to why it broke out, and what each side was fighting for and against, depends somewhat on perspective, and the timing of the question. To British proponents, the war was argued as necessary to keep control of an important strategic location, which also happened to have some impressive gold and diamond reserves, and to protect the rights of British subjects resident in the republics, who were being oppressed by a government that also oppressed its Black population. On the other side, it was, a little more clearly, about preserving territorial integrity and the Boer way of life, whatever the merits of that might be, against the encroachments of British interest and control in South Africa.[10] Neither side considered the opinion of the Africans who lived there and whose bodies would be marked by the scarcity and violence created by the war. As both Tatiana Konrad and Bonnie Miller show in this volume, imperialism's consuming hunger seldom considered the physical bodies of those it was drawing resources from. The War in South Africa was an entirely lopsided contest in favour of the British Empire, although the republics declared war first, enabling Britain to treat this as a defensive, and thus defensible, conflict. The presentation of the war was angled so that it supported the honourable, chivalric intentions with which an expanding empire justified itself.

The conflict was popular at its outset, and widely understood as a righteous war. Prime Minister Wilfrid Laurier's address to the first contingent of volunteers as they prepared to board the *Sardinian* on 30 October 1899, emphasized the nobility of their task: "The cause for which you men of Canada are going to fight is the cause of justice, the cause of humanity, of civil rights and religious liberty. This is not a war of conquest … The object is not to crush out the Dutch population, but to establish in that land … British sovereign law, to assure to all men an equal share of liberty."[11] Newspaper and government rhetoric echoed these sentiments, representing the conflict as just and thus appropriately fought by the flower of the British Empire's manhood.

Bodies as Symbols

The bodies of the volunteer soldiers selected to enforce the empire's will were read as evidence of its superiority. War correspondent Stanley McKeogh Brown wrote of the Royal Canadian Regiment that "they went as the representatives of ideal Canadian manhood, while mentally and physically they well upheld the honour of the country whose best sons they were."[12] That it was a small force that was sent over, especially compared with the world wars that followed, and potential volunteers were more numerous than places in the contingent, meant that military authorities could be selective about the physical characteristics of those recruited. This included a preference for taller men, though height restrictions were unofficial. Alexander Stearns McCormick described his comrades (and himself) in glowing, although anecdotal, terms. "The finest class of men, well-educated, of good families, who left good business positions, professions or universities … Physique exceptional; fifty per cent being six feet or more, few less than five feet nine."[13] While these numbers are unsubstantiated and probably generous, John Cranfield and Kris Inwood have shown that the soldiers who went to South Africa were indeed probably somewhat taller than average Canadian men in this time period.[14] Height is read, in much newspaper reporting of the time, and later memoirs such as McCormack's, as a kind of visual shorthand for health and manliness. Newspapers described the Canadian contingent as composed of "fine, strapping fellows, broad-shouldered, clean-limbed and blue-eyed."[15] While the recruits were not weighed when they enlisted, a certain boyish lightness was an integral part of the image the press perpetuated about the Canadians in South Africa asserting, "They have, as a rule, a light, springy, devil-may care sort of swagger."[16]

Newspapers and government rhetoric presented Canadian soldiers as a recognizable physical type. These men served as representatives of prescriptive manliness to Canadians reading about their exploits, and as foils for the images of the Boers against whom they were fighting.[17] The importance of corporeal representations of national characteristics meant that the Boers were described with a similar emphasis on their physicality. In a history explaining the necessity of British expansion in South Africa, J. Castel Hopkins wrote, "Physically and mentally … the Dutch farmer is much the same everywhere in South Africa – tall, raw-boned, awkward in manner, slow of speech, fond of hunting whenever and wherever possible, accustomed to the open air, lazy as regards work, but active in pursuits involving personal pleasure."[18] The argument that the inhabitants of the South African republics, with their Calvinist religious beliefs and countenancing of slavery, were backwards and stood in the way of inevitable British progress was directly inscribed on their "raw-boned" bodies.

Descriptions of Boer women also emphasized their physical lassitude. Like the men, they were portrayed as slow and heavy, in obvious contradistinction to the portrayals of the active, alert Canadian volunteers who had been sent to rout them. The physical descriptions (by writers who had never met them, nor even been to South Africa) highlighted the women's unattractiveness, as well as the sexual inequality of their society. Hopkins wrote, "The women of the republics are very ignorant, and as mentally feeble as might be expected from their surroundings and history. Physically, stoutness is the end aim of female ambition, and to weigh two, or even three hundred pounds is the greatest pride of the Dutch women of the veldt. They are invariably treated as the inferior sex, and even eat apart from the men."[19] Presenting the women as physically large served to emasculate the Boer men as femininity was increasingly being associated with thinness in much of western society. As well, the Victorian era was a time when societies with greater gender differentiation were perceived to be more civilized, so that this description of the Afrikaner woman as so different from the ideal, delicate, "angel of the house" added support to the social Darwinist interpretation of the inevitable and proper demise of less civilized societies before superior British-Canadian culture. The war was justified by using the bodies of its participants as symbols, with the fat bodies of the Afrikaners evidence of the propriety of their relegation in the face of the light active bodies of the soldiers opposing them.

Letters Home

In the face of such enemies, then, the Canadians went to war confident in the righteousness of their cause, the splendour of their appearance, the fitness of their bodies, and the heroism and adventure that awaited them there. But the bodies in this war were, of course, not only symbols. The war was fought by men who marched and rode and shot at each other, who slept and ate and bled, and its depredations shaped the physical bodies of all involved. If the Canadians went in expecting adventure and easy victory, the war's reality, including British unpreparedness and a more wily and determined enemy than expected, soon disillusioned many soldiers. It also often took a toll on their bodies in a way that was different from the vague but manly "hardening" they had been led to expect in their military training. Noble Jones, perhaps feeling his deprivation a little more closely on a Christmas Eve far from home, wrote to his sister.

> I tell you people at home has no idea what a soldiers life means on active service I tell you it is not camp and 5 hrs a day drill look nice & clean it means 24 miles a days March with hardly anything to eat then a lye down in the trenches take a little sleep if you can with your harness & ammunition bullets whistling all around you no fun.[20]

Despite proponents' arguments about the salubrious effects the war would have for the Canadian volunteers, food and water were often insufficient and unhealthy. Disease, including dysentery, measles, and typhoid, were rampant, and more soldiers died of illness than in combat. The shedding of any extraneous body weight was almost inevitable in such circumstances.

Word filtered home about the privations soldiers faced in the war. Letters were shared, and published in local newspapers. War was meant to be an antidote to the dangerous ease of urban life, and some hardship was to be expected, was even part of the adventure. But problems of food had significant emotional resonance for families. The volunteers serving overseas tended to be young men, and in letters parents and siblings often expressed their concern that their boys were getting enough to eat. Edith Maveety wrote to her brother Douglas, who was serving with Strathcona's Horse, anxious to know whether he was well fed and taken care of.

> There are dozens and dozens of questions I would like to ask. Are you kicking about your grub tin? George Goodfellow – he went in 2nd Contingent – said that they starved a man and his people say he would not kick unless it was pretty bad.[21]

Food is part of the language of care within families and its lack concerned those whose brothers and sons had sailed far from home. Edith's letter also gives evidence of the informal networks through which neighbours and friends shared information to try to learn more about the situation of their far-away loved ones. Just as Lynn Kennedy demonstrates in chapter 3, that weight became a marker of health in infant development, so discussions of weight gain or loss became a way for families to assess the well-being of their soldiers overseas. While soldiering was promoted partly because it was thought to accustom a young man to more hardship than civilian city life presented, and thus lead him to hearty manliness, this might go too far if it involved actual deprivation. This was a danger often at the forefront of correspondents' minds. Family letters show their efforts to gain insight into the conditions their loved ones were living under by discussing both what they ate, and changes in their physical bodies.

Fat as Health

The soldiers' letters home, along with revealing their developing ambivalence about the war, often used discussion of food, weight, and fatness to describe their experiences and emotions to distant correspondents. Art Galoska's letter to his friend Robert Robinson expressed homesickness, and some dissatisfaction with elements of wartime life, but countered that negativity with talk of weight gain.

> I would like to know how the regatta came off, (I'll bet there were two or three surprises), and how the club is doing. I hope Ernie Morissette's arm is all right again. I often think of what old Jack Clarke said to me about being foolish for volunteering – especially when I was seasick or when doing guard or outpost on a cold night. But it must agree with me, as I stand it all right and I weigh 165 lbs. – which is a lot more than I have ever done before. I am not sorry I came, but you can bet I'll never do it again.

Gaining weight was understood to be a sign of health, both physical and mental. Weighing "a lot more than I have ever done before" was an assertion of Galoska's robustness at a time when being underweight was more of a concern for many, especially outside of the upper and middle classes, and especially for soldiers.[22] Along with an increase in bulk being a widely understood shorthand for men's physical well-being, declaring weight gain also served as a reassurance of emotional solidity. A loss of appetite was associated with a nervous temperament, and perhaps a certain effeminacy. A hearty appetite offered reassuring evidence of manly emotional stoicism as well as self-sufficiency. Asserting one's fatness countered familial worries about mental along with physical health.

Sometimes the effort to both describe and reassure, and the multiple interpretations ascribed to fat, made for complicated letters. George Smith wrote to Lewis, who seems to be a younger brother, in a tone that shifts back and forth between reassurance and complaint.

> I am quite well now and free of sickness of anysort & weigh 167 lbs. every body says that I am getting fat I hope so. We have a Baboon with us now & the Boys say it is hard to tell us apart. You know Happy McIlroy[?] he got of 2 hours cells for looting to-day if you could see some of England's crack regiments to-day you would laugh every body looks tired & weary & ragged unwashed & unshaved. I used to wonder why they always pictured a tramp with an empty corn can. I know now for many is the time that I have boiled some tea in an empty jam tin & cooked a piece of meat on a sheet of tin & made soup in a 4lb corn beef tin, I'll show you how to eat a square meal when I get home.[23]

George's physical description of himself and his fellow soldiers is a telling counter to the image of the well-groomed, energetic, and morally upright volunteer that the Canadian and British press had made so much of. It also repeats a theme frequent in their letters home, in which descriptions of hunger and deprivation are paired with commentary about their good health, with fat offered as the evidence of that robustness.

Another letter from Smith, this time to his parents, also offered up his weight gain as evidence of vigorous health, and a reason for his loved ones not to be concerned about him. He ended a 1900 missive: "Now the Mail Man is waiting for the letters so I close. I was never in better health & am gaining in weight and weigh about 155 lbs now my foot is Perfectly strong yesterday I entered a house & got about a kilo of Honey & 2lbs of butter 5lbs of dripping & a lot of soap[?] so I'm living high."[24] George is reassuring his parents that he is doing well. His injured foot is better and he is gaining weight. And yet, it is unlikely that these soldiers on active duty, often marching far ahead of their baggage trains, and in a time when weigh-scales were still rare, could actually access anything to measure their increased weight with. The different numbers George asserts as a measure of his increased mass seem more likely to be estimates, the numbers themselves plucked out of the air. Expressing his growth in such quantified terms though, rather than just saying he is heavier, makes the weight gain seem more substantial and less subjective. It is another example of the increasing shift toward measuring and quantified expressions of weight, especially as it was connected to health and fitness, that took place over the course of the nineteenth century, as discussed by Conor Heffernan in chapter 4 of this collection. Smith's letter also follows another common trope, in which letters that discuss, often in painful detail, a lack of food and water, and complain about the hardships of long marching, insufficient shelter, and annoying officers, close with a statement of never having been in better health. It is a contrary enough statement to be startling at times. The contradiction can perhaps be understood partly as a letter-writing convention of the day, so that by the end of the nineteenth century weight had become a trope with a specified meaning, and letters should properly end with a statement of robust, well-fed health, regardless of whether that was actually the case.

Fat as Power and Strategy

If fat was used as a language of reassurance, comforting distant family and friends with evidence of health, it was also an element of other kinds of discourse during this conflict. In soldiers' letters describing the way they have been able to access sufficient food, they are not just comforting worried parents, they are also bragging. George Smith, and the many others who served with the British and Canadian regiments and write in this vein, has gathered food through looting Afrikaner homes and farms, something he clearly does not see as shameful.[25] The letter itself, he tells his parents, was written on pages torn out from a notebook he had taken from a local farmhouse. Having food is a sign of success, both in the war itself, and in its contributions to building the empire. When soldiers like Smith write in their letters home about how they are becoming physically bigger, they are using their fatter bodies as clear evidence of their achievements in this role. Like the political cartoons Bonnie Miller discusses in chapter 9, in which Uncle Sam grows fat from the land he is ingesting, imperial success is demonstrated on the bodies of the victors in the war in South Africa. In this case, on a quite literal, individual level, the letter-writer's weight gain, and his access to food, is clear physical evidence that he has the upper hand and is on the road to victory.

If fat was a sign of power and imperial success, taking food from the enemy was also satisfying in other ways. This was a war that, like many wars, was often frustrating and boring; there was much waiting, and much fruitless marching around after a more mobile enemy. Having a farm to turn one's attention to was different, and active, and an interaction with an at least somewhat more tangible enemy. Charlie Tweddell wrote in his diary about his brigade "capturing" food from the civilians in a way that shows he found it interesting and rewarding.

> We arrived at Jacobsdal about 10 00 a.m. & bivouacked outside the town. As soon as the brigade was dismissed all hands ran towards the little town & captured all the Cattle, Sheep, Pigs & Fowl they could lay hands on. It was a sight of a lifetime to see the Kilties & all the other regmts. capturing & butchering fresh meat for our dinners. Some made for the gardens & rooted up all they could find. Water cress, Water melons, Corn & fruit in small quantities. Treggett & I went to a well & got our bottles full of lovely cool water then we strolled round the town & got some fruit off the trees (I think they were appricots) a small Water melon & some corn.[26]

While his diary entries also mention taking household items as souvenirs, gathering food from their opponents, and burning their crops is usually the main focus of references to looting in the diaries and letters.

The focus on food as a means of control and a measure of success was not just a characteristic of the conflict on the level of the individual soldier, it was also how the entire war, particularly its last two years, was fought. Control over food became a key element of strategy, and the goal, to a large extent, on which the conflict hinged. The first part of the War in South Africa was a series of surprising defeats for the British, but, partly thanks to large numbers of reinforcements and new leadership, they reversed their earlier losses, and took Pretoria and Bloemfontein, the capitals of the two small republics. It was assumed by the British military and political leadership that this would mean the imminent end of the war, but many inhabitants of the Transvaal and the Orange Free State fought on. It was a mobile, guerrilla campaign and the Boer "commandos" seemed impossible to tell apart from the civilians, who also were assumed to be aiding and feeding them.[27]

In response to attacks on railway lines, the British commander-in-chief Frederick, Lord Roberts instituted a scorched earth policy. Roberts issued a proclamation on 16 June 1900, stating that, for every attack on a railway line the closest homestead would be burned down. As this did not stop the "bitter enders" (those who rejected a negotiated peace after the taking of the capitals), another proclamation in September of that year stated that all homesteads would be burned in a radius of 16 kilometers of any attack, and that all livestock would be killed or taken away and all crops destroyed. This policy was intensified dramatically when Lord Kitchener took over from Roberts as commander of the British forces in November 1900. Homesteads and whole towns were burned down even if there had been no recent attack on any railway. In this way, by the end of the war almost all Boer homesteads – about 30,000 in all – had been razed to the ground and thousands of livestock killed.[28]

This was part of the work of the Canadian soldiers in the war, and it is striking that their references to burning homes, destroying crops, and pillaging tend to be fairly open and conversational. Many mention it in their diaries and letters as simply part of the work of the day, without any evident introspection about this behaviour's distance from the lofty war aims they might have enlisted for. Malcolm Rial's diary entry in mid-January of 1901 is typical.

> 16 January 1901 Remain Oozaak. 3.30am gun-fire coffee [with rum or brandy]. About 4am Captain Bartrum and self with half Companies of B&F start off for Modderfontein straight across country sending wagons by road to bring in families. Our orders are to bring in all families and destroy all foodstuffs and ovens. We get off two houses-full in two journeys by 11.30. … There are several more families in front. The fruit at this season is mainly pomegranates, peaches and apples with a few lemons here and there. We get some kidney beans and cabbages. We burn all wheat, oats and hay and then return to camp driving 4 wee pigs in front of us getting in about 12.30. Put Boer families in 3 tents.[29]

The destruction was all in a day's work, and worthy of no more commentary than what sort of fruit was in season. The destruction of foodstuffs and of the country's capacity to quickly produce more led to widespread hunger across the Afrikaner and Black African populations both during and for years after the war.[30]

Historian Carman Miller acknowledges that looting, particularly of food, was common. "To hungry soldiers, looting food appeared to be both a lark and a necessity akin to pilfering from the quartermaster."[31] Part of this can be related to necessity. Feeding its troops was an enormous logistical task, and one that the British command found overwhelming enough that it permitted a certain degree of "living off the land." It took about a ton of provisions daily to keep a hundred men on active service. Supplies from imperial sources had to cross an ocean, make their way slowly through crowded ports, and come overland via a single-track railway and wagons. And they had to contend with locals also anxious for supplies. Days after a massive shipment of 3,000 oxen, 30,000 forage rations, and 150,000 soldiers' rations was ambushed, Lord Roberts told officers to use local resources "to the fullest extent," and to appropriate them if they were not for sale or seemed unowned.[32] This official policy was combined with a certain willingness to look away when soldiers took unauthorized food, though the Canadians' letters also report receiving punishments for unauthorized looting.

That this looting comes across so openly in letters is evidence partly that the British and colonial soldiers saw themselves as just following orders, with no responsibility for the consequences. But also, especially since Canadian looting sometimes went beyond what their officers mandated, a further explanation seems required. That capturing food sometimes necessitated subterfuge shows a connection to the "frontier" elements of nineteenth-century Canadian manliness that can be compared with the pacifying of the country's western frontier only a few years earlier.[33] Indeed, that looting was an aspect of the war that sometimes felt like adventure, even fun, is evident in the often jocular tone the soldiers use when describing their actions. There were also nationalistic connotations. Canadians highlighted the food and other goods they gained possession of as evidence of manly self-sufficiency and an active initiative that they sometimes presented as evidence of the superiority of colonial masculinity compared with the tendency of British "Tommies" to wait passively for orders.

Fatness in this war, as a discursive marker of backwardness, or health, or power, was intrinsically tied to the food that sustained it. Taking food for themselves, or destroying it so that it could not support the enemy, was a key part of how Britain and its colonies waged the War in South Africa. Helen Bradford puts this in a less particular context, seeing the looting and farm burnings not as idiosyncratic manifestations of frustration but rather as expressions of longer-term British policies of colonial pacification. She argues that, although the scorched earth policy is often treated as an unpleasant but necessary anomaly in what has been called "the last of the gentlemen's wars," it should be understood as fitting easily into the larger picture of British colonial pacification in other imperial ventures, for example Rhodesia and Afghanistan.[34]

Concentration Camps

Connected to the farm burnings was the mass transfer of those who had lived on these homesteads into concentration camps. Men of fighting age were sent to prisoner of war camps, which were sometimes quite distant, in St Helena and Bermuda. Women and children were moved by soldiers to large camps throughout South Africa. This process was presented by the British as a sign of their civilization; they were not leaving their enemies unsheltered and unfed (again, food becomes an important element of the power structure in this conflict). Relocating people was also intended to solve the problem of farmers offering covert support to the commandos, and to discourage the Afrikaners enough that they stopped their resistance. The concentration camps have been generally judged as unsuccessful on all of these counts. They were angrily decried, at the time and since, as cruel and dangerous, and historians have often argued that the destruction of their domestic life actually stiffened Boer resolve.[35] While they were not intended as Nazi-style extermination camps, they were crowded, badly run, and unhygienic. Thousands of people died, more in the separate camps for Black South Africans. The camps where non-whites were sent offered insufficient shelter and were unprovisioned, with inmates, whose protection was one of the ostensible reasons for the war, expected to grow their own food to eat despite being interned on barren, desolate ground.[36]

There was some domestic dissent against these means of waging war. British activist Emily Hobhouse visited some camps and sent back damning descriptions of the deprivation there. In a similar way to the images of starvation that helped motivate the American population to war with Spain that Miller discusses in this volume, these drew emotional responses among some circles in Britain and the colonies. Future British Prime Minister Henry Campbell-Bannerman famously decried the "methods of barbarism" his country was using against the Boers. In Canada, the prominent journalist Goldwin Smith tried, with little success, to arouse his countrymen to outrage over the "domestic murder" of the farm burnings.[37] Atrocities against Black South Africans went largely unprotested.

Conclusion

The War in South Africa ended in British victory with the Treaty of Vereeniging in 1902. In trying to understand why that conclusion took so much more time and resources than expected, soul-searching in the United Kingdom after the war often turned back on the bodies of its undernourished urban working class as the reason for the empire's poor showing.[38] The empire required fatter, better-fed citizens if it was going to keep up its strength and global dominance.

Food is a common theme in soldiers' letters home, and in the missives they received from their loved ones. This is not surprising. The correspondence back and forth across the ocean was an effort to maintain bonds of kinship and friendship over great distances. Families eat together. They also talk about food together, with memories of special events and dishes, shared recipes, and plans for future celebratory meals being important means of connection.[39] This theme is heightened by the particularities of wartime. The men, along with suffering from homesickness, were often bored, with food a highlight in an otherwise uneventful day.

The letters to and from Canadian soldiers during the South African War though, use food in a way that is not just timeless, but also quite specific to their context. They reveal food being used sometimes as comfort and a reassurance of safety, and sometimes as evidence of a power over the land on which lived the people against whom they were fighting. Into this discourse, fat, as clear evidence of sufficient food, became a shorthand for strength. In a war in which men's bodies were symbols of the superiority of their empire and nation, and which was fought using access to food as a weapon, fat and its absence became a key part of the language of victory and defeat.

Looking at fat in this war, then, offers insight into the ways imperialism at the end of the nineteenth century was understood. Fat was part of the symbolic language of the war, with imperial expansion justified discursively through the "heavy, backwards bodies" of the Afrikaners, contrasted with the tall, "clean-limbed" troops of the empire. The study of this war also highlights the slipperiness and contingent nature of fat as a marker of identity. Fat, among Canadians during the War in South Africa, was understood differently according to the bodies that possessed it, or suffered from its lack. Fatness among Boer women was a sign of primitiveness, while among Canadian soldiers it showed health, power, and masculine initiative and self-reliance. As the other chapters in this volume have shown, fat was an intersectional marker of identity, read differently according to gender, class, and race.

Fatness was also both individual and embedded in relationships. The soldiers' letters home show that fatness was part of the language of connections within a family; that looting food and teasing about weight was part of the comraderie with one's fellow soldiers; and that access to food, and the ability to acquire it for oneself and destroy it for others, was a key aspect of being part of the British Empire. For the military body at the end of the nineteenth century, fat was important, both symbolically and in real physical terms, but its meaning was not fixed, or simple.

NOTES

1 Letter from Noble John Jones to Joe Jones, 30 March 1900. Canadian Letters and Images Project. https://www.canadianletters.ca/content/document-7711?position=19&list=P0YEbRlA629GBwZ7zuzoZZhQJeh4phCD-Z71BBQ_brw.

2 See, for example, Christina Jarvis, *The Male Body at War: American Masculinity during World War II* (Northern Illinois University Press: DeKalb, 2004).

3 Bernard Lightman draws together some important contemporary interpretations of Darwinism and social Darwinism in Darwin and the Popularization of Evolution. *Notes and Records of the Royal Society of London* 64, no. 1 (20 March 2010), 5–24.

4 For a discussion of Canadian manifestations of this concern, see Mark Moss, *Manliness and Militarism: Educating Young Boys in Ontario for War* (Don Mills, ON: Oxford University Press), 112.

5 See George Parkin's description of international affairs as a struggle between nations and races to be resolved according to the rule of survival of the fittest. George R. Parkin, *Imperial Federation: The Problem of National Unity* (London: MacMillan, 1894).

6 J.L. Cranfield, "Chivalric Machines: The Boer War, the Male Body, and the Grand Narrative in the *Strand Magazine*." *Victorian Literature and Culture* (2012), 40, 550. John Tosh, "Masculinities in an Industrializing Society: Britain, 1800–1914," *Journal of British Studies*, April 2005 44, no. 2 (April 2005), 330–42, 341–2.

7 Carl Berger, *The Sense of Power: Studies in the Ideas of Canadian Imperialism, 1867–1914* (Toronto, 1971).

8 Carman Miller has shown that the soldiers tended to be urban, white-collar workers. Carman Miller, "A Preliminary Analysis of the Socio-economic Composition of Canada's South African War Contingents," *Social History /Histoire Sociale*. Nov. 75 8, no. 16, 219–37.

9 Gordon Heath, *A War with a Silver Lining: Canadian Protestant Churches and the South African War, 1899–1902* (Montreal & Kingston: McGill-Queen's University Press, 2009), 86.

10 See Arthur Keppel-Jones, "A Test Case for Protection by the Mother Country;" John A. Hobson, "A Small Confederacy of International Mine Owners;" and J.S. Marais, "The Threat of an Independent South Africa," in *The Anglo: Boer War: Why was it Fought? Who was Responsible?*, ed. Theodore C. Caldwell (Boston: D.C. Heath and Co.), 1965.

11 Cited in Robert Page, *Imperialism and Canada 1895–1993* (Toronto: Holt, Rinehart, and Winston, 1972), 13.

12 Stanley McKeown Brown, *With the Royal Canadians* (Toronto: The Publishers' Syndicate, 1900), 6.

13 *The Royal Canadians in South Africa, 1899–1902* [nd, np].

14 John Cranfield and Kris Inwood, "The Great Transformation: A Long-Run Perspective on Physical Well-Being in Canada," *Economics and Human Biology* 5 (2007), 204–28.

15 S.M. Brown, *With the Royal Canadians* (Toronto 1900), 6.

16 Public Archives of British Columbia, "British Columbia Scrapbook," quoted in Miller, 76.

17 Amy Shaw, "The Boer War, Masculinity, and Citizenship in Canada, 1899–1902" in *Contesting Bodies and Nation in Canadian History*, ed. Patrizia Gentile and Jane Nicholas (Toronto: University of Toronto Press, 2013).
18 J. Castell Hopkins and Murat Halstead, *South Africa and the Boer-British War: Comprising A History of South Africa and Its People, Including the War of 1899 and 1900* (Toronto: John Winston and Co, 1900), 167.
19 Hopkins and Halstead, *South Africa and the Boer-British War*, 174.
20 Noble John Jones to Maggie Jones, 24 December 1899. https://www.canadianletters.ca/content/document-7583?position=5&list=iYQHJMIv_3D_9WQ7Dbv0JMaBZ6j1dgUJIZflcSYDElQ.
21 Canadian War Museum, Edith Maveety to J. Douglas Maveety, 8 May, 1900. File 58A 1 137.15.
22 Karl E. Friedl, "Body Composition And Military Performance: Origins Of The Army Standards," in *Body Composition and Physical Performance: Applications For the Military Services*, ed. B.M. Marriott and J. Grumstrup-Scott (Washington, DC: National Academies Press, 1990), 31.
23 George Smith to Lewis, Bloemfontein, 4 August 1900. LAC MG29 E100.
24 Letter from George Smith to his parents, 9 May 1900. Library and Archives Canada, George Smith Correspondence MG29 E100.
25 Black Africans, having already been dispossessed of most of their wealth by this time, were not explicit targets of looting.
26 C.H. Tweddell, *Charlie's First War: South Africa, 1899–1900*, ed. Carman Miller (Montreal & Kingston: McGill-Queen's University Press, 2014), 126–7.
27 Keith Surridge "'All you soldiers are what we call pro-Boer': The Military Critique of the South African War, 1899–1902," *History* 82, no. 268 (October 1997), 582–600.
28 Fransjohan Pretorius, *Scorched Earth* (Cape Town: Tafelberg, 2017).
29 Malcolm Riall, *Boer War: The Letters, Diaries and Photographs of Malcolm Riall from the War in South Africa 1899–1902*, ed. Nicholas Riall (London: Brassey's, 2000), 124.
30 Floris Van der Merwe, *The Boer War Show of St. Louis* (Stellenbosch: FJG Publikasies, 1904), 3.
31 Miller, 84.
32 S.B. Spies, *Methods of Barbarism?: Roberts and Kitchener and Civilians in the Boer Republics, January 1900–May 1902* (Cape Town: Human & Rousseau, 1977), 31; Pakenham, *Boer War*, 381.
33 Amy Shaw, "Fathers and Sons of Empire: Domesticity, Empire, and Canadian Participation in the Anglo-Boer War" in *Fighting with the Empire Canada, Britain, and Global Conflict, 1867–1947*, ed. Steve Mardi and William John Pratt (Vancouver: University of British Columbia Press, 2019).

34 Helen Bradford, "Gentlemen and Boers: Afrikaner Nationalism, Gender, and Colonial Warfare in the South African War," in *Writing a Wider War: Rethinking Gender, Race, and Identity in the South African War, 1899–1902*, ed. Greg Cuthbertson, Albert Grundlingh, and Mary-Lynn Suttie. Ohio University Press, Athens, 2002, 39.
35 Aidan Forth, *Barbed-Wire Imperialism: Britain's Empire of Camps, 1876–1903* (Oakland: University of California Press, 2017).
36 Nosipho Nkuna, "Black Involvement in the Anglo-Boer War, 1899–1902," *Military History Journal* 11 no. 3 (October 1999).
37 Amy Shaw, "Dissent in Canada against the Anglo-Boer War," in *Worth Fighting For: Canada's Tradition of War Resistance from 1812 to the War on Terror*, ed. Lara Campbell, Michael Dawson, and Catherine Gidney (Toronto: Between the Lines, 2015).
38 Miller, 436.
39 Ishiguro talks about food and family in the context of immigrant letters home around this time. Laura Ishiguro, *Nothing to Write Home About: British Family Correspondence and the Settler Colonial Everyday in British Columbia* (Vancouver: University of British Columbia Press, 2019), 126.

Conclusion

Discussions of the fat body are ubiquitous in contemporary society. Medical discourse and popular culture across the western world offer stark warnings about the dangers of the "obesity epidemic." The Centers for Disease Control and Prevention in the United States warns that "Obesity is a common, serious and costly chronic disease." Health Canada identifies obesity as "a risk factor in a number of chronic diseases," while Britain's National Health Service terms it "a common problem." Popularly connected to the consumption of energy-dense food and a more sedentary lifestyle, the "problem" has international scope. The World Health Organization asserts that obesity has nearly tripled since 1975, with as many as 1.9 billion adults considered overweight. Obesity in this context is defined in uncomplicatedly negative terms "as abnormal or excessive fat accumulation that may impair health." Equally important, these organizations assert that "obesity is preventable." This, of course, indicates that the fat body is a problem, something that should be prevented or cured. This labelling of fat as a growing epidemic also presents the fat body as a new, recent concern, created by the luxurious idiosyncrasies of contemporary life. To this interpretation, the fat body has little historical heft; before the twentieth century, it was, at most, a medical anomaly without much social, cultural, or political salience. Our predecessors, it suggests, were healthier and wiser, untroubled by the problems we have brought on ourselves through a sedentary and junk-food-fuelled lifestyle.[1]

Self-identified fat advocates and scholars in the field of Fat Studies fundamentally reject the medicalization implied not only in the idea of an epidemic, but in the very terms "obesity" and "overweight." Marilyn Wann, in her foreword to *The Fat Studies Reader*, subtitled "An Invitation to Revolution," asserts that "Calling fat people 'obese' medicalizes human diversity. Medicalizing diversity inspires a misplaced search for a 'cure' for naturally occurring difference. Far from generating sympathy for fat people, medicalization of weight fuels anti-fat prejudice and discrimination in all areas of society." Fat studies scholars instead encourage an examination of the "power arrangements that are based on weight" within society, and reject the practice of viewing the fat body as a problem that needs to be solved.[2] Interestingly, despite their otherwise nearly polarized opposition, this perspective also tends to present the nineteenth century as a more positive era in its views about fat. Laura Fraser, in an essay on the history of fat in the United States, for example, asserts that "a hundred years ago, a beautiful woman had plump cheeks and arms … women were *sexy* if they were heavy. In those days, Americans knew that a layer of fat was a sign that you could afford to eat well and that you stood a better chance of fighting off infectious diseases than most people."[3] The fat body in this envisioning of the past was thus linked to aesthetic beauty and social and physical success. Our predecessors, it suggests, were healthier and wiser, untroubled by the anxieties we have brought on ourselves by insisting on a singular, thin, body type.

Neither of these perceptions of past views on adipose bodies is entirely wrong, but both tend to create an overly simplified vision of the meaning of fatness (or thinness) in the nineteenth century. In truth, many different assessments existed over the course of the nineteenth century, changing both over time and according to the perspective of the observer. Amy Erdman Farrell in *Fat Shame* traces the changes that had already begun to occur by the mid-nineteenth century, as understandings of fat began to shift from frequently being seen as a mark of wealth and health to being more generally associated with negative characteristics such as greed, gluttony, and even stupidity and ugliness.[4] Adding further nuance, the identity of the body being judged was crucial, with factors such as gender, age, race, class, and ethnicity significantly determining the way in which fatness or thinness might be assessed. The process through which identities modified perceptions of fat was particularly complex when intertwined with concerns of power, politics and, particularly as the nineteenth century progressed, ideas about colonialism and imperialism.

Its shifting interpretations meant that fat had multiple, overlapping, and sometimes contradictory meanings in the nineteenth-century English-speaking world. It was not singularly negative or positive. It signified success for soldiers, advocates of empire, and new mothers. But it also showed weakness, and a lack of control over one's body. Fat was a sign of savagery but also of the dangers of over-civilization, corrupted into an effeminate decadence. It could mean health and attractiveness, or be a signifier of capitalist or imperialist exploitation. Fat, then, was intrinsic to how groups of people understood and presented themselves and how they perceived others. Understanding fat is necessary to understanding the nineteenth century. This book has taken steps in that direction.

Section I shows how philosophers and social theorists in the nineteenth century identified very different ways of seeing the fat body, linking "excess adiposity" to moral rather than physical health. And yet the growing interest in science and measurement in the nineteenth century, and the increasing authority of the medical profession, meant that the trend from qualitative to quantitative assessments of the body became an increasingly important part of the narrative. Section II provides insight into how the growing availability of scales and standardized charts indicating average or normative sizes were increasingly applied in all stages of life, from infant growth charts to actuarial insurance tables that assessed the healthy weight of middle-aged men and women. Physical culturists took this trend a step further, using exercise and diet to manipulate their body size in the pursuit of health. Yet, despite the growing emphasis on measurement that would become tied to a sense of fat as a problem in the twentieth century, very little is known about the actual weight of most individuals in the nineteenth century. The increasing number of charts and graphs suggested averages (and the growing tyranny of the "normal") but most individuals remained un-weighed, and even fewer had their weights recorded for the edification of future historians. Specific populations such as soldiers and prisoners have provided an intriguing sample of bodies that were measured, but as the essays in this collection suggest, there are a number of challenges with trying to weigh the historical body.

Perhaps equally notable in the methodological challenges of measuring weight is the fact that this was not the way that most people during most of the nineteenth century thought about their own bodies. They thought of weight gain or loss in terms of health or illness rather than as a number on a scale, and cultural representations suggested a much more complex understanding of the fat body than merely its weight. Section III explores these diverse cultural representations. Nineteenth-century culture, for example, celebrated Daniel Lambert for his immense girth, as an exceptional example of humanity rather than a mere oddity or an example of unhealthy obesity. Another figure often linked to the fat body in the nineteenth century, and mentioned in two chapters in this collection, was Sarah (also known as Saartjie) Baartman, her body put on display for European audiences. Baartman's experiences draw into sharp relief how the ideas of gender, race, and colonialism all became written on the body and in discussions of fat. Representations from literature to anthropological studies reflected these complex understandings of beauty, race, control, and culture. These views of fat could also become political. Section IV examines the intersection of the body, access to resources, and imperialism, making the body, fat or thin, symbolic of larger power relations.

This book has introduced just some of the complex and frequently shifting ways that fat was perceived in the long nineteenth century, offering a number of different lenses through which historians might understand both the physical realities and the symbolic meanings of these bodies. The emphasis on weight as a measurable thing indicating health or lack thereof has become so central to the narrative in the twentieth and twenty-first centuries that it has flattened out the discussion, rendering the many other perspectives on fat and the body virtually invisible. Bringing the many interpretations of the fat body in the long nineteenth century into the conversation offers new ways of understanding identity and power relations in that period, and new ways of looking at fat and the body in the current debate over the "obesity epidemic."

NOTES

1 CDC.gov/obesity/adult; www.canada.ca/en/health-canada/services/healthy-living/your-health/lifestyles/obesity; www.nhs.uk/conditions/obesity; https://www.who.int/news-room/fact-sheets/detail/obesity-and-overweight.

2 Marilyn Wann, "Foreword: Fat Studies: An Invitation to Revolution," in *The Fat Studies Reader*, ed. Esther Rothblum and Sondra Soloway (New York: New York University Press, 2009), xi, xiii.

3 Laura Fraser, "The Inner Corset: A Brief History of Fat in the United States," in *The Fat Studies Reader*, ed. Esther Rothblum and Sondra Soloway (New York: New York University Press, 2009), 11.

4 Amy Erman Farrell, *Fat Shame: Stigma & the Fat Body in American Culture* (New York: New York University Press, 2011), 4 and 30.

Bibliography

Published Primary Sources

An American Matron. *The Maternal Physician: A Treatise on the Nurture and Management of Infants, from the birth until two years old.* Philadelphia: Lewis Adams, Clark & Raser, 1818.

Atwood, Margaret. *Lady Oracle.* New York, Simon and Schuster, 2012.

Banting, William. *Letter on Corpulence,* 4th ed. London: Harrison, 1869.

Barker, Anthony. *Physical Culture for Fat People.* Anthony Barker: New York, 1903.

Blaikie, William. *How to Get Strong and Stay So.* New York: Harper & Brothers, 1879.

Brown, Stanley McKeown. *With the Royal Canadians.* Toronto: The Publishers' Syndicate, 1900.

Callcott, Margaret Law, ed. *Mistress of Riversdale: The Plantation Letters of Rosalie Stier Calvert, 1795–1821.* Baltimore: Johns Hopkins University Press, 1991.

Conrad, Joseph. *Heart of Darkness,* 1899. London: Arcturus, 2017.

Cromie, W.M.J. "Inactivity Means Death." *Physical Culture,* 4, no. 2 (1900): 80–1.

– "Why Should we Exercise?" *Physical Culture,* 3, no. 2 (1900): 77–8.

Crozer, J.P. *The Care of the Baby: A Manual for Mothers and Nurses,* 3rd ed. Philadelphia: W. B. Saunders & Co., 1903.

Crupper, Christopher. "Love and Beauty – Sartjee the Hottentot Venus." October 1811. Library of Congress. https://www.loc.gov/pictures/item/2007680266/.

Dewees, William P. *Treatise on the Physical and Medical Treatment of Children,* 3rd ed., Philadelphia: Carey, Lea & Carey, 1829.

Dowd, D.L. *Physical Culture for Home and School, Scientific and Practical.* New York: D.L. Dowd, 1895.

Drakard, J. *The Life of Daniel Lambert, With an Account of Men Noted for Their Corpulency.* Stamford, 1809.

Duncan, T.C. *The Feeding and Management of Infants and Children, and the Home Treatment of the Diseases.* Chicago: Duncan Bros., 1880.

– *How to be Plump: or Talks on Physiological Feeding.* Chicago: Duncan Bros., Pub, 1878.

Ewell, Thomas. *Letters to Ladies, Detailing Important Information Concerning Themselves and Infants.* Philadelphia: W. Brown, 1817.

Fletcher, Ella Adelia. *The Philosophy of Rest.* New York: Dodge Publishing Company, 1900.

– *The Woman Beautiful.* New York: W.M. Young & Co., Publishers, 1899.

Gillray, James. *Following the Fashion.* n.p., 1794.

Gould, Benjamin A. *Investigations in the Military and Anthropological Statistics of American Soldiers.* Cambridge: Riverside Press, United States Sanitary Commission, 1869.

Harrison, Eliza Cope, ed. *Best Companions: Letters of Eliza Middleton Fisher and Her Mother, Mary Hering Middleton, from Charleston, Philadelphia, and Newport, 1839–1846.* Columbia: University of South Carolina Press, 2001.

Hellam, Julia Clark. *Studies in Child Development: A Manual for Mothers and Mothers' Clubs.* Chicago: Row, Peterson & Co., 1913.

Hopkins, J. Castell, and Murat Halstead. *South Africa and the Boer-British War: Comprising A History of South Africa and Its People, Including the War of 1899 and 1900.* Toronto: John Winston and Co, 1900.

Joyce, James. *Ulysses.*1920; Reprint, London: Bodley Head 1960.

Keppler, Udo J. "Putting the Screws on Him." November 1904. Library of Congress. https://www.loc.gov/item/2011645581/.

Leary, Getz & Co. *Lives of great and celebrated characters of all ages and countries: comprising heroes, conquerors, jugglers and other curiosities of human nature.* Philadelphia: Leary, Getz & Co, 1860.

Lee, Fitzhugh, and Joseph Wheeler. *Cuba's Struggle Against Spain with the Causes for American Intervention and a Full Account of the Spanish-American War, Including Final Peace Negotiations.* New York: The American Historical Press, 1899.

Lombroso, Cesare, and William Ferrero, *The Female Offender.* New York: D. Appleton & Company, 1895.

King, Wilma, ed. *A Northern Woman in the Plantation South: Letters of Tryphena Blanche Holder Fox, 1856–1876.* Columbia: University of South Carolina Press, 1993.

Macfadden, Bernarr. *The Miracle of Milk: How To Use The Milk Diet Scientifically at Home.* New York: The Macfadden Company, 1923.

– *Physical Culture Cookbook.* New York: The Macfadden Company, 1901.

– *MacFadden's Physical Training.* New York: The Macfadden Company, 1900.

– *The Power and Beauty of Superb Motherhood.* New York: The Macfadden Company, 1901.

Maclaren, Archibald. "Military Gymnasia." *Royal United Services Institution*, 8, no. 31 (1864): 217–30.

Mathews, A. *The life and correspondence of Charles Mathews, the elder, Comedian.* London: Routledge, Warne and Routledge, 1860.

O'Rell, Max. [Pseud.]. *John Bull and His Island.* Translated from French. New York: Charles Scribner's Sons, 1889.

Parkin, George R. *Imperial Federation: The Problem of National Unity.* London: MacMillan, 1894.

Pett, Lionel Bradley. "A Canadian Table of Average Weights for Height, Age, and Sex." *American Journal of Public Health* 45 (1955): 862–8.

– "Malnutrition in Canada." *Canadian Medical Association Journal* 50 (1944): 9–14.

Pett, L.B., and G.F. Ogilvie. "The Canadian Weight-Height Survey." *Human Biology* 28 (1956): 177–88.

– "The Report on Canadian Average Weight, Height and Skinfolds," *Canadian Bulletin on Nutrition* 5 (1957): 1–81.

Pringle, Elizabeth W. Allston. *Chronicles of Chicora Wood.* New York: Charles Scribner's Sons, 1922.

Pye, Henry Chavasse. *Advice to a Mother on the Management of Her Children, and on the Treatment on the Moment of Some of Their More Pressing Illnesses and Accidents*, 9th ed. London: John Churchill & Sons, 1868.

The Royal Canadians in South Africa, 1899–1902 [nd, np].

Sandow, Eugen. *Sandow on Physical Training: A Study in the Perfect Type of the Human Form.* London: JS Tait & Sons, 1894.

– *Strength and How to Obtain It.* London: Gale & Polden, 1897.

Sigourney, L.H. *Letters to Mothers.* 2nd ed. New York: Harper & Bros, 1839.

Smith, Hugh. *The Female Monitor, Consisting of a Series of Letters to Married women on Nursing and the Management of Children.* Wilmington, Peter Brynberg, 1801.

Sozinskey, Thomas. *The Care and Culture of Children: A Practical Treatise for the Use of Parents.* Philadelphia: H.C. Watts Co, 1880.

Starr, Louis. MD. *Hygiene of the Nursery.* 4th ed. Philadelphia: P. Blakiston, Son & Co., 1894.

Talbot, D.A. *Woman's Mysteries of a Primitive People: The Ibibio of Southern Nigeria.* London: Casel and Company, 1915.

Tracy, Stephen, MD. *The Mother and Her Offspring.* New York: Harper & Bros., Pub., 1853.

Van der Merwe, Floris. *The Boer War Show of St. Louis.* Stellenbosch: FJG Publikasies, 1904.

Wilson, G.H. *The Eccentric Mirror.* London, 1806.

Archival Collections

Bridgeman Image Library
British Columbia Archives
British Museum
Canadian Letters and Images Project
Canadian War Museum
Library and Archives Canada
National Portrait Gallery, London
New York Historical Society
Ontario Archives
Provincial Archives of Saskatchewan
Public Archives of New Brunswick
South Carolina Historical Society
Southern Historical Collection, University of North Carolina
Stark Center, University of Texas at Austin
Tulane University Special Collections
Victorian & Albert Museum
Wellcome Collection, London.

Newspapers and Periodicals

Anaconda Standard
Atlanta Constitution
Biloxi Daily Herald
Boston Daily Globe
Boston Herald
Chicago Tribune
Christian Science Monitor
Des Moines Daily News
Indianapolis News
Indianapolis Sentinel
Hamilton Evening Democrat
Judge
Life
Los Angeles Sunday Times
Literary Digest
Minneapolis Journal
New York Herald
New York Journal
New York World
Newark Daily Advocate

Philadelphia Inquirer
Richmond Times
San Francisco Call
Seymour Daily Republican
Sunday Oregonian
Washington Post

Secondary Sources

Addison, Heather. *Hollywood and the Rise of Physical Culture.* New York: Routledge, 2003.

Afigbo, A. "The Eastern Provinces under Colonial Rule." In *Groundwork of Nigerian History,* edited by O. Ikimi. Ibadan: Heinemann Educational Books, 2004.

Anderson, John P. *Conrad's* Heart of Darkness*: Rebirth of Tragedy.* Boca Raton: Universal Publishers, 2005.

Anderson, M., and L. Aronson. "Jonathan A. Green: An African Photographer Hiding in Plain Sight." *African Arts* 44, no. 2 (2011).

Antonie, Luiza, Kris Inwood, Dan Lizotte, and J. Andrew Ross. "Tracking People over Time in 19th Century Canada." *Machine Learning* 96 (2014): 129–46.

Apple, Rima D. "'Advertised by our Loving Friends': The Infant Formula Industry and the Creation of New Pharmaceutical Markets, 1870–1910." *Journal of the History of Medicine and Allied Sciences* 41 (Jan. 1986): 3–23.

– "'To Be Used Only Under the Direction of a Physician': Commercial Infant Feeding and Medical Practice, 1870–1940," *Bulletin of the History of Medicine* 54 (Fall 1980): 402–17.

Ayandele, A. "External Relations with Europeans: Explorers, Missionaries and Traders" in *Groundwork of Nigerian History,* edited by O. Ikimi, 367–89. Ibadan: Heinemnn Educational Books, 1980.

Bacon, Lindo. *Health At Every Size: The Surprising Truth About Your Weight.* 2nd ed. Dallas, TX: BenBella Books, 2010.

Baecque, Antonio de. *The Body Politic: Corporeal Metaphor in Revolutionary France, 1770–1800.* Translated by Charlotte Mandell. Stanford: Stanford University Press.

Bank, Andrew. "Anthropology and Portrait Photography: Gustav Frisch's 'Natives of South Africa', 1863–1872." *Kronos: Journal of Cape History,* Special Issue: Visual History, no. 27.

Banta, Martha. *Barbaric Intercourse: Caricature and the Culture of Conduct, 1841–1936.* Chicago: University of Chicago Press, 2003.

Bascom, W., and M. Herskovits. "The Problem of Stability and Change in African Culture." In *Continuity and Change in African Cultures,* edited by W. Bascom and M. Herskovits. Chicago: University of Chicago Press, 1959.

Baten, Joerg, et al. "Evolution of Living Standards and Human Capital in China in the 18th–20th Centuries: Evidence from Real Wages, Age-Heaping." *Explorations in Economic History* 47 (2010): 347–59.

Beauvoir, Simone. *Le deuxième sexe*. Paris: Editions Gallimard, 1949.

Bederman, Gail. *Manliness and Civilization: A Cultural History of Gender and Race in the United States, 1880–1917.* Chicago: University of Chicago Press, 1995.

Bemis, Samuel F. "The Great Aberration of 1898." In *American Imperialism in 1898*, edited by Theodore P. Greene. Boston: D.C. Heath and Co., 1955.

Berg, M.E., and E. Eger, eds. *Luxury in the Eighteenth-Century: Debates, Desires and Delectable Goods.* Basingstoke: Palgrave Macmillan, 2002.

Berger, Carl. *The Sense of Power: Studies in the Ideas of Canadian Imperialism, 1867–1914.* Toronto: University of Toronto Press, 1971.

Bodenhorn, Howard, T. Guinanne, and T. Mroz. "Sample-Selection Biases and the Industrialization Puzzle." *Journal of Economic History* (2017): 171–207.

Bodenhorn, Howard, and Gregory N. Price. "Crime and Body Weight in the Nineteenth-Century: Was There a Relationship between Brawn, Employment Opportunities and Crime." *Économies et Sociétés, Série AF, Historie Economique Quantitative* 41 (January 2010), 1–20.

Bondeson, J. *Freaks: The Pig-Faced Lady of Manchester Square & Other Medical Marvels.* Stroud: Tempus Publishing, 2006.

Bordo, Susan. *Unbearable Weight: Feminism, Western Culture, and the Body.* Berkeley, CA: University of California Press, 1993.

Boritch, Helen. "The Criminal Class Revisited: Recidivism and Punishment in Ontario, 1871–1920." *Social Science History* 29 (2005): 137–70.

Boyd, Robert. *The Coming of the Spirit of Pestilence: Introduced Infectious Diseases and Population Decline among Northwest Coast Indians, 1774–1874.* Seattle and Vancouver: University of Washington Press and UBC Press, 1999.

Bradford, Helen. "Gentlemen and Boers: Afrikaner Nationalism, Gender, and Colonial Warfare in the South African War." In *Writing a Wider War: Rethinking Gender, Race, and Identity in the South African War, 1899–1902*, edited by Greg Cuthbertson, Albert Grundlingh, and Mary-Lynn Suttie, 37–66. Athens: Ohio University Press, 2002.

Branson, Susan. "Phrenology and the Science of Race in Antebellum America." *Early American Studies: An Interdisciplinary Journal* 15, no. 1 (2017): 164–93.

Bray, George A. "Obesity: Historical Development of Scientific and Cultural Ideas." *International Journal of Obesity* 14 (1990): 909–26.

Brewer, John. *The Common People and Politics, 1750–1790s.* Cambridge: Chadwyck-Healey, 1986.

Brewer, J., and R. Porter, eds. *Consumption and the World of Goods.* London: Routledge, 1993.

Brink, P. "The Fattening Room among the Annang of Nigeria." *Medical Anthropology* 12 (1999).

– "Fertility and Fat: The Annang Fattening Room." In *Social Aspects of Obesity*, edited by I. de Garine and N. Pollock. Amsterdam: Overseas Publishers Association, 1995.

Brosco, Jeffrey P. "Weight Charts and Well Child Care: When the Pediatrician Became the Expert in Child Health." In *Formative Years: Children's Health in the United States, 1880–2000*, edited by A.M. Stern & H. Markel, 91–120. Ann Arbor, MI: University of Michigan Press, 2002.

Brown, Alan, and G. Albert Davis. "The Prevalence of Malnutrition in the Public School Children of Toronto." *Canadian Medical Association Journal* 11 (1921): 124–6.

Brown, Bill "Thing Theory." *Critical Inquiry* 28, no. 1 (Things), (Autumn, 2001): 1–22.

Brown, Jennifer. *Cannibalism in Literature and Film*. London: Palgrave Macmillan, 2013.

Budd, Michael Anton. *The Sculpture Machine: Physical Culture and Body Politics in the Age of Empire*. New York: NYU Press, 1997.

Campbell, John. "Work, Pregnancy, and Infant Mortality among Southern Slaves." *Journal of Interdisciplinary History* 14 (Spring 1984): 793–813.

Campbell, Mary and Gordon Campbell. *The Pen, Not the Sword*. Nashville: Aurora Publishers Inc., 1970.

Campos, Paul. *The Obesity Myth: Why America's Obsession with Weight is Hazardous to Your Health*. New York: Gotham Books, 2004.

Canguilhem, Georges. *The Normal and the Pathological*. Translated by Carolyn R. Fawcett and Robert S. Cohen. New York: Zone Books, 1991 [1972].

Canning, Charlotte. *The Most American Thing in America: Circuit Chautauqua as Performance*. Iowa: University of Iowa Press, 2005.

Carl, LeRoy M. "Political Cartoons: 'Ink Blots' of the Editorial Page." *Journal of Popular Culture* 4 (1970): 39–45.

Carroll, H. *Visualising Elite Political Women in the Reign of Queen Charlotte, 1761–1818*. Unpublished PhD thesis. Edinburgh: University of Edinburgh, 2017.

Carson, Scott. "Biology, Complexion, and Socioeconomic Status: Accounting for 19th Century US BMIs by Race." *Australian Economic History Review* 55 (2015): 238–55.

– "The Body Mass Index of Blacks and Whites in the United States during the Nineteenth Century." *Journal of Interdisciplinary History* 42 (2012): 371–91.

– "Body Mass Index Through Time: Explanations, Evidence, and Future Directions." In *The Oxford Handbook of Economics and Human Biology*, edited by John Komlos and Inas R. Kelly, 133–51. Oxford: Oxford University Press, 2016.

– "Body Mass, Wealth, and Inequality in the 19th Century: Joining The Debate Surrounding Equality and Health." *Economics and Human Biology* 11 (2013): 90–4.

– "Body Weight and United States Economic Development 1840–1940." CESIFO working paper 7573 (2019).
– "Nineteenth Century Race, Body Mass, and Industrialization: Evidence from American Prisons." *Journal of Interdisciplinary History*, 42 (2012): 371–91.
– "Statures of 19th century Chinese Males in America." *Annals of Human Biology* 34 (2007): 173–82.
Cassata, Francesco. *Building the New Man*. Budapest: Central European University Press, 2011.
Caswell, Lucy Shelton. "Drawing Swords: War in American Editorial Cartoons." *American Journalism* 21 no. 2 (2004): 13–45.
Chapman, David L. *Sandow the Magnificent: Eugen Sandow and the Beginnings of Bodybuilding*. Chicago: University of Illinois Press, 1994.
Checkley, Edwin. *A Natural Method of Physical Training*. New York: William C. Bryant, 1895.
Christen, Peter. *Data Matching: Concepts and Techniques for Record Linkage, Entity Resolution, and Duplicate Detection*. Springer-Verlag Berlin Heidelberg, 2012.
Clarke, Nic, John Cranfield, and Kris Inwood. "Fighting Fit? Diet, Disease, and Disability in the Canadian Expeditionary Force, 1914–18." *War and Society* 33 (2014): 80–97.
Cohen, Patricia Cline. *A Calculating People: The Spread of Numeracy in Early America*. Chicago: University of Chicago Press, 1982.
Coltman, V. "Im-material Culture and History of Art(efacts)." In *Writing Material Culture History*, edited by A. Gerritsen and G. Riello, 232–48. London: Bloomsbury, 2014.
Conrad, Peter. *The Medicalization of Society: On the Transformation of Human Conditions into Treatable Disorders*. Baltimore, MD: John Hopkins University Press, 2007.
Cozzi, Annette. *The Discourses of Food in Nineteenth-Century British Fiction*. New York: Palgrave Macmillan, 2010.
Crais, Clifton C., and Pamela Scully. *Sara Baartman and the Hottentot Venus: A Ghost Story and a Biography*. New Jersey: Princeton University Press, 2009.
Cranfield, J.L. "Chivalric Machines: The Boer War, the Male Body, and the Grand Narrative in the *Strand Magazine*." *Victorian Literature and Culture* (2012).
Cranfield, John, and Kris Inwood, eds. "Genes, Class or Culture? French-English Height Differences in Canada." In *Lives in Transition: Longitudinal Research from Historical Sources*, 233–53. Montreal and Kingston: McGill-Queen's University Press, 2015.
– "The Great Transformation: A Long-Run Perspective on Physical Well-Being in Canada." *Economics and Human Biology* 5 (2007): 204–28.

– "A Tale of Two Armies: Comparative Growth in the Mirror of World War One." *Australian Economic History Review* 55 (2015): 212–33.

Cranfield, John, Kris Inwood, and J. Andrew Ross. "Before the Obesity Epidemic: The Body Mass Index of Canadians in World War One and World War Two." *Canadian Bulletin of Medical History* 32 (2015): 319–35.

Crosby, Alfred W. *The Measure of Reality: Quantification and Western Society, 1250–1600.* Cambridge: Cambridge University Press, 1997.

Czerniawski, Amanda M. "From Average to Ideal: The Evolution of the Height and Weight Table in the United States, 1836–1943." *Social Science History* 31 no. 2 (Summer 2007): 273–96.

Daschuk, James. *Clearing the Plains: Disease, Politics of Starvation, and the Loss of Indigenous Life.* Regina: University of Regina Press, 2013.

Davis, Lennard, ed. "Introduction: Normality, Power, and Culture." In *The Disability Studies Reader.* 4th Ed. 1–14. New York: Routledge, 2013.

Day, C. *Consumptive Chic: A History of Beauty, Fashion and Disease.* London and New York: Bloomsbury Academic, 2017.

De La Peña, Carolyn Thomas. *The Body Electric: How Strange Machines Built the Modern American.* New York: NYU Press, 2003.

– "Dudley Allen Sargent: Health Machines and the Energized Male Body." *Iron Game History,* 8, no. 2 (2003): 3–19.

Depauw, Ewout. "There and Back Again: The Selectivity of Recidivism in Belgian Prisons." *Social Science History 44* (2020): 445–62.

Donald, Diana. *The Age of Caricature: Satirical Prints in the Reign of George III.* New Haven and London: Yale University Press, 2006.

Duchan, J.F., and D. Kovarsky, eds. *Diagnosis as Cultural Practice.* Berlin: Mouton de Gruyter, 2005.

DuPuis, E. Melanie. *Dangerous Digestion: The Politics of American Dietary Advice.* California: University of California Press, 2015.

Dye, Nancy Schrom, and Daniel Blake Smith. "Mother Love and Infant Death, 1750–1920." *Journal of American History* 73 (Sept. 1986): 329–53.

Edwards, E. "Photography and the Performance of History." *Kronos* (Special Issue: Visual History), *Journal of Cape History,* no. 27 (2001): 15–29.

Essien, A. "The Sociological Implication of the Worldview of the Annang People: An Advocacy for Paradigm Shift." *Journal for Emerging Trends in Educational Research and Policy Studies* (JETERAPS) 1, nos. 11, 31.

Eveleth, Phyllis B., and J.M. Tanner. *Worldwide Variation in Human Growth.* Cambridge: Cambridge University Press, 1976.

Farrell, Amy Erdman. *Fat Shame: Stigma and the Fat Body in American Culture.* New York: New York University Press, 2011.

Fay, F. A. *Fashioning Faces: The Portraitive Mode in British Romanticism.* Hanover and London: New Hampshire University Press, 2010.

Feir, Donna, Rob Gillezeau, and Maggie Jones. "The Slaughter of the Bison and Reversal of Fortunes on the Great Plains." *Federal Reserve Bank of Minnesota Working Paper* January 2019.

Fildes, Valerie A. *Breasts, Bottles and Babies: A History of Infant Feeding.* Edinburgh: Edinburgh University Press, 1986.

Firth, John. "History of Tuberculosis. Part 1 - Phthisis, Consumption and the White Plague." *Journal of Military and Veterans' Health* 22 (June 2014): 29–35.

Fischer, Roger A. "Political Cartoon Symbols and the Divergence of Popular and Traditional Cultures in the United States." In *Dominant Symbols in Popular Culture*, edited by Ray B. Browne, Marshall W. Fishwick, and Kevin O. Browne, 181–208. Bowling Green: Bowling Green State University Popular Press, 1990.

Floud, Roderick, and Kenneth W. Wachter. "Poverty and Physical Stature: Evidence on the Standard of Living of London Boys 1770–1870." *Social Science History* 6 (1982): 422–52.

Forth, Aidan. *Barbed-Wire Imperialism: Britain's Empire of Camps, 1876–1903.* Oakland: University of California Press, 2017.

Forth, Christopher E. *Fat: A Cultural History of the Stuff of Life.* London: Reaktion Books, 2019.

– "Fat, Desire and Disgust in the Colonial Imagination." In *History Workshop Journal* no. 73 (Spring 2012): 211–39.

Foucault, Michel. *The Archaeology of Knowledge.* Translated by A.M. Sheridan Smith. London: Routledge, 1989 [London: Tavistock, 1972].

– *The Birth of the Clinic: An Archaeology of Medical Perception.* New York: Pantheon, 1973.

– *The History of Sexuality: An Introduction* (vol. 1). Translated by Robert Hurley. New York: Vintage Books, 1990. New York: Pantheon Books, 1978.

– *The Order of Things: An Archaeology of the Human Sciences.* New York: Pantheon Books, 1970.

– *"Society Must Be Defended": Lectures at the Collège de France, 1975–1976.* Translated by David Macey. New York: Picador, 2003.

Fraser, Laura. "The Inner Corset: A Brief History of Fat in the United States." In *The Fat Studies Reader*, edited by Esther Rothblum and Sondra Soloway, 11–14. New York: New York University Press, 2009.

Friedl, Karl E. "Body Composition And Military Performance: Origins Of The Army Standards." In *Body Composition and Physical Performance: Applications For the Military Services*, edited by B.M. Marriott and J. Grumstrup-Scott, 31–56. Washington, DC: National Academies Press, 1990.

Fyson, Donald, and François Fenchel. "Prison Registers, Their Possibilities and Their Pitfalls: The Case of Local Prisons in Nineteenth-century Quebec." *The History of the Family* 20 (2015): 163–88.

Gabbidon, Shaun L. *Crimininological Perspectives on Race and Crime.* New York: Routledge, 2010.

Gagan, David, and Rosemary Gagan. "Working-Class Standards of Living in Late-Victorian Urban Ontario: A Review of the Miscellaneous Evidence on the Quality of Material Life." *Journal of the Canadian Historical Association* 1 (1980): 171–93.

Gagen, Elizabeth A. "Making America Flesh: Physicality and Nationhood in Early Twentieth-Century Physical Education Reform." *Cultural Geographies* 11, no. 4 (2004): 417–42.

Galinsky, A.D., K. Hugenberg, C. Groom, and G. Bodenhausen. "The Reappropriation Of Stigmatizing Labels: Implications For Social Identity." *Identity Issues in Groups Research on Managing Groups and Teams,* 5 (2003): 221–56.

Gallati, Barbara Dayer. "The Shattuck Family: Aaron Draper Shattuck's Experiment in Narrative Content." *The American Art Journal* 20, no. 3 (1988): 36–47.

Galton, David J. "Greek Theories on Eugenics." *Journal of Medical Ethics* 24 no. 4 (August 1998): 263–7.

Gard, Michael, and Jan Wright. *The Obesity Epidemic: Science, Morality and Ideology.* London: Routledge, 2005.

Gear, Josephine. "The Baby's Picture: Woman as Image Maker in Small Town America." *Feminist Studies* 13 (Summer 1987): 419–42.

Geipel, John. *The Cartoon: A Short History of Graphic Comedy and Satire.* Newton Abbot: David & Charles, 1972.

Geloso, Vincent. "Distinct within North America: Living Standards in French Canada, 1688–1775." *Cliometrica* 13 (2019): 277–321.

Geloso, Vincent, and Peter Lindert. "Relative Costs of Living, for Richer and Poorer, 1688–1914." *Cliometrica* 14 (2020): 417–42.

Gilman, Sander L. *Fat: A Cultural History of Obesity.* Cambridge: Polity Press, 2008.

– "Fat as Disability: The Case of the Jews." *Literature and Medicine* 23 (2004): 46–60.

– *Fat Boys: A Slim Book.* Lincoln: University of Nebraska Press, 2004.

– "How Fat Detectives Think." In *Cultures of the Abdomen,* edited by Christopher Forth and Ana Carden-Coyne, 221–37. Palgrave Macmillan, New York, 2005.

– *Obesity: The Biography.* Oxford: Oxford University Press, 2013.

– *Picturing Health and Illness: Images of Difference.* Baltimore: The Johns Hopkins University Press, 1995.

Golden, Janet. *A Social History of Wet Nursing in America: From Breast to Bottle.* Cambridge: Cambridge University Press, 1996.

Golden, Janet, and Lynn Weiner. "Reading Baby Books: Medicine, Marketing, Money and the Lives of American Infants." *Journal of Social History* 44 (Spring 2011): 667–87.

Green, Alan, Mary MacKinnon, and Chris Minns. "Conspicuous by Their Absence: French Canadians and the Settlement of the Canadian West." *Journal of Economic History* 65 (2005): 822–49.

Haines, Michael. "Growing Incomes, Shrinking People: Can Economic Development be Hazardous to Your Health." *Social Science History* 28 (2004): 249–70.

Harris, Bernard. *The Health of the Schoolchild.* Buckingham: Open University Press, 1995.

Heath, Gordon. *A War with a Silver Lining: Canadian Protestant Churches and the South African War, 1899–1902.* Montreal and Kingston: McGill-Queen's University Press, 2009.

Heffernan, Conor. "Strength Peddlers: Eddie O'Callaghan and the Selling of Irish Strength." *Sport in History*, 38, no. 1 (2018): 23–45.

Hess, Stephen, and Sandy Northrop. *Drawn and Quartered: The History of American Political Cartoons.* Montgomery: Elliot & Clark Publishing, 1996.

Heywood, Leslie. *Dedication to Hunger: The Anorexic Aesthetic in Modern Culture.* Berkeley: University of California Press, 1996.

Higgs, Edward. *The Information State in England: The Central Collection of Information on Citizens since 1500.* Basingstoke: Palgrave Macmillan, 2004.

Hobson, John A. "A Small Confederacy of International Mine Owners." In *The Anglo: Boer War: Why was it Fought? Who was Responsible?* edited by Theodore C. Caldwell, 18–24. Boston: D.C. Heath and Co., 1965.

Hoppa, R.D., and T.N. Garlie. "Secular Changes in the Growth of Toronto Children During the Last Century." *Annals of Human Biology* 25 (1998): 553–61.

Horrell, Sara, David Meredith, and Deborah Oxley. "Measuring Misery: Body Mass, Ageing and Gender Inequality in Victorian London." *Explorations in Economic History* 46 (2009): 93–119.

Huff, Joyce L. "A 'Horror of Corpulence': Interrogating Bantingism and Mid-Nineteenth-Century Fat-Phobia." In *Bodies Out of Bounds: Fatness and Transgression*, edited by J. E. Braziel and K. LeBesco, 39–59. Berkeley: University of California Press, 2001.

Hulme, Peter. "Introduction: The Cannibal Scene." In *Cannibalism and the Colonial World*, edited by Francis Barker, Peter Hulme, and Margaret Iversen. Cambridge: Cambridge University Press, 1998.

Hunt, Tamara L. *John Bull: Political Caricature and National Identity in Late Georgian England.* Burlington, VT: Ashgate Publishing, 2003.

Hunt, William R. *Body Love: The Amazing Career of Bernarr Macfadden.* Wisconsin: Popular Press, 1989.

Hurren, Elizabeth T. *Dying for Victorian Medicine: English Anatomy and Its Trade in the Dead Poor, c.1834–1929.* Hampshire and New York: Palgrave Macmillan, 2012.

Hutson, David J. "Plump or Corpulent?: Lean or Gaunt? Historical Categories of Bodily Health in Nineteenth-Century Thought." *Social Science History* 41, no. 2 (Summer 2017): 283–303.

Hyman, Gwen. *Making a Man: Gentlemanly Appetites in the Nineteenth-Century British Novel.* Athens: Ohio University Press, 2009.

Ignacio, Abe, Enrique de la Cruz, Jorge Emmanuel, and Helen Toribio. *The Forbidden Book: The Philippine-American War in Political Cartoons.* San Francisco: T'Boli Publishing, 2004.

Imeh, I. *Daughters of Seclusion: The Revelation of the Ibibio "Fattened Bride" as the Icon of Beauty and Power.* New York: Lang Publishing 2012.

Inwood, Kris, and Evan Roberts. "'Indians are the Majority of the Prisoners'? Historical Variations in Incarceration Rates for Indigenous Women and Men in British Columbia." *The Howard Journal of Criminal Justice* 59 (2020): 350–69.

– "Longitudinal Studies of Human Growth and Health: A Review of Recent Historical Research." *Journal of Economic Surveys* 24 (2010): 801–40.

Inwood, K., R. Kippen, H. Maxwell-Stewart, and R. Steckel. "The Short and the Tall: Comparing Stature and Socio-Economic Status for Male Prison and Military Populations." *Social Science History* 44 (2020): 463–83.

Inwood, Kris, and Hamish Maxwell-Stewart. "Selection Bias and Social Science History." *Social Science History* 44 (2020): 411–16.

Inwood, Kris, Hamish Maxwell-Stewart, Deborah Oxley, and Jim Stankovich. "Growing Incomes, Growing People in Nineteenth-century Tasmania." *Australian Economic History Review* 55 (2015): 187–211.

Inwood, Kris, Hamish Maxwell-Stewart, and J. Stankovich. "The Prison and the Colonial Family." *History of the Family,* 20, no. 2 (2015) 231–48.

Ishiguro, Laura. *Nothing to Write Home About: British Family Correspondence and the Settler Colonial Everyday in British Columbia.* Vancouver: University of British Columbia Press, 2019.

Jarvis, Christina. *The Male Body at War: American Masculinity during World War II.* Northern Illinois University Press: DeKalb, 2004.

Jeffreys, M. "The Nyama Society." *African Studies* 15, no. 1 (1956): 15–28.

Jones, Kathleen W. "Sentiment and Science: The Late Nineteenth Century Pediatrician as Mother's Advisor." *Journal of Social History* 17 (Autumn 1983): 79–96.

Jordan, Thomas E. *The Degeneracy Crisis and Victorian Youth.* Albany: SUNY Press: 1993.

Kaplan, Amy. "Left Alone with America: The Absence of Empire in the Study of American Culture." In *Cultures of United States Imperialism,* edited by Amy Kaplan and Donald E. Pease, 3–21. Durham: Duke University Press, 1993.

Kassan, John F. *Houdini, Tarzan and the Perfect Man: The White Male Body and the Challenge of Modernity in America.* New York: Hill and Wang, 2001.

Katzmarzyk, Peter T. "The Canadian Obesity Epidemic: An Historical Perspective." *Obesity Research* 10 (2002): 666–74.

Kelm, Mary-Ellen. *Colonizing Bodies: Aboriginal Health and Healing in British Columbia 1900–1950.* Vancouver: UBC Press, 1998.

Kemnitz, Thomas Milton. "The Cartoon as a Historical Source." *Journal of Interdisciplinary History* 4 (Summer 1973): 85.

Kendall, Ora, Tammy Lipskie, and Shauna MacEachern. "Canadian Health Surveys 1950–1977." *Chronic Diseases in Canada* 18 (1997): 70–90.

Keppel-Jones, Arthur. "A Test Case for Protection by the Mother Country." In *The Anglo: Boer War: Why was it Fought? Who was Responsible?*, edited by Theodore C. Caldwell, 2–11. Boston: D.C. Heath and Co. 1965.

Ketchum, Alton. *Uncle Sam: The Man and the Legend.* New York: Hill and Wang, 1969.

Klein, Dorie. "The Etiology of Female Crime: A Review of the Literature." *Issues in Criminology*, 8, no. 2 (Fall 1973).

Komlos, John, and Brian A'Hearn. "Clarifications of a Puzzle: The Decline in Nutritional Status at the Onset of Modern Economic Growth in the United States." *Journal of Economic History* 79 (2019): 1129–53.

Komlos, J., and M. Brabec. "The Trend of Mean BMI Values of US Adults, Birth Cohorts 1882–1986 Indicates that the Obesity Epidemic Began Earlier Than Hitherto Thought." *American Journal of Human Biology*, 22 *(2010):* 631–38.

– "The Trend of BMI Values of US Adult by Deciles, Birth Cohorts 1882–1986 Stratified by Gender and Ethnicity." *Economics and Human Biology*, 9 (2011), 234–50.

Laqueur, Thomas. *Making Sex: Body and Gender from the Greeks to Freud.* Cambridge, MA: Harvard University Press, 1992.

LeBesco, Kathleen. *Revolting Bodies? The Struggle to Redefine Fat Identity.* Amherst: University of Massachusetts Press, 2004.

Levy-Navarro, E. *The Culture of Obesity in Early and Late Modernity: Body Image in Shakespeare, Jonson, Middleton & Skelton.* London: Palgrave Macmillan, 2008.

Lightman, Bernard. "Darwin and the Popularization of Evolution." *Notes and Records of the Royal Society of London* 64, no. 1 (20 March 2010): 5–24.

Litoff, Judy Barrett. *American Midwives, 1860 to the Present.* Westport, CT: Greenwood Press, 1978.

Lux, Maureen. *Medicine That Walks: Disease, Medicine and Canadian Plains Native People, 1880–1940.* Toronto: University of Toronto Press, 2001.

MacFadden, Mary Williamson, and Emile Gauvreau. *Dumbbells and Carrot Strips: The Story of Bernarr MacFadden.* New York: Holt, 1953.

Marais, J.S. "The Threat of an Independent South Africa." In *The Anglo: Boer War: Why was it Fought? Who was Responsible?*, edited by Theodore C. Caldwell, 79–84. Boston: D.C. Heath and Co. 1965.

Marsh, Leonard C. *Health and Unemployment: Some Studies of Their Relationships.* Toronto: Oxford University Press, 1936.

Maxwell-Stewart, Hamish and James Bradley. "'Behold the Man': Power, Observation and the Tattooed Convict." *Australian Studies*, 12, no. 1 (1997): 71–97.

May, Ernest R. *Imperial Democracy: The Emergence of America as a Great Power* (New York: Harcourt, Brace, and World, 1961.

McCormick, M.C. "The Contribution of Low Birth Weight to Infant Mortality and Childhood Morbidity." *New England Journal of Medicine* 312(2) (10 Jan. 1985): 82–90.

McKendrick, N., J. Brewer, and J.H. Plumb. *The Birth of a Consumer Society: The Commercialization of Eighteenth-Century England.* Bloomington, Indiana: Indiana University Press, 1982.

McKenzie, Shelly. *Getting Physical: The Rise of Fitness Culture in America.* Lawrence: University Press of Kansas, 2013.

McMillen, Sally. "Mothers' Sacred Duty: Breast-Feeding Patterns among Middle- and Upper-Class Women in the Antebellum South." *Journal of Southern History* 51 (Aug. 1985): 333–56.

McPhail, Deborah. *Contours of the Nation: Making Obesity and Imagining Canada, 1945–1970.* Toronto: University of Toronto Press, 2017.

Meckel, Richard A. *Save the Babies: American Public Health Reform and the Prevention of Infant Mortality, 1850–1929.* Baltimore: Johns Hopkins University Press, 1990.

Medhurst, Martin J., and Michael A. Desousa. "Political Cartoons as Rhetorical Form: A Taxonomy of Graphic Discourse." *Communication Monographs* 48 (September 1981): 197–236.

Messenger, J., and B. Messenger. "Sexuality in Folklore in a Nigerian Society." *Central Issues in Anthropology* 3, no. 1 (1981): 29–50.

Miller, Bonnie M. *From Liberation to Conquest: The Visual and Popular Cultures of the Spanish-American War of 1898.* Amherst: University of Massachusetts Press, 2011.

Miller, Carman. "A Preliminary Analysis of the Socio-economic Composition of Canada's South African War Contingents." *Social History /Histoire Sociale* 8, no. 16 (Nov 1975): 219–37.

Miller, Kelsey. "The Completely Bonkers History of the Bathroom Scale." *Elemental*, 15 Feb. 2021. elemental.medium.com.

Millward, Robert, and Frances Bell. "Infant Mortality in Victorian Britain: The Mother as Medium." *The Economic History Review* 54 (Nov. 2001): 699–733.

Mitchinson, Wendy. *Fighting Fat: Canada, 1920–1980.* Toronto: University of Toronto Press, 2018.

Mol, Annemarie. *The Body Multiple: Ontology in Medical Practice.* Durham: Duke University Press, 2002.

Monaghan, Lee F. "Big Handsome Men, Bears, and Others: Virtual Constructions of 'Fat Male Embodiment.'" In *Sociology of the Body: A Reader*, edited by Claudia Malacrida and Jacqueline Low, 57–64. Don Mills, ON: Oxford University Press, 2008.

Morais, Dominic G. "Branding Iron: Eugen Sandow's 'Modern' Marketing Strategies, 1887–1925.'" *Journal of Sport History*, 40, no. 2 (2013): 193–214.

Morgan, Stephen. "Stature and Economic Development in South China, 1810–1880." *Explorations in Economic History* 46 (2009): 53–69.

Morin, A. Arsenault, V. Geloso, and V. Kufenko. "The Heights of French-Canadian Convicts, 1780s to 1820s." *Economics & Human Biology* 36 (2017): 126–36.

Moss, Mark. *Manliness and Militarism: Educating Young Boys in Ontario for War.* Don Mills, ON: Oxford University Press.

Muldrew, C. *Food, Energy and the Creation of Industriousness: Work and Material Culture in Agrarian England, 1550–1780.* Cambridge: Cambridge University Press, 2011.

Mullins, Greg. "Nudes, Prudes, and Pigmies: The Desirability of Disavowal in Physical Culture." *Discourse*, 15, no. 1 (1992): 27–48.

Murray, Thomas E. "The Language of Bodybuilding." *American Speech*, 59, no. 3 (1984): 195–206.

Noakes, A. *Ben Marshall, 1768–1835.* Leigh-on-Sea: F. Lewis, 1978.

Nicholas, Jane, and Patrizia Gentile, eds. "Introduction." In *Contesting Bodies and Nation in Canadian History*, 3–30. Toronto: University of Toronto Press, 2013.

Nicholson, Robin. *Bonnie Prince Charlie and the Making of a Myth: A Study in Portraiture, 1720–1892.* Lewisburg, PA: Bucknell University Press, 2002.

Nkuna, Nosipho. "Black Involvement in the Anglo-Boer War, 1899–1902." *Military History Journal* 11, no. 3 (October 1999).

Northrop, C. "Satirical Prints and Imperial Masculinity: Johnny Newcome in the West Indies." *Nineteenth-Century Gender Studies*, 14, no. 2.

Nuttall, Frank Q. "Body Mass Index: Obesity, BMI, and Health: A Critical Review." *Nutrition Today* 50 (2015), 117–28.

Oliver, J. Eric. *Fat Politics: The Real Story Behind America's Obesity Epidemic.* New York: Oxford University Press, 2006.

Oliver, Peter. *"Terror to Evil-doers": Prisons and Punishment in Nineteenth-Century Ontario.* Toronto: University of Toronto Press and Osgoode Society, 1998.

Orbach, S. *Fat is a Feminist Issue.* London: Arrow Books, 2016.

Owens, Erica, and Bronwyn Beistle. "Eating the Black Body: Interracial Desire, Food Metaphor, and White Fear." In *Body/Embodiment: Symbolic Interaction and the Sociology of the Body*, edited by Phillip Vannini and Dennis D. Waskul, 201–12. Burlington, VT: Ashgate, 2006.

Page, Robert. *Imperialism and Canada 1895–1993*. Toronto: Holt, Rinehart, and Winston, 1972.

Parsons, Joanne Ella. "Eating Englishness and Causing Chaos: Food and the Body of the Fat Man." In "Jorrocks's Jaunts and Jollities, Handley Cross, and Hillingdon Hall," edited by R.S. Surtees. *Nineteenth-Century Contexts* 36, no. 4 (2014): 335–46.

Pearson, Susan J. "'Infantile Specimens': Showing Babies in Nineteenth-Century America." *Journal of Social History* 42 (Winter 2008): 346–7.

Pérez, Jr., Louis A. *The War of 1898: The United States and Cuba in History and Historiography*. Chapel Hill: University of North Carolina Press, 1998.

Philippe, Robert. *Political Graphics: Art as a Weapon*. New York: Abbeville Press, 1980.

Pieterse, Jan Nederveen. *White on Black: Images of Africa and Black in Western Popular Culture*. Yale University Press, 1995.

Piva, Michael J. *The Conditions of the Working-Class in Toronto, 1900–1921*. Ottawa: University of Ottawa Press, 1979.

Pollack, Benjamin and Janice Todd. "Before Charles Atlas: Earle Liederman, the 1920s King of Mail-Order Muscle." *Journal of Sport History* 44, no. 3 (2017): 399–420.

Ponce, Rachel N. "'They Increase in Beauty and Elegance': Transforming Cadavers and the Epistemology of Dissection in Early Nineteenth-Century American Medical Education." *Journal of the History of Medicine and Allied Sciences* 68, no. 3 (July 2013): 331–76.

Porter, Roy. *Bodies Politic: Disease, Death and Doctors in Britain, 1650–1900*. Ithaca, NY: Cornell University Press, 2001.

Press, Charles. *The Political Cartoon*. Toronto: Associated University Presses, Inc., 1981.

Pretorius, Fransjohan. *Scorched Earth*. Cape Town: Tafelberg, 2017.

Price, Gregory. "Obesity and Crime: Is There a Relationship?" *Economics Letters* 103 (2009): 149–52.

Probyn, Elspeth. *Carnal Appetites: FoodSexIdentities*. London: Routledge, 2000.

Rafter, Nicole. "Lombroso's Reception in the United States" in *The Eternal Recurrence of Crime and Control: Essays in Honour of Paul* Rock, edited by David Downes, Dick Hobbs, and Time Newburn. Oxford: Oxford University Press, 2010.

Raschke, Debrah. *Modernism, Metaphysics, and Sexuality*. Selinsgrove: Susquehanna University Press, 2006.

Reich, J. "The World's Most Perfectly Developed Man: Charles Atlas, Physical Culture, and the Inscription of American Masculinity." *Men and Masculinities*, 12, no. 4 (2010): 444–61.

Reggiani, Andrés Horacio. "Physical Culture, Athletic Performance and Hygiene of the Nation: The Rise of Sports Medicine in Argentina (1930–1940)." *Historia Crítica*, 61 (2016): 65–84.

Riall, Malcolm. *Boer War: The Letters, Diaries and Photographs of Malcolm Riall from the War in South Africa 1899–1902*, edited by Nicholas Riall. London: Brassey's, 2000.

Riess, Steven A. *Sport in Industrial America, 1850–1920.* New York: John Wiley and Sons, 2012.

Rodan, Debbie, and Katie Ellis. *Disability, Obesity and Ageing: Popular Media Identifications.* New York: Routledge, 2016.

Rogers, W.G. *Mightier Than the Sword: Cartoon, Caricature, Social Comment.* New York: Harcourt, Brace and World, Inc., 1969.

Sahoo, Krushnapriya et al. "Childhood Obesity: Causes and Consequences." *Journal of Family Medicine and Primary Care* (India) 4, no. 2 (2015): 187–92.

Salmon, Marylynn. "The Cultural Significance of Breastfeeding and Infant Care in Early Modern England and America." *Journal of Social History* 28 (1994): 247–69.

Santolin, C., and Luiz C. Rigo. "The Birth of Pathologizing Discourse of Obesity." *Movimento, Porto Alegre* 21, no. 1 (2015): 81–94.

Schiebinger, Londa. *Nature's Body: Gender in the Making of Modern* Science. Boston: Beacon Press, 1993.

Schneider, Eric C. *In the Web of Class: Delinquents and Reformers in Boston, 1810s–1930s.* New York: NYU Press, 1993.

Schwarz, Hillel. *Never Satisfied: A Cultural History of Diets, Fantasies and Fat.* New York: The Free Press, 1986.

Schwenk, Achim, and Derek C. Macallan. "Tuberculosis, Malnutrition and Wasting." *Current Opinion in Clinical Nutrition and Metabolic Cure* 13, no. 4 (July 2000): 285–91.

Seneca. *Moral and Political Essays, Book 1, XV.* Translated by J. Cooper. Cambridge: Cambridge University Press, 1995.

Shaw, Amy. "The Boer War, Masculinity, and Citizenship in Canada, 1899–1902." In *Contesting Bodies and Nation in Canadian History*, edited by Patrizia Gentile and Jane Nicholas, 97–114. Toronto: University of Toronto Press, 2013.

– "Dissent in Canada against the Anglo-Boer War." In *Worth Fighting For: Canada's Tradition of War Resistance from 1812 to the War on Terror*, edited by Lara Campbell, Michael Dawson, and Catherine Gidney. Toronto: Between the Lines, 2015.

– "Fathers and Sons of Empire: Domesticity, Empire, and Canadian Participation in the Anglo-Boer War." In *Fighting with the Empire Canada,*

Britain, and Global Conflict, 1867–1947, edited by Steve Mardi and William John Pratt. Vancouver: University of British Columbia Press, 2019.

Shepherd, Roy J. "How Should We Assess Body Fatness?" *The Health and Fitness Journal of Canada, 10* (2017): 23–44.

Shimkin, Michael S. "The Numerical Method in Therapeutic Medicine." *Public Health Reports* 79, no. 1 (Jan. 1964): 1–12.

Shoemaker, Robert, and Richard Ward. "Understanding the Criminal: Record-Keeping, Statistics and the Early History of Criminology in England." *British Journal of Criminology* 57 (2017): 1442–61.

Shortt, S.E.D. "Physicians, Science, and Status: Issues in the Professionalization of Angle-American Medicine in the Nineteenth Century." *Medical History* 27 (1983): 51–68.

Shprintzen, Adam D. *The Vegetarian Crusade: The Rise of an American Reform Movement, 1817–1921.* North Carolina: University of North Carolina Press Books, 2013.

Silver, Anna Krugovoy. *Victorian Literature and the Anorexic Body.* Cambridge: Cambridge University Press, 2002.

Sinha, Mrinalini. *Colonial Masculinity.* New York: Manchester University Press, 1995.

Sivulka, Juliann. *Soap, Sex, and Cigarettes: A Cultural History of American Advertising.* Boston: Cengage Learning, 2011.

Smith, Andrew F. *New York City: A Food Biography.* Lanham: Rowman and Littlefield, 2013.

Somers, Paul. *Editorial Cartooning and Caricature: A Reference Guide.* Westport: Greenwood Press, 1998.

Spies, S.B. *Methods of Barbarism?: Roberts and Kitchener and Civilians in the Boer Republics, January 1900–May 1902.* Cape Town: Human & Rousseau, 1977.

Stahl, Saul "The Evolution of the Normal Distribution." *Mathematics Magazine* 79 (2006): 96–113.

Stearns, Peter N. *Fat History: Bodies and Beauty in the Modern West.* New York: New York University Press, 1997.

Steckel, Richard H. "Biological Measures of the Standard of Living," *Journal of Economic Perspectives* 22 (2008): 129–52.

– "Birth Weights and Infant Mortality among American Slaves." *Explorations in Economic History* 23 (Apr. 1986): 173–98.

– "Heights and Human Welfare: Recent Developments and New Directions." *Explorations in Economic History* 46 (2009): 1–23.

– "Inequality amidst Nutritional Abundance: Native Americans on the Great Plains." *Journal of Economic History* 70 (2010): 265–86.

Steckel, Richard H., and J.M. Prince. "Tallest in the World: Native Americans of the Great Plains in the Nineteenth Century." *American Economic Review* 91 (2001): 287–94.

Steinitz, Lesley. "The Language of Advertising: Fashioning Health Food Consumers at the Fin de Siècle." In *Food, Drink, and the Written Word in Britain, 1820–1945*, edited by Mary Addyman, Laura Wood, and Christopher Yiannitsaros, 135–63. London: Routledge, 2017.

Strange, Carolyn. *The Velvet Glove: Maternalistic Reform at the Andrew Mercer Ontario Reformatory for Females 1874–1927.* Unpublished MA thesis, Ottawa: University of Ottawa Press, 1983.

Street, R. *The Daniel Lambert Picture Book.* Dorset: Artesius Publications, 2019.

Strings, Sabrina. *Fearing the Black Body: The Racial Origins of Fat Phobia.* New York: New York University Press, 2019.

Surel, Jeannine. "John Bull." In *Patriotism: The Making and Unmaking of British National Identity*, Volume III National Fictions, edited by Raphael Samuel, 3–25. London: Routledge, 1989.

Surridge, Keith. "'All you soldiers are what we call pro-Boer': The Military Critique of the South African War, 1899–1902." *History* 82, no. 268 (October 1997): 582–600.

Talairach-Vielmas, Laurence. *Moulding the Female Body in Victorian Fairy Tales and Sensation Novels.* Aldershot: Ashgate, 2007.

Tanner, James M. *A History of the Study of Human Growth.* Cambridge: Cambridge University Press, 1981.

Taylor, Miles. "John Bull and the Iconography of Public Opinion in England c.1712–1929." *Past & Present*, no. 134 (February 1992): 93–128.

Thompson, R. *Flash of the Spirit: African and Afro-American Arts and Philosophy.* New York: Knopf Doubleday Publishing 1984.

Todd, Jan. "Bernarr MacFadden: Reformer of Feminine Form." *Journal of Sport History* 14, no. 1 (1987): 61–75.

– *Physical Culture and the Body Beautiful: Purposive Exercise in the Lives of American Women, 1800–1870.* Macon: Mercer University Press, 1999.

– "The Strength Builders: A History of Barbells, Dumbbells and Indian Clubs." *The International Journal of the History of Sport*, 20, no. 1 (2003): 73–5.

Tompkins, Kyla Wazana. *Racial Indigestion: Eating Bodies in the 19th Century.* New York: New York University Press, 2012.

Torrance, G.M., M.D. Hooper, and B.A. Reeder. "Trends in Overweight and Obesity among Adults in Canada (1970–1992): Evidence from National Surveys Using Measured Height and Weight." *International Journal of Obesity* 26 (2002): 797–804.

Tosh, John. "Masculinities in an Industrializing Society: Britain, 1800–1914." *Journal of British Studies* 44, no. 2 (April 2005).

Tweddell, C.H. *Charlie's First War: South Africa, 1899–1900*, edited by Carman Miller. Montreal and Kingston: McGill-Queen's University Press, 2014.

Urquhart, M.C. "New Estimates of Gross National Product, Canada, 1870–1926: Some Implications for Canadian Development." In *Long-Term*

Factors in American Economic Growth, edited by Stanley Engerman and Robert Gallman. Chicago: University of Chicago Press, 1986.

Vertinsky, Patricia. "'Weights and Means': Examining the Surveillance of Fat Bodies through Physical Education Practices in North America in the Late Nineteenth and Early Twentieth Centuries." *Journal of Sport History* 35, no. 3 (Fall 2008): 449–68.

Vester, Katharina. "Regime Change: Gender, Class, and the Invention of Dieting in Post-Bellum America." *Journal of Social History*, 44, no. 1 (2010): 39–70.

Vigarello, Georges. *The Metamorphoses of Fat: A History of Obesity*. Columbia: Columbia University Press, 2013.

Wahrman, D. "Percy's Prologue: From Gender Play to Gender Panic in Eighteenth-Century England." *Past and Present*, 159, no. 1 (1998): 113–60.

Walden, K. "The Road to Fat City: An Interpretation of the Development of Weight Consciousness in Western Society." *Historical Reflections / Réflexions Historiques* 12, no. 3 (1985): 331–73.

Waller, David. *The Perfect Man: The Muscular Life and Times of Eugen Sandow, Victorian Strongman*. London: Victorian Secrets, 2011.

Wann, Marilynn. "Foreward: Fat Studies: An Invitation to Revolution." In *The Fat Studies Reader*, edited by Esther Rothblum and Sondra Solovay, xi–xxvi. New York: New York University Press, 2009.

Ward, W. Peter. "Stature, Migration and Human Welfare in South China, 1850–1930." *Economics and Human Biology* 11 (2013): 488–501.

Ward, W. Peter, and Patricia C. Ward. "Infant Birth Weight and Nutrition in Industrializing Montreal." *American Historical Review* 89 (Apr. 1984), 324–45.

Warner, Deborah. "Weighing the Baby," National Museum of American History, 10 July 2017. americanhistory.si.edu/blog/weighing-baby.

Weaver, John. *Crimes, Constables and Courts: Order and Transgression in a Canadian City, 1816–1970*. Montreal and Kingston: McGill-Queen's University Press, 1995.

Weaver, Lawrence T. "In the Balance: Weighing Babies and the Birth of the Infant Welfare Clinic." *Bulletin of the History of Medicine* 84 (Spring 2010): 30–57.

Wertz, Richard, and Dorothy Wertz. *Lying-In: A History of Childbirth in America*. New Haven, CT: Yale University Press, 1989.

West, E., and R.J. Knight. "Mother's Milk: Slavery, Wetnursing, and Black and White Women in the Antebellum South." *Journal of Southern History* 83 (2017): 37–68.

West, Shearer. "Wilkes's Squint: Synecdochic Physiognomy and Political Identity in Eighteenth-Century Print Culture." *Eighteenth-Century Studies*, 33, no. 1 (Fall, 1999): 65–84.

Whorton, James C. "Historical Development of Vegetarianism." *The American Journal of Clinical Nutrition*. 59, no. 5 (1994): 1103S–1109S.

Wilker Jackson, *Eyen Akpabuyo Mme ma Ido Afo*: https://www.youtube.com/watch?v=kqy6oCi18ig&start_radio=1&list=RDEMiDza5crckbvoNr69mQkbEw.

Wilson, R. *Barnum: An American Life*. New York: Simon and Schuster, 2019.

Wolf, Jaqueline H. *Don't Kill Your Baby: Public Health and the Decline of Breastfeeding in the Nineteenth and Twentieth Centuries*. Columbus: Ohio State University Press, 2001.

Wolfgang, Marvin E. "Pioneers in Criminology: Cesare Lombroso (1825–1909)." *Journal of Criminal Law and Criminology* 52, no. 4 (November–December 1961): 361–91.

Young, James Allen. "Height, Weight, and Health: Anthropometric Study of Human Growth in the Nineteenth-Century American Medicine." *Bulletin of the History of* Medicine 53, no. 2 (Summer 1979): 214–43.

Zimran, Ariel. "Sample-Selection Bias and Height Trends in the Nineteenth-Century United States." *Journal of Economic History* 79 (2019): 99–138.

Contributors

Luiza Antonie is an associate professor in the School of Computing Science at the University of Guelph. She is a specialist in machine learning and data mining with applications to labour markets, medicine, and history.

Wesley R. Bishop is an assistant professor of American and Public History at Jacksonville State University, Alabama. His research focuses on social movements and public sphere studies. He is the co-author of *Liberating Fat Bodies: Social Media Censorship and Body Size Activism* (2024), and is the founding and managing editor of North Meridian Press.

Kristen Hardy is an interdisciplinary researcher and educator whose published work explores relations among bodies, minds, and systems of power. She has taught in departments of sociology, anthropology, religion, gender studies, and disability studies. She is currently sessional faculty at the University of Winnipeg, and an Adjunct Professor (Health Studies) and Associate Member of Graduate Studies at Brandon University.

Conor Heffernan is a lecturer in the Sociology of Sport at Ulster University. He has published several books on physical culture, his latest being *Indian Club Swinging and the Birth of Global Fitness* (2023). Conor's research interests span British, American, and Irish health cultures in the late nineteenth and early twentieth centuries.

Freya Gowrley is a scholar of the cultural lives of images and objects based at the University of Bristol. She writes about the relationship between art and identity from the early modern period to the present day, particularly focusing on the home, the body, and the collaged object.

Her book on the visual culture of fatness, *Unseemly: A Visual History of the Fat Body*, will be published in 2026.

Kris Inwood is a professor in Economics and History at the University of Guelph. He publishes on the economic history of Canada and related economies.

Lynn Kennedy is an associate professor and chair in the Department of History and Religion at the University of Lethbridge, where she teaches American history. Her research focuses on issues of domesticity and household formation in the nineteenth-century South, including childbirth and motherhood, sewing and fashion, and divorce. She is the author of *Born Southern: Childbirth, Motherhood and Social Networks in the Old South* (2010).

Tatiana Konrad is a postdoctoral researcher at the University of Vienna and has written and edited numerous books on climate change, war and media, and disability studies including, most recently, *Climate Change Fiction and Ecocultural Crisis: The Industrial Revolution to the Present* (2024); *Disability, the Environment, and Colonialism* (2024); *Imagining Air: Cultural Axiology and the Politics of Invisibility* (2023), and *Plastics, Environment, Culture, and the Politics of Waste* (2023).

Hamish Maxwell-Stewart is a professor of Heritage and Digital Humanities at the University of New England, Australia. He has a particular interest in the digitisation and analysis of historical record series, especially criminal justice records. His most recent book (co-written with Michael Quinlan) is *Unfree Workers: Insubordination and Resistance in Convict Australia 1788–1860* (2022).

Bonnie Miller is a professor of History at the University of Massachusetts Boston, specializing in the history of U.S. imperialism, visual culture, and food studies. She is author of *From Liberation to Conquest: The Visual and Popular Cultures of the Spanish American War of 1898* (2011). She has also published numerous articles and book chapters on Spanish-American War journalism, the politics of display at U.S. world fairs, and food history.

Bessie Rigakos is the vice president and dean at Marian University's Saint Joseph's College, Indianapolis. Her research focuses on medical sociology, specifically sex, gender, and sexuality. She has published various works, including a peer-reviewed article on scientific process visualization and a book chapter on modern health standards. She is currently working on a manuscript about social media censorship and body-size activism.

Amy Shaw is an associate professor in the Department of History and Religion at the University of Lethbridge. She has written and edited several books and articles in the area of war and society, gender, and citizenship, the latest book being *Making the Best of It: Women and Girls of Canada and Newfoundland during the Second World War* (2020).

Nsima Udo is a doctoral fellow at the Centre for Humanities Research, University of the Western Cape. His research examines African Indigenous cultures, festivals, and performance in history and their sociocultural complexities and symbolism in relation to gender, ethics, aesthetics, and vocation. His MA thesis, "Visualizing the Body: Photographic Clues and the Cultural Fluidity of Mbopo Institution, 1914–2014," won the African Thesis Award in 2019.

Index

Page references to illustrations and figures are in *italic*.